Evidence for Health

From Patient Choice to Global Policy

Evidence for Health

From Patient Choice to Global Policy

Anne Andermann
Associate Professor, Department of Family Medicine,
Associate Member, Department of Epidemiology, Biostatistics and Occupational Health, and
Research Associate in Public Health and Primary Health Care, St Mary's Research Centre,
McGill University, Montreal, Canada

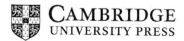
CAMBRIDGE
UNIVERSITY PRESS

CAMBRIDGE UNIVERSITY PRESS
Cambridge, New York, Melbourne, Madrid, Cape Town,
Singapore, São Paulo, Delhi, Mexico City

Cambridge University Press
The Edinburgh Building, Cambridge CB2 8RU, UK

Published in the United States of America by Cambridge University Press, New York

www.cambridge.org
Information on this title: http://www.cambridge.org/9781107648654

First published 2013

Printed and bound in the United Kingdom by the MPG Books Group

A catalogue record for this publication is available from the British Library

Library of Congress Cataloguing in Publication data
Andermann, Anne, 1972–
Evidence for health : from patient choice to global policy / Anne Andermann.
     p.   ;   cm.
Includes bibliographical references and index.
ISBN 978-1-107-64865-4 (pbk.)
I. Title.
[DNLM: 1. Public Health.   2. Decision Making.   3. Evidence-Based Practice.   4. Health
Policy.   5. Outcome Assessment (Health Care)   6. World Health. WA 100]
362.1–dc23

                                                                    2012024120

ISBN 978-1-107-64865-4 Paperback

I have written this book for Lara and Ben, with the hope that promoting evidence-informed decisions will allow them to live in a healthier and more equitable world.

Contents

Foreword

Tikki Pang

Visiting Professor, Lee Kuan Yew School of Public Policy,
National University of Singapore, Singapore and formerly
Director, Research, Policy and Cooperation, World Health Organization,
Geneva, Switzerland

In an age of financial crises, diminishing resources and competing priorities, Anne Andermann's book is very timely and fills an important gap in the critical area of developing sound and sustainable health policies. While many books and manuals have been written on the use of evidence in the development of clinical practice guidelines, there have been very few attempts at a treatise on the use of evidence in policy formulation. Written as a practical guide to evidence-informed decision-making, this book will be an invaluable tool for policy-makers and others, including health practitioners, enabling and empowering them to make rational decisions and better withstand vested interests and political, economic and even ideological pressures, which are so pervasive in the policy sphere.

Based on her own extensive experience, the author takes us systematically through the strategies commonly used to improve health, and the more difficult topic of how decisions are made which impact health outcomes. She then tackles the practical issue of producing evidence and the critical bottleneck which exists between the production and use of evidence. Often, a major challenge is the lack of understanding between researchers and policy-makers, which, I believe, can be overcome to a large extent by giving attention to the issues highlighted in this book. In the chapter on evidence production, the author highlights, for example, the increasing importance of implementation research, which aims to develop strategies for optimising the delivery, uptake and use of new or existing interventions by populations in need. This type of research is particularly important in supplying the kind of evidence which policy-makers appreciate and understand more readily than basic biomedical or even clinical research. The chapter also highlights the importance of evaluating the impact of policy, and how such research can feed back into the "knowledge loop" in an iterative, reinforcing manner. The final chapter cogently tackles the oft-neglected final step of how evidence-informed decisions are actually made, highlighting the necessity of coming up with various options which take into account ethical, social, legal and cultural issues, and the sensitivities and concerns of interested parties who may be affected by the decision.

This book is valuable for three reasons.

First, is its pragmatic, realistic and empathetic approach. Relating her ideas to her own personal experiences, which make the book feel vibrant and "alive", the author highlights the reality that policy-making is inherently complex and challenging, with evidence being only one factor which has to be integrated with a myriad of others. In the words of Sir Michael Marmot, the reality is that "scientific findings do not fall on blank minds that get made up as a result. Science engages with busy minds that have strong views about how things are and ought to be".

Second, is its implicit message that the need to understand the importance of evidence is as relevant and important for a doctor, a nurse, or an individual patient and consumer, as it is for senior policy-makers at national or global levels. All of these people must, ultimately, make decisions pertaining to the health of human beings, be it at the level of an individual or whole populations, both in developed and developing countries.

Third, is that it offers many universal lessons and recommendations on the importance and use of evidence, which are applicable beyond the health sector to other sectors that nonetheless have a direct or indirect influence on human health. The book thus speaks to the reality of an increasingly globalised world where health challenges are transnational, multidimensional and multi-sectoral.

In addition to its obvious value as a practical "A to Z" guide for decision-makers, the book should be compulsory reading at the postgraduate level in the fields of public policy and public administration, where future decision-makers need to be sensitized to the thoughts of Goethe, who famously said "knowing is not enough, we must apply; willing is not enough, we must act".

I have no doubt that this landmark publication will go a long way in advancing the cause of evidence-informed decision-making, which is the foundation for creating and maintaining strong and sustainable health systems. Robust health systems can then achieve their ultimate goal of improving the health status and lives of the people they serve in an ethical, equitable and sustainable manner.

Preface

The idea for this book came to me when I was teaching a course on epidemiology to graduate students in the Health and Health Policy (HHP) Programme at Princeton University's Woodrow Wilson School for Public and International Affairs. Many of my students were completing a Master's degree in Public Administration (MPA) or Public Policy (MPP). They had already worked in government or for well-known international non-governmental organisations (NGOs) and had been involved in making decisions that could affect the health of hundreds of thousands of people. Yet for the most part they did not have any formal education or training in health sciences upon which to base these decisions. With undergraduate degrees in political science, management and economics, the process of producing, appraising and using scientific evidence was a "black box" that was unveiled during the course so that the students could be more critical readers of the research literature (or even of reports of the literature published in the media, which is where most people read about scientific evidence). Even health practitioners working on the frontlines – including doctors, nurses, midwives, lay health workers and others – are not always well versed in research methods and how research findings can be used to improve health. While evidence is certainly not the only "ingredient" that goes into decision-making for health, making decisions without evidence is like sailing the seas without a map and compass. Therefore, to foster more evidence-informed decision-making, I thought it would be important to write a book targeted towards practitioners and policy-makers that demystifies the process of knowledge production and illustrates the complexity of decision-making so that knowledge users are better able to incorporate the scientific evidence into decisions, to thereby influence health outcomes in a more strategic and informed way. This is by no means an epidemiology textbook, but rather a practical guide to evidence-informed decision-making with the goal of improving health and reducing health inequities.

My main argument throughout this book is that the health of individuals and populations is a product of the many decisions that we make on a daily basis. If our world has enormous (and some might say highly unethical) health inequities whereby some people can expect to die at age 40 whereas in other parts of the world people live on average to age 80, it is because we make it so and we allow these disparities to continue. These are not laws of nature. There are just people, like you and me, making a series of decisions that have consequences for health – even when these decisions are being made outside of the health sector. The flip side of this is that we also have the power to change the health landscape, or even our own health, but this depends upon using the best available scientific evidence to inform decision-making, and ensuring that decisions are not thwarted by vested interests or lack of political will.

Indeed, making evidence-informed decisions is not a straightforward process. I recall my experiences as a researcher in a health technology assessment (HTA) agency. The role of this organisation, at arm's length from the Ministry of Health, was to provide government with evidence-informed recommendations for improving health services, and ultimately for improving health. My role was to develop a process for evidence-informed decision-making with regard to genetic screening that also made explicit the underlying value judgements and ethical considerations. However, there was a clash with the economist on the Board of Directors who strongly believed that all considerations can be incorporated into a cost-effectiveness analysis and who disagreed that cost issues are just one aspect – rather than the central aspect – of decision-making. On another occasion, there was a clash with a fellow researcher – a devout Catholic and anti-abortionist – who was developing recommendations for prenatal screening that would affect the entire population. To what extent should her own personal values be permitted to influence recommendations made in a multicultural society where citizens do not share the same values? How can we ensure that value judgements are made explicit rather than pretending that they do not exist? Even risk tolerance varies from person to person. How to choose a threshold for an entire population when some people would be comfortable with a risk of 1 in 100 of carrying an affected fetus, and others would be unable to sleep at night if they had a risk of 1 in 1,000? This book illustrates that decision-making for health is a highly complex and contentious area where even experts can disagree on the best process for making these decisions – and quite often, there isn't a systematic or explicit process being used at all.

While there is no single, universally accepted approach to decision-making, this book provides an algorithm that uses a series of questions for arriving at evidence-informed decisions that take into consideration the multiple complexities and value judgements involved. In many ways, the process (i.e. being participatory and involving stakeholders, as well as being explicit in justifying why a certain decision is made) is just as important as the product (i.e. the final decision made).

From my later experiences working as a public health consultant for another government agency that provides technical assistance to local health regions, I witnessed first-hand how decisions made by government can be very poorly received when certain stakeholders do not understand how these decisions were made and feel that the decisions are unfair. Quite literally there were fists thumping on tables and cries of injustice, followed by vehement accusations that the government was simply trying to save money and ration services. This was true decision-making in action. Not for the faint of heart. My role was to chaperone the process of revisiting the decision, which was done in a systematic, evidence-informed and participatory way. Everyone walked through the process together and various experts were called in as needed to clarify certain issues. The key was that everyone was on the same page and could appreciate the multiple complexities and considerations involved. While the local stakeholders still wanted to lobby for their cause, they were much more understanding the second time around when the government made the exact same decision – because this time there was also a clear explanation and understanding of why this decision was made. Of course, this does not mean that it was a straightforward case. Indeed, when the policy-maker from the Ministry asked for my opinion prior to making their decision public, I had to admit that it was a bit of a grey zone. On the one hand, offering this new preventive service to the region could be justified on the basis that this region has a somewhat higher prevalence of the health problem in question. On the other hand, this would be one of the first jurisdictions worldwide to offer such a service outside of a research context, there are many known technical and ethical ramifications involved in introducing this service, and the health problem is also fairly common in other neighbouring jurisdictions (although not quite as prevalent), which would lead to inequities in terms of access to services (also known as the "postcode lottery"). Thus, there were reasons given that clearly explained why the government chose not to go ahead with the introduction of this service – it was not simply a case of rationing health care and saving money. Moreover, as the knowledge base and the context evolve, this decision could certainly be revisited over time to see whether these reasons still apply in future. The more I am involved in decision-making at a political level, the more I empathise with the challenges involved in integrating so many diverse considerations and viewpoints, and the more I believe in the value of a systematic approach that makes these multiple factors explicit.

Reflecting these experiences, the scope of this book is very broad, from the personal decisions that individual patients make about their own health to global policy decisions that can impact the health of millions of people worldwide. As a graduate student at Oxford University, the focus of my doctoral research was to better understand the expectations and information needs of women presenting to primary care, and what factors could promote evidence-informed patient choice. Later, as a family doctor, I experienced the daily challenges of helping my own patients make difficult decisions about their health: for instance, whether to undergo surgery that can improve quality of life but entails a certain risk of dying during the procedure or to forego surgery and live as long as possible with increasingly impaired function. As a public health physician working to promote the health of an Aboriginal population in the North of Canada (for public health physicians, the "patient" is the population), I was involved in examining the Health Impact Assessments of economic development projects and making recommendations on how to balance the needs of various disadvantaged populations in the North in a way that is fair and maximises benefits while minimising harm. As well, while working at the World Health Organization (WHO) in Geneva, I advocated for universal access to primary health care worldwide as an important method of social protection and lever for tackling health inequities. Currently, I combine public health practice at the local and national level, clinical work in a university-affiliated teaching hospital serving a diverse multi-cultural community, supervision and training of medical students and residents, and global health research aimed at empowering frontline health workers to tackle the social causes of poor health. I therefore write this book wearing several "hats": as a policy-maker, a researcher, an educator, a health practitioner and even as a patient.

As one moves from patient choice to global policy, the level of complexity increases significantly. Yet, all decisions fundamentally entail various trade-offs when considering the different options and balancing the overall benefits and harms of choosing one option over another. Through this book, I hope that I can help policy-makers and practitioners to make more evidence-informed decisions for improving health. In particular, with the growing emphasis on the upstream social determinants of health, I hope that this book will also reach decision-makers outside of the health sector, as decisions made in areas such as education, employment, housing, gender equality and so forth are fundamental to tackling the major health inequities of our time. To make progress in reducing these inequities, we need evidence-informed decisions that consider the health impact of all policies, not just those involving the health care system. Better-informed decisions can lead to healthier and more equitable societies. It is up to us to choose.

Endorsements

"To enable individuals to be in control of their lives, action is needed on the social circumstances in which people are born, grow, live, work, and age. Evidence for Health: From Patient Choice to Global Policy is an innovative and timely book that provides important insight on how to make more transparent and informed decisions that will result in healthier individuals and more equitable societies."

Professor Sir Michael Marmot, Director, UCL Institute of Health Equity, London, UK, and formerly Chair, WHO Commission on the Social Determinants of Health

"Evidence for health seems self-evident, however, Andermann in her thought-provoking book, points not only to the value of evidence, but also to the imperative to learn how to integrate it more systematically in all decisions related to health from local to global. Progress on this front would certainly contribute to better decisions and better health."

Dr. Timothy Evans, Dean, BRAC School of Public Health, Dhaka, Bangladesh, and formerly Assistant Director General of the World Health Organization, Geneva, Switzerland

"Public health has too often focused on making recommendations about what people ought to do rather than considering what changes behaviours and policies. Drawing from multiple disciplines, Andermann thoughtfully addresses this challenge, reviewing how we make decisions that affect health – from the individual to the global level – and detailing how we can generate and best make use of evidence to reduce health inequities and improve people's health."

Dr. Kumanan Rasanathan, Health Section, United Nations Children's Fund (UNICEF), New York, USA

"This book addresses key questions confronted by policymakers, health practitioners and the population at large. Written in a very simple and user-friendly manner, Evidence for Health will be a highly valuable tool for understanding and addressing health inequities in both developed and developing countries."

Mr. Saeed Awan, Director, Centre for the Improvement of Working Conditions & Environment, Department of Labour and Human Relations, Government of Punjab, Lahore, Pakistan

"A fresh, thoughtful, and panoramic look at the role of evidence in health. This book should be of interest to any student of public health or public policy."

Dr. Peter Singer, Professor of Medicine and Director, Sandra Rotman Centre, University Health Network and University of Toronto

"Decision-making is a complex process, particularly in medicine and public health. It frequently implies the simultaneous display of technical abilities, political appraisals, and moral judgements. Anne Andermann's book, Evidence for Health: From Patient Choice to Global Policy, makes this process accessible to all. I have no doubt that it will become an invaluable tool for health professionals working in clinical, management, and public health settings."

Dr. Julio Frenk, Dean of the Faculty, Harvard School of Public Health, and former Minister of Health of Mexico

About the author

Dr. Anne Andermann is a family physician, a public health specialist and a former Rhodes Scholar. Her doctoral studies at Oxford University focused on the impact of new genetic and genomic technologies in primary care, and she later worked for the Quebec Health Technology Assessment Agency (formerly AETMIS) on developing guidance for population-based genetic screening policy-making. Dr. Andermann has also worked at the World Health Organization (WHO) in Geneva on research capacity strengthening in low- and middle-income countries. During that time, she was a member of the WHO Research Ethics Review Committee and a main contributing author to the *World Health Report 2008* on increasing universal access to primary health care. Dr. Andermann is currently an Associate Professor in the Department of Family Medicine at McGill University, Regional Medical Officer for Health Canada's First Nations and Inuit Health Branch (FNIHB), Public health physician for the Cree Board of Health and Social Services of James Bay Northern Quebec (CBHSSJB), Chair of the public health theme for the new undergraduate medical curriculum at McGill's Faculty of Medicine, practising physician and Chair of the Community-Oriented Primary Care (COPC) Committee at St Mary's Hospital, and founder of an international research collaboration that aims to provide guidance and support for frontline health workers so that they can play a greater role in addressing the social causes of poor health and reducing health inequities. Her main area of interest is promoting the health of vulnerable and marginalised populations, including women and child health, Aboriginal health, global health and the health of families with rare and orphan genetic diseases. In 2011, she received the Canadian Rising Stars in Global Health Award from Grand Challenges Canada. This is her first book.

Acknowledgments

I would like to thank my colleagues, friends and family members who have helped me over the years in preparing this book, from debating the merits of vertical versus horizontal approaches to reading and editing draft chapters. In particular, I would like to thank Eva and Fred Andermann, Itamar Katz, Lilah Moore and Jean-Francois Boivin for their helpful comments. As well, I am grateful to Nisha Doshi and Richard Marley at Cambridge University Press for their guidance, to Tikki Pang for kindly agreeing to write the foreword, and to Marguerite Pigeon for doing a final read-through of the completed manuscript. I am greatly indebted to Karen and Kayleigh since without high-quality child care this book would not have been possible. Finally, I would like to thank my husband, Carlos Fraenkel, who encouraged me from the start to take on this project and stood by me through to its completion.

* * *

I have written this book in memory of my late grandmother, Dr. Mina Deutsch, who instilled in me a strong sense of social justice and taught me that even seemingly insurmountable challenges can be endured and overcome. I have also written this book in memory of my late DPhil (PhD) thesis supervisor, Dr. Joan Austoker, who set me on the path of public health and evidence-informed decision-making.

People themselves must have responsibility for the development and change of the world in which they live.

Amartya Sen

If our goal is to improve health, those within the health sector must move outside classrooms, laboratories, and hospital walls to embrace a broader approach to health.

Mary Ann Mercer

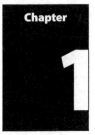

Introduction

The purpose of this book is to better understand how to improve the health of individuals, populations and the global community. What are the major threats to health? What are the causes of poor health? What works to improve health? How do we know that it works? What are the barriers to implementation? What are the measures of success? These are some of the key questions that will be addressed in this book. The aim is to provide health practitioners and policy-makers with a broad overview of how to improve health and reduce health inequities, as well as the tools to make more evidence-informed decisions that will have a positive influence on health.

Indeed, countless decisions that affect health are made every day, whether at the level of individual health choices made by patients and the general public, population health policies and programmes made by politicians and public health officials, or global health strategies and recommendations made by an increasing number of players at the international level, including civil servants, non-governmental organisations (NGOs), philanthropists, academics, public–private partnerships and so forth. For instance, a mother takes time off from work to bring her child to the local clinic to be vaccinated. A student buys a fruit for an afternoon snack rather than potato chips. A 28-year-old woman who carries the *BRCA* gene for hereditary breast-ovarian cancer undergoes preventive surgery to remove her breasts and ovaries. A government passes a bill to extend parental leave to one year and to increase funding for early childhood development programmes. The World Health Organization (WHO) recommends increasing universal health coverage and social protection by strengthening primary health care as the foundation for all health systems. In each of the above examples, people were faced with a choice (i.e. to vaccinate or not, to eat a fruit or chips, to have preventive surgery or enhanced screening, to finance social programmes or reduce taxes, to promote vertical programming that focuses on preventing and treating a single disease or a more comprehensive approach based on primary health care), and a decision was made that will either improve or impair health outcomes.

The health status of individuals, populations and the global community is shaped by these decisions. However, despite a growing body of scientific evidence on how to best improve health, decisions often do not incorporate this evidence. At times the reasons for disregarding the scientific evidence are strategic, economic or political. More often, it is due to a lack of awareness and understanding, as well as issues of logistics and timing. Having the right information at the right time in the right format is critical to incorporating evidence into decision-making.

In practice, this is not as straightforward as it seems, and an entire field of knowledge translation has stemmed from trying to address the widening "know–do" gap (i.e. the gap between what we know about how to improve health and what we decide to do to make it happen). There are often important knowledge gaps that make it difficult to find adequate evidence to incorporate into decision-making. And, even when evidence does exist, it is necessary but not sufficient, since other factors including contextual issues and value judgements must also be incorporated and made explicit as part of the decision-making process.

This book therefore attempts to demystify the notion of evidence for health and to create realistic expectations about the role of evidence in decision-making by explaining why evidence is useful, how it is produced, and how it can be better packaged and communicated to help people in making more evidence-informed decisions – from patient choice to global policy.

If the ultimate goal of all health decisions is to improve health outcomes and to reduce health inequities, it is important to know what these terms mean, to know where we want to go, and how to know when we get there. Chapter 2 therefore begins by providing an overview of the concepts of health and health inequities. This is followed by the current thinking on risk factors and determinants of health (i.e. what causes poor health), as well as the continuum of strategies that are used in the field of public health for improving health and reducing health inequities (from treatment and rehabilitation to disease prevention, health promotion and addressing the underlying social determinants of health).

Similarly, to influence health decisions, it is important to better understand what such decision-making entails. Chapter 3 therefore provides an introduction to the many factors that influence decision-making for health at the individual, population and global levels. At the individual level, for instance, decisions are shaped by the sources and quality of information available, personal values, prior experience with the health condition in question, and risk perceptions regarding the various possible outcomes of action or inaction. At the population level there are added layers of complexity, as these decisions must also take into account the multiple implications of proposed policies and programmes for individuals, target groups and the population overall. This includes balancing the needs of competing stakeholder groups, each with their own vested interests, and considering issues of opportunity costs and accountability when using public resources. Finally, at the global level, there are even more layers of complexity since health threats do not respect national borders, multilateral trade agreements and diplomatic considerations become important, and an ever-growing arena of public and private players with their own opinions and interests apply pressure to influence global policy, often bypassing existing fora and structures intended to ensure good global governance. All three levels of decision-making are inextricably linked since global treaties and national policies have an enormous influence on individual-level decisions, while, collectively, individual-level decisions have an important impact on population and global health.

Next, Chapter 4 discusses why evidence is important for informing health decisions and how this evidence is generated. The chapter begins with a brief history outlining the origins of the growing "evidence-based" movement in the health sector, including the initial resistance by physicians followed by the widespread acceptance of using evidence in clinical decision-making, and the extension of the "evidence-based" model to many other health-related disciplines, from nursing and dentistry to public health and health policy. Chapter 4 also describes what counts as evidence and how evidence is produced through a discussion of the different types of research studies that can be used to answer different types of research questions at each stage in the "research cycle". For instance, at the first stage, qualitative research and descriptive studies, such as cross-sectional surveys, can be used to determine the relative importance and frequency of various health problems (e.g. what do people in the community consider to be the most important health problems? how many people in the community have HIV, depression, heart disease or cancer?). At the next stage, observational studies, including case-control and cohort studies, can be used to better understand the causes of priority health problems (i.e. the risk of developing heart disease is 50% higher for those who smoke, the distribution of smokers in the population is related to gender and socio-economic status, etc.). Randomised controlled trials or other experimental study designs can then be used to test the efficacy of interventions in acting on the various causes to prevent or reduce the burden of disease (e.g. prescribing the nicotine patch can increase smoking cessation rates by 30%). Finally, after large-scale implementation of interventions, quasi-experimental studies such as pre–post studies or natural experiments can be used to evaluate effectiveness in impacting population health (e.g. one year after anti-smoking laws and regulations were passed, the number of smokers was reduced by 40%, and within five years the number of new cases of heart disease was reduced by 10%).

Chapter 5 then discusses the facilitators and barriers to using evidence in decision-making. Facilitators to evidence-informed decisions include finding, critically appraising and synthesising the relevant research literature in a timely way to provide a more accurate appreciation of the wider body of evidence. Indeed, task forces, health technology assessment agencies and international networks are important means of reliably synthesising and disseminating the evidence. As well, it is important to package the main messages using media that are suitable and accessible to the intended audiences – whether decision aids for patients, online evidence portals for busy health practitioners, or policy briefs for politicians – thus encouraging the uptake and use of evidence in day-to-day practice. Nonetheless, the barriers to using evidence in decision-making are many, ranging from knowledge gaps and decision-making in the face of uncertainty, to vested interests undermining the existing evidence base to push forward their own agenda.

Given these barriers, and the sheer complexity involved, a systematic approach can be helpful in identifying and integrating the different types of evidence, contextual consid-erations and value judgements that are an inherent part of decision-making. While there is no single way of summarising or ordering the various elements involved, Chapter 6 provides an algorithm that lays out many of the key issues that should be considered to facilitate better-informed and more transparent decisions for improving the health of individuals and populations. The main steps of this algorithm include: (1) defining the priority health problems, (2) understanding the underlying causes, (3) listing the options to improve health, (4) assessing whether there is an added benefit that outweighs the harms, (5) determining whether the options are acceptable to those involved, (6) calculating the costs and opportunity costs, (7) determining whether the options are feasible in a given context, (8) exploring the ethical, legal and social issues, (9) identifying what different stakeholders stand to gain or lose, and (10) making a summative assessment of which options improve health most while minimising the harms and ensuring an equitable distribution of benefits and harms. While at the end of the day a judgement must still be made, at the very least, following the algorithm ensures that the key evidence and con-textual issues have been considered, and that the various trade-offs and opportunity costs are clearly laid out, so that when it comes time to make value judgements, it is far easier to document the reasons underlying the decisions made.

Chapter 7 concludes the book by discussing the importance of a fair, transparent and participative process for decision-making at all levels. Indeed, the process is part of the product by promoting a shared understanding among all stakeholders of: (1) the evidence, (2) the implications, and (3) the intended outcomes. This shared understanding serves to promote informed choices, as well as reduce conflict and future "undoing" of decisions made, while still permitting decisions to be revisited over time as the knowledge base and/or context evolves. Chapter 7 also addresses the many challenges for making this systematic approach to promoting evidence-informed decision-making work in practice, and for documenting progress both in terms of the process and the outcomes. These include identifying and involving the key stakeholders and decision-makers from the outset, ensuring that the best available evidence has been reliably collected and synthesised, helping people to better understand probabilistic information through the use of pictures and stories rather than statistics, avoiding potential bias when framing the information, and ensuring that the evidence is accessible during the critical window of opportunity so that it can be incorporated into decision-making. A final challenge is documenting the extent to which evidence was used to inform health decisions, but even more importantly, the degree to which this has resulted in improved health outcomes. The book therefore ends with a discussion of ways to evaluate the decision-making process, and particularly the impact that these decisions have on improving health.

Throughout the book I argue that people make choices at various levels that have an impact on health. Therefore, the health status of individuals, populations and the global community is to a large extent determined by the choices that are made – for better or for worse. We therefore have the power to improve health on a large scale by influencing these choices. While there are a number of technical barriers (i.e. not knowing what works, poor quality data, etc.), these problems can generally be overcome through further research and a more nuanced understanding of the issues. However, competing interests and a lack of political will pose the real barriers. Nonetheless, these problems too can be overcome through greater transparency, advocacy and the engagement of civil society to pressure policy-makers into being less complacent about the inequities of our world. These inequities are man-made, and they can also be undone by making better-informed decisions that improve health and reduce health inequities. Geoffrey Rose once said that "the primary determinants of disease are mainly economic and social, and therefore its remedies must also be economic and social. Medicine and politics cannot and should not be kept apart".[1] We live in a world where threats to health are pervasive and far-reaching – from oppressive military regimes and colonial legacies to institutionalised violence and insufficiently regulated economies. Yet we can choose the society we want to live in by influencing the choices that shape our society. This book provides some insight into how to go about creating this much-needed change.

References

1. Rose G. *Rose's Strategy of Preventive Medicine*. Oxford: Oxford University Press, 2008.

Strategies for improving health

Almost 40 years ago, the *Declaration of Alma-Ata* set forth the aspirational goal of "health for all".[1] While a great deal of progress has been made in recent decades,[2] there remain many important decisions still to be made if we want to come even closer to achieving this goal. However, if the aim of making more evidence-informed decisions is to improve health, it would be helpful to first know what health is. While this appears to be a rather straightforward question, as Socrates found over two millennia ago, many people, when pressed, have difficulty defining even the most fundamental concepts – like knowledge and justice – that are central to their everyday lives. Similarly, health and health inequities are also basic concepts that should be explored further from the outset. What is health? Why should we want to improve health? What are the most effective strategies for improving health? How can we measure whether there have been health improvements? This chapter provides an overview of the concepts of health and health inequities, of the causes of poor health, and of the various strategies to improve health and reduce health inequities.

Health and health inequities

Health is a complex concept that can be examined and defined in many different ways. A widely used definition is inscribed in the 1948 constitution of the World Health Organization (WHO), which considers health to be "a state of complete physical, mental and social well-being and not merely the absence of disease or infirmity".[3] This definition moves away from a strictly biomedical model of health that focuses only on the disease or disability. Instead, the WHO definition adopts a wider bio-psycho-social model to better integrate the importance of the psychological and social dimensions of health. One might go even further and include a spiritual dimension of health. According to the Canadian Royal Commission on Aboriginal Peoples, many indigenous communities consider health to be "a state of balance and harmony involving body, mind, emotions and spirit. It links each person to family, community and the earth in a circle of dependence and interdependence, described by some in the language of the Medicine Wheel".[4] Health is therefore a holistic and multidimensional concept that must be explored from different angles and perspectives to be fully understood (Fig. 2.1).[5]

Health as the absence of disease and disability

Even the narrow and simple definition of health – i.e. "the absence of disease and disability" – is not as straightforward as it seems. Medical anthropologist Arthur Kleinman ascribes distinct meanings to the terms disease, illness and sickness.[6] Disease entails a physiological dysfunction.

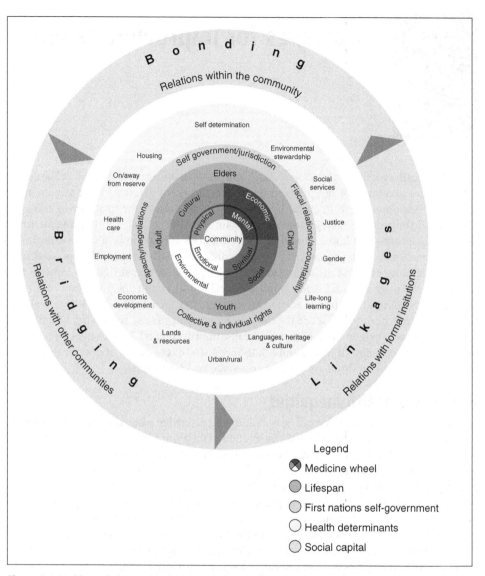

Figure 2.1 Health as a holistic and multidimensional concept.
Reproduced with permission from Reading J, Kmetic A, Gideon V. *First Nations Wholistic Policy and Planning Model: Discussion Paper for the World Health Organization Commission on the Social Determinants of Health.* Ottawa: Assembly of First Nations, 2007.

For example, when a blood clot travels to the brain and causes a blockage of a small blood vessel depriving the brain of oxygen, this results in brain damage, also known as a stroke. People who suffer a stroke often become paralysed on one side of the body or lose the ability to speak. This constitutes a physiological dysfunction. Illness, however, is the subjective perception of this dysfunction. Do these people consider themselves to be unwell? How are they affected by their dysfunction? One individual with only mild tingling in the fingers of one hand may consider themselves to be very ill, whereas another person with complete paralysis on one side of the body may adapt by learning to use a computer with their functioning hand and not feel ill at all.

Finally, sickness is whether or not the person is able to fulfil their social role. In spite of the physiological dysfunction, are they nonetheless able to fulfil their role as a parent, as an employee, as a friend? Thus while the physiological dysfunction occurs at a biological level, the experience of illness is at a psychological level, and how the dysfunction impacts one's life is at a social level (hence the bio-psycho-social model).

A similar hierarchy of terms exists for disabilities as defined by the WHO *International Classification of Impairment, Disability and Handicap*, more recently called the *International Classification of Functioning, Disability and Health*, which distinguishes between impairment at the biological or body function level, disability, which restricts the activity of the individual, and handicap, which is the disadvantage in fulfilling one's social role and fully participating in society.[7] Even if modern medicine is able to repair the impairment and reduce the disability, the degree of handicap very much depends on the extent to which we as a society are able to reintegrate persons with disabilities and adapt the physical and social environment to maximise opportunities for them to contribute in their social role. Therefore, improving health requires more than addressing the problem at the biological level by prescribing a medication or performing a surgery. It is also necessary to address the emotional, social and spiritual dimensions that are invariably associated with the health problem.

Health as the number and quality of years lived

Most people have an intuitive sense of what it means to be unwell and what it means to be healthy. At one extreme, when a person is very unwell, the worst health outcome is death (although some argue that there are certain health states which produce extreme suffering that are even worse than death).[8] It is therefore not surprising that some of the first measures developed to assess the health of populations were derived from death records.

For example, in 1662, John Graunt published one of the first analyses of vital statistics based on records of births and deaths collected by the Church.[9] Using this data he was able to compare death rates of people living in the country versus the city (i.e. London) and also to better understand the causes of death, ranging from "bit by a mad dog" to fever, consumption and old age. Among the most important causes of death at the time (in addition to frequent plagues) were diseases of infancy and childhood. Graunt calculated that about one-third of children died before their fifth birthday, which in today's terminology would be equivalent to a childhood mortality rate of 333 deaths per 1,000 live births. He also developed the first life tables, which illustrated that three-quarters of the population did not live beyond their 26th birthday and only 1% survived to their 77th birthday.

These vital statistics may be somewhat crude measures of health, but they are nonetheless very useful and continue to be important tools for measuring health status to this day. According to recent data, the average life expectancy in Organisation for Economic Co-operation and Development (OECD) countries (representing over 30 member countries that are among the wealthiest in the world) rose from 68.5 years in 1960 to 79.1 years in 2007.[10] Correspondingly, the average infant mortality rate in these countries dropped from 30 deaths per 1,000 live births in 1970 to 5 deaths per 1,000 live births in 2005. However, there are unfortunately still countries, particularly those in poor and politically unstable parts of the world, with vital statistics that are not much better than in the days of John Graunt. According to the *World Health Statistics Report 2010*, while the average life expectancy worldwide is 68 years, the number was much lower in some places (e.g. 42 years in Afghanistan and Zimbabwe, 46 years in Angola and Chad) and much higher in other places (e.g. 83 years in Japan and San

Marino).[11] Therefore, people in some low-income and politically unstable countries live on average 40 years less than people in the richest and most stable countries in the world.

Similarly, while childhood mortality rates have been on the decline over the last two decades in most countries, Afghanistan continues to have a staggeringly high rate of 257 deaths under five years of age per 1,000 live births. Angola, Chad and Somalia also have over 200 deaths per 1,000 live births (i.e. at least 20% of children in these countries die before their fifth birthday). As well, 30 other countries, mostly in Sub-Saharan Africa, have between 100 and 199 deaths per 1,000 live births (i.e. at least 10% of children under five die). This is in stark contrast to countries such as Finland, Greece, Iceland, Japan, Luxembourg, Norway, Singapore, Sweden and Slovenia, where there are only 3 deaths per 1,000 live births (0.3%), demonstrating that almost all childhood deaths are preventable and therefore needless human tragedies.

Health as a state of complete physical, mental and social well-being

While there is already significant complexity in the concept of "the absence of disease and disability", the definition of health as "a state of complete physical, mental and social well-being" is perhaps even more elusive. The term "well-being" is used in different disciplines to mean different things. It is wrapped up with notions of health, happiness, wealth and success. Well-being is also closely related to the concept of quality of life – yet another broad and elusive term. Many different theoretical frameworks and scales exist to better understand and measure health-related quality of life. Health economists, for instance, use methods such as rating scales, time trade-off and standard gamble techniques to assess the quality of life associated with a given health condition.[12] The time trade-off technique, for example, asks a person to imagine a hypothetical scenario where they could choose how many years of life they would be willing to give up to avoid living with a particular health condition for a specified period of time. The person may choose to live until the age of 60 years rather than 80 years (20 years less) to avoid spending 5 years in a persistent vegetative state where they can neither move nor speak and are kept alive using a respirator and a feeding tube. Or they may choose to live until age 77 years rather than 80 years (3 years less) to avoid living 15 years with diabetes, which involves taking multiple medications each day and attending regular medical visits to avoid premature heart attack, stroke, amputation, kidney failure or blindness. Thus the quality of life or utility of being in a persistent vegetative state would be considered much worse than living with diabetes. These utilities are then used to help develop more sophisticated composite measures of health as compared to the more straightforward life expectancy and mortality rates described earlier. For instance, Quality-Adjusted Life Years (QALYs) and Disability-Adjusted Life Years (DALYs) balance the length of life with the quality of life. Thus the goal in improving health is not only to increase the number of years lived, but also to improve the quality of these years. Therefore, in future, one would want the Health-Adjusted Life Expectancy at Birth (HALE) to be a very close approximation of Life Expectancy at Birth (LE) and, thus, most of the years lived would be lived in good health.

Health as a resource for individuals and for society

Although we have only scratched the surface in terms of understanding and measuring health, an important question that often follows is why do we care about health, and, even more importantly, why should others care about improving our health? Particularly as many of the determinants of health are found outside the health sector, as we shall explore further in the next section, it is important to make a strong argument as to why people working to improve education, to protect the environment or to increase profits for shareholders should care about making decisions that can also maximise health outcomes.

One approach would be to use the humanitarian argument. This approach, which is often successful in soliciting charitable donations for non-governmental organisations (NGOs), calls upon people to take action to prevent or, more often, to intervene and attempt to alleviate, the pain and suffering of others. However, while somewhat effective in certain arenas, the humanitarian argument is not always a powerful tool when there are competing interests involved that can override the desire to be altruistic. Therefore, it is also necessary to use alternative approaches that make a more self-interested argument for health (i.e. what's in it for me?).

For instance, according to the *Ottawa Charter for Health Promotion*, health is "a resource for everyday life, not the objective of living".[13] People do not live with the sole goal of being healthy, but desire to be healthy so that they can pursue other goals in life – such as raising a family, fostering a career, making a difference in the world, making money and enjoying life, leaving a legacy for the future and so forth. At a societal level, health can also contribute to greater economic growth, human development, peace and security.[14] Therefore it can be shown that health has an inherent as well as an instrumental value, both for individuals and also for society.

Perhaps the most persuasive approach is the self-preservation argument. In our globalised world, where there is increased travel across borders, it is apparent that emerging infectious diseases and environmental threats are on the rise and do not respect national boundaries. Without concerted international efforts, there may be grave impacts on all countries. No matter how wealthy or powerful they may be, no country is 100% safe, as epidemics such as SARS and the ongoing threat of avian influenza have demonstrated. These self-interest and self-preservation arguments may ultimately be more convincing than humanitarian arguments, although one would hope that world leaders, and not just philanthropists, care about alleviating human suffering by improving health.

Healthy individuals and healthy populations

When thinking about health, it is also important to consider *whose* health. Often our focus is more personal. Will my child be able to get emergency care in case of an injury? Will my father be able to have surgery to avert another heart attack? However, while this individual perspective is clearly important, it can inadvertently lead to health inequities since some people have greater resources for health than others. As well, focusing on the personal perspective often drives us to consume greater and greater amounts of costly health services and to develop more and more expensive health technologies to treat health problems, rather than focusing on prevention. According to the Naylor Report that was released following the SARS pandemic, public health efforts are chronically underfunded and receive less than 3% of the overall spending on health.[15] Therefore, in addition to the individual perspective, it is also necessary to adopt a population perspective to better understand how to protect and promote health on a large scale.[16]

Populations, however, are rarely homogeneous. They are often composed of different groups with a variety of health needs that are being met, to a greater or lesser extent, by the health and social systems in place. The differences in health status between different groups are commonly referred to as health inequities. Often, these health inequities are a reflection of underlying social inequities that exist between groups. Social inequities are measured in different ways. For instance, one of the most commonly used techniques is the Gini coefficient that measures the distribution of income, ranging from 0 (total equality where every citizen has the same income) to 1 (total inequality where one citizen has 100% of the national income).

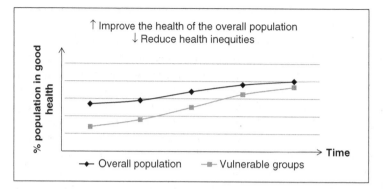

Figure 2.2 The dual goal of population health is to improve health and to reduce health inequities.

Less-equal countries such as Haiti and South Africa have Gini coefficients around 0.60, whereas more-equal countries such as Denmark, Finland, Norway, Sweden and Japan have Gini coefficients closer to 0.20.[17] In contrast, health inequities are generally demonstrated by the gradient in health outcomes from the poorest to the richest quintiles (one-fifth) of the population or by comparing the "gap" in health outcomes between two distinct groups (i.e. Aboriginal versus non-Aboriginal, women versus men, migrant workers versus non-migrant workers, etc.). The goal of population health is therefore twofold: to improve the health of the population overall and to reduce health inequities within and between groups (Fig. 2.2).

For example, in Australia, the average life expectancy of Aboriginal peoples is almost 20 years less than for non-Aboriginal Australians.[18] In Canada, the life expectancy gaps between Aboriginal and non-Aboriginal groups are approximately six to eight years.[19] Similar health gaps are also found in many other countries around the world. The population health goal would therefore be to increase the life expectancy of all citizens while reducing the life-expectancy gap between Aboriginal and non-Aboriginal groups. This example uses life expectancy as the health outcome, but any health outcome may be used here. For instance, the goal could be to reduce the incidence of obesity or cancer or suicide for all members of the population while also reducing the gap between specific vulnerable groups and the population average. Throughout this book, when I refer to improving health, I always have in mind this dual goal of improving the overall health of the population and reducing health inequities.

Risk factors and determinants of health

Being able to improve health outcomes requires first understanding the factors that lead to poor health (i.e. the causes), and then being able to intervene effectively (Fig. 2.3).

For hundreds, if not thousands, of years there have been various theories on what causes poor health, ranging from "bad air" or miasmas to demons and evil spirits. In 1884, the German physician and scientist Robert Koch demonstrated the microbial aetiology of certain diseases using a set of four criteria that are now known as Koch's postulates.[20] By extracting bacteria from diseased organisms, growing the bacteria in culture, inoculating healthy organisms, which then became ill, and then re-extracting the bacteria, Koch was able to show that the microscopic bacteria, which are not visible to the human eye, are the causal agents of certain diseases. Koch was thus the first to provide experimental evidence of the germ theory of disease that revolutionised the prevention and treatment of communicable diseases. However, such

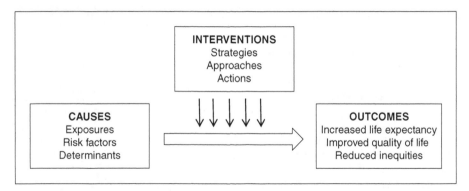

Figure 2.3 Causes, interventions and outcomes.

experimental methods would now be considered unethical in human subjects (and some would argue in animals as well), thus other approaches to determining causality were needed. As well, many important causes of death and disease, such as carcinogens, do not act immediately but rather take effect over extended periods of time, and therefore a longer follow-up is required to demonstrate causality, depending on the health problem in question.

Risk factors associated with disease

While infectious agents such as bacteria and viruses generally have very short incubation periods lasting only a few hours, days or weeks from the time of exposure to the development of symptoms,[21] many common chronic diseases such as cancer and heart disease involve many years of exposure to a variety of risk factors before symptoms appear.

One of the first landmark, population-based studies that provided strong evidence for an association between a specific risk factor (i.e. smoking) and a negative health outcome (i.e. lung cancer) was the cohort study of Sir Richard Doll and colleagues, which followed a group of British doctors for over 50 years.[22] Another classic cohort study that identified multiple modifiable risk factors for heart disease (i.e. high blood pressure, high blood cholesterol, smoking, obesity, diabetes and physical inactivity) was the Framingham Heart Study, which has been ongoing since 1948.[23]

Thus, for many decades, the main focus was on identifying the various risk factors, such as smoking, sedentary lifestyle and unhealthy diet, that are associated with chronic disease. It was assumed that reducing exposure to these risk factors would thereby prevent disease and premature death. Yet, multiple-risk-factor interventions using counselling and educational methods aimed at behaviour change have not been successful at reducing mortality.[24] Therefore, perhaps these risk factors are just markers of other more deeply rooted causes of poor health.

Upstream determinants of health

Increasingly it is being recognised that risk factors are not evenly distributed within populations. Certain subgroups, particularly those of lower socio-economic status (SES), have been found to have a larger proportion of risk factors and, consequently, suffer from poorer health. This is especially the case in the absence of pro-poor interventions such as progressive taxation and income transfers that can redistribute wealth and markedly reduce the Gini coefficient, thus narrowing the gap between the rich and the poor and mitigating the negative impact of poverty on health (Box 2.1).[25]

Box 2.1   What determines health?

Why is Jason in the hospital?
> Because he has a bad infection in his leg.

But why does he have an infection?
> Because he has a cut on his leg and it got infected.

But why does he have a cut on his leg?
> Because he was playing in the junk yard next to his apartment building and there was some sharp, jagged steel there that he fell on.

But why was he playing in a junk yard?
> Because his neighbourhood is kind of run down. A lot of kids play there and there is no one to supervise them.

But why does he live in that neighbourhood?
> Because his parents can't afford a nicer place to live.

But why can't his parents afford a nicer place to live?
> Because his dad is unemployed and his mom is sick.

But why is his dad unemployed?
> Because he doesn't have much education and he can't find a job.

But why . . .?

Reproduced with permission from *Toward a Healthy Future: Second Report on the Health of Canadians*. Ottawa: Minister of Public Works and Government Services Canada, 1999.

Indeed, for a wide range of health outcomes from disease incidence to hospitalisation and mortality, it has been shown that richer quintiles (i.e. the richest one-fifth of the population) have better health than the poorer quintiles (i.e. the poorest one-fifth of the population). Moreover, the intermediate quintiles have gradually worsening health the poorer they get, often referred to as the "social gradient".

While one could target the poorer groups and attempt to reduce their exposure to specific risk factors, the focus has shifted to better understanding why these discrepancies exist between groups and what could be done about the underlying "upstream" factors such as income, social status, education, early childhood development and so forth that influence these differences.[26] These "upstream" factors are known collectively as the social determinants of health. Following the recent publication of the final report of the WHO Commission on Social Determinants of Health entitled *Closing the Gap in a Generation*,[27] social determinants are currently a major focus of research on the causes of poor health, particularly since inequities in health have been growing rather than diminishing. This shift from a risk-factor approach to a social determinants approach has been increasingly gaining in momentum over the last few decades.

The health care system is not the only determinant of health

Many people still believe that pouring more money into bloated health care systems is the best way to improve health. Yet in 1974 there was a major shift in our collective thinking brought about by a landmark report entitled *A New Perspective on the Health of Canadians*, written by the then Canadian Minister of Health, Marc Lalonde.[28] Although Canada had just launched their publicly funded Medicare system, which provides universal access to health care services for all Canadians, Lalonde argued that the provision of health services is only one determinant of health, and certainly not the most important one. He considered that there were three other determinants of health (which he called "health fields") that were equally or

Box 2.2 Moving from putting on "band-aids" to prevention

I first learned about the power of prevention as a medical student. One of my few "out-of-hospital" learning experiences involved taking a walk with a social worker through a poor neighbourhood served by a local community clinic. We passed by people sleeping on the street and a park which was commonly frequented by injection drug users, but I was particularly struck by our visit to an elderly woman with no children or relatives who was living alone in a small apartment on the ground floor of an ordinary-looking residential building. The previous year she had slipped in the bath and had broken her hip – a common occurrence among the elderly, particularly elderly women with osteoporosis (brittle bones). As a result, she spent three months in acute care to undergo hip replacement surgery, which was complicated by infection, then another six months in a rehabilitation centre building up her muscle strength and relearning how to walk with her new prosthesis. At $1,000 per day in hospital, plus the surgery and medication costs, the government had spent over $100,000 for the acute care stay alone and at least another $50,000 for the lengthy rehabilitation, not to mention the emotional and physical trauma that this caused the elderly woman. How much would it have cost to have prevented this injury in the first place? Someone from social services could have made a home visit and helped the woman to equip her bathroom with a handrail and non-slip bathmat and chair. As well, having identified her as being at high risk, an attendant could have visited her home twice a week to help her with her bath, as well as attending to any other health matters or related issues. This would have certainly cost far less than $150,000, even over the course of many years of follow-up. The moral imperative should therefore be to avoid preventable health problems and to rethink how we are spending our resources, which could be better spent in other ways, both at home and abroad. How many thousands of children in low-income countries could be vaccinated for $150,000? Multiply that by 10 preventable hip surgeries or by 100. We do not lack the resources but we need to take a broader view on the causes of poor health to guide how we spend these resources.

even more important than health care services. These included human biology (i.e. a person's genetic endowment), lifestyle factors (i.e. whether the person smokes, exercises, has a healthy diet, etc.) and the environment (i.e. including both the physical and social environment). Therefore, while most health budgets are spent on expensive medical services and technologies fuelled by the moral imperative of acute care medicine (i.e. how can you deny services to this person in need?), there is very little focus on addressing the upstream causes of poor health. Yet acute care medicine generally provides a "band-aid" or a quick-fix solution when ideally one could prevent many health problems from occurring in the first place (Box 2.2).

Many determinants of health lie outside the health sector

The visionary 1986 *Ottawa Charter for Health Promotion* expanded on Lalonde's health field concept by identifying many more determinants of health, most of which lie outside the health sector. These "prerequisites for health" include: peace, shelter, education, food, income, a stable ecosystem, sustainable resources, social justice and equity. Some might believe that these prerequisites are only threatened in poor countries. However, even in wealthier countries, the basic necessities of life (i.e. food, shelter, sanitation, etc.) are still unmet for large segments of the population, and thus present important barriers to health. Of course, in politically unstable countries where there is war and oppression, the situation is even worse. In the International Red Cross and Red Crescent Museum in Geneva there is a room with a plaque for each year going back over a century. Each plaque bears the names of the nation states around the world at war that year. In some years there is a long list with dozens of countries at war, and in other years the list is shorter, but the number never goes down to zero. Decades of infrastructure development and efforts to improve health can be wiped out by even short bouts of political instability, sometimes requiring generations to recover. While we tend to focus our energy and resources on trying to tackle specific diseases and risk factors, we often lose sight of the bigger picture. Indeed politics matters to the health of citizens. Social justice and equity are key values in public health.[29] Unfortunately, the societies in which we live do not always share these values (to which the Gini coefficients can attest). Many countries have a small group of people – the elite ruling class – who control the majority of the country's wealth. Given this imbalance, it is therefore not surprising that political stability is often elusive. Social democracies that truly serve their citizens by providing them with economic, social and political rights including a range of social protection safety nets, such as publicly funded universal health care coverage and unemployment insurance, are better equipped to promote health and reduce health inequities, which in turn contributes to greater political stability. A similar argument can be made for improving global governance and redressing the imbalance between rich and poor countries, as the legacy of colonisation and the ongoing exploitation of poor countries further restricts the capacity of many national governments to adequately provide for the well-being of their citizens.

A framework for describing the determinants of health

While several different frameworks and models exist for describing the determinants of health, the Hamilton and Bhatti integrated model of population health and health promotion includes what are currently held to be among the main determinants (Fig. 2.4).[30]

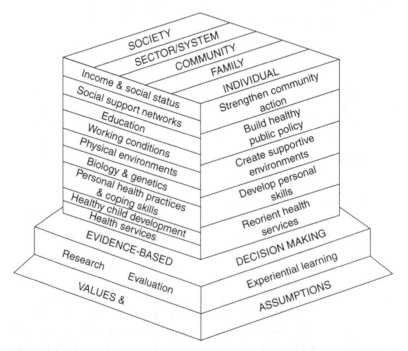

Figure 2.4 Integrated model of population health and health promotion.
Reproduced from Hamilton N, Bhatti T. *An Integrated Model of Population Health and Health Promotion.* Ottawa: Health Canada, 1995, with the permission of the Minister of Public Works and Government Services Canada, 2012.

Lalonde's original "health fields" are included in this list, as are income and education, two of the major "prerequisites for health" from the Ottawa Charter. Other determinants that have been identified more recently as being important are social support, working conditions and early childhood development. Not included on this list but equally important are gender and culture. Of course, understanding the many complex and inter-related causes of poor health is only the first step. Being able to take action to improve population health outcomes is a whole other challenge.

Strategies for improving health

One of the main strategies that has long been used to improve health is centred on the clinical encounter (e.g. the doctor–patient relationship), whereby the patient seeks care from a health care provider and an attempt is made to improve health one individual at a time through diagnosis, treatment and rehabilitation. For instance, when a person is sick, they go to see a health practitioner (i.e. doctor, nurse, community health worker, traditional healer, etc.), who makes an assessment of the health problem (i.e. a diagnosis) and then recommends one or more ways to improve health (i.e. treatments). These recommendations may include a healthier diet, more exercise, quitting smoking, reducing the intake of alcohol and drugs, attending individual or group therapy, taking a medication or spiritual healing. While providing acute care in a clinical setting is certainly important, as discussed previously, it is also necessary to apply a public health lens and use a broader range of strategies if we want to make an impact on improving health at the population level.

Indeed, improving health at the population level requires planning (Fig. 2.5). However, instead of focusing on individual patients, the starting point is the population. And rather than seeking advice one-on-one, health planners are the "healers" of the entire population. Whether they are public health experts, consultants, community leaders or even health practitioners (as in the community-oriented primary care model), health planners make a "diagnosis" of the main health problems in the population and recommend ways to improve the health of the population. For instance, their recommendations may include establishing a nurse home-visitation programme for all first-time parents of newly born babies to reduce child abuse and neglect, partnering with the education and labour sectors to improve educational attainment and employment rates, promoting policies for wealth redistribution and the provision of high-quality, low-cost housing, or creating supportive environments to

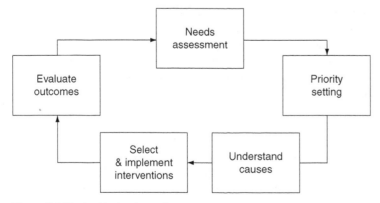

Figure 2.5 The health planning cycle.

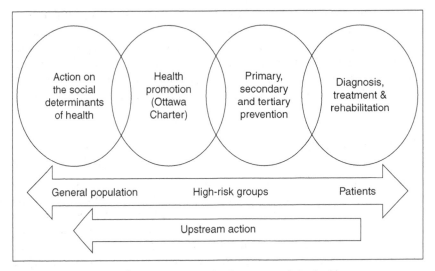

Figure 2.6 A continuum of strategies is required to improve population health.
Reproduced from Andermann A. Screening for abdominal aortic aneurysm: should we lower the intervention cut-off point? *BMJ* 2012: 344:e3111, with permission from BMJ Publishing Group Ltd.

increase physical activity. Health planning therefore entails better understanding the health needs of the population, choosing appropriate strategies for addressing priority health problems, as well as evaluating whether the strategies that have been implemented were effective in improving health.

An important key to successful health planning is choosing an appropriate complement of strategies that address the priority health problems and are well suited to the local context. Similar to baking a cake, if you do not use the right ingredients you are unlikely to get a good outcome. Therefore the choice of which strategies to use is particularly important.

A continuum of strategies for improving health

There is no single best way to improve health. In his seminal article, "Sick individuals and sick populations", Geoffrey Rose discusses the pros and cons of taking a "population approach" (i.e. interventions aimed at improving the health of the entire population) versus a "high-risk approach" (i.e. interventions targeted towards those with risk factors or disease).[31] In reality, however, it is rarely a question of either–or, but rather a continuum of strategies is required. These strategies range from the treatment and rehabilitation of people who are acutely ill to disease prevention, health promotion and action on the upstream determinants of health (Fig. 2.6).[32] I will describe each of these briefly here.

Treatment and rehabilitation

Treatment and rehabilitation are fairly straightforward concepts. A patient is sick or hurt. The patient seeks help from the formal or informal health care system. Different remedies are tried until the patient is healed or can at least be reintegrated into society and return to their former functioning and social roles insofar as possible. For most people, this is what comes to mind when there is a discussion about improving health. Improving health is often equated with health care services, although, as we have seen previously in this chapter, there are also many other important strategies further upstream.

Disease prevention

Disease prevention has been defined in Last's *Dictionary of Epidemiology* as "actions aimed at eradicating, eliminating or minimizing the impact of disease and disability".[33] Generally, disease prevention is categorised as primary, secondary or tertiary prevention according to the timing of action in the natural history of the disease (Fig. 2.7).

Primary prevention

Primary prevention involves taking action to reduce potential exposure to risk factors before people develop the disease, with the aim of reducing the incidence of disease (i.e. the number of new cases). For instance, a programme to prevent teenagers from becoming smokers would be a primary prevention strategy to reduce the number of new cases of lung cancer over the next 30 to 40 years. Many public health recommendations are forms of primary prevention, ranging from reducing sun exposure (to prevent skin cancer) and brushing your teeth (to prevent dental caries) to eating a healthy diet and being physically active (to prevent obesity, diabetes and heart disease). Ideally one would want to prevent disease before it happens, yet, politically, it is often difficult to secure funding for programmes where it may take many years or even decades before the impact can be detected.

Secondary prevention

Another form of prevention in which the impact can be detected in a much shorter time frame is secondary prevention or screening. In secondary prevention, people already have an

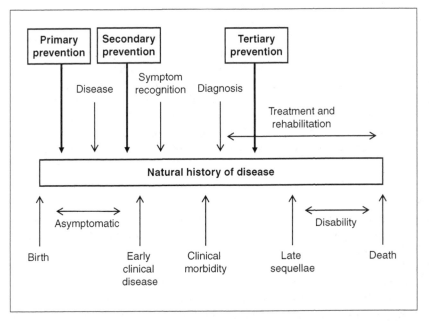

Figure 2.7 Prevention strategies according to the timing of action in the natural history of disease.

early form of the disease and it is possible to detect the disease at a pre-symptomatic stage to cure or prevent progression with greater success than if diagnosed clinically once the disease becomes symptomatic. Unlike in primary prevention, the natural history of the disease has progressed such that people already have the disease, and therefore the aim is to reduce the prevalence of the disease (i.e. the total number of cases) through early treatment and cure. A common example of secondary prevention is population-based screening for cancer, whereby people who have early markers of disease (e.g. pre-cancerous lesions such as colon polyps or cervical dysplasia) but do not yet have any obvious signs or symptoms, are screened using a variety of tests (i.e. colonoscopy for colon cancer, Papanicolaou test for cervical cancer, mammography for breast cancer, etc.). Those with a positive screen test often undergo confirmatory diagnostic testing (e.g. a biopsy examined by a pathologist to detect the presence of cancerous cells), and those who are found to have the disease are then treated. While screening can be a powerful preventive strategy, large-scale screening programmes are costly and labour intensive. As well, there are invariably those who test positive and even undergo invasive treatments when they do not have the disease (false positive) and, even worse, those who are reassured that they are healthy when they in fact do have the disease, delaying diagnosis and treatment (false negative). Thus while secondary prevention is a popular strategy for improving health, we would ideally want to prevent the disease before it occurs (primary prevention). Of course, if early detection leads to improved outcomes (which is not always the case and must be supported by the evidence), then it is better than waiting until symptoms appear.

Tertiary prevention

Tertiary prevention is not intended to reduce the incidence (number of new cases) or prevalence (total number of cases), but simply to reduce the impact of the disease. In tertiary prevention the natural history of the disease has progressed such that people already have clinical manifestations of the disease (e.g. they have suffered a heart attack or stroke). In these cases, tertiary prevention is used to avoid further complications (including death) so that people are able to reintegrate more easily back into their usual functioning and social roles. For instance, beta-blocker medication is given to people who have suffered a heart attack to prevent further heart attacks and to reduce overall mortality.[34] Similarly, elderly patients who have had a fall often receive physical and occupational therapy to strengthen their muscles and to make their home environment safer to prevent further falls that could result in disability or even death.[35] Thus tertiary prevention is closer to the realm of medical treatment and care, whereas primary prevention is closer to the realm of health promotion as defined by the Ottawa Charter.

Health promotion

The first International Conference on Health Promotion was held in Ottawa, Canada in 1986 and led to the signing of the Ottawa Charter, which laid out an overall framework for improving the health of populations. This framework is still highly respected and widely used today. Indeed, the 2005 Bangkok Charter reaffirmed the action areas of the Ottawa Charter and proposed additional measures for promoting health in an increasingly globalised world, notably by focusing on the need for increased partnerships and intersectoral action to tackle the upstream determinants of health, which largely lie outside the health sector.

The Ottawa and Bangkok charters define health promotion as "the process of enabling people to increase control over their health and its determinants, and thereby improve their health".[36] The five main health promotion action areas articulated in the Ottawa Charter are:

(1) build healthy public policy,
(2) create supportive environments,
(3) strengthen community action,
(4) develop personal skills, and
(5) reorient health services.

Developing personal skills is perhaps most closely related to the concept of primary prevention. For instance, when doctors advise their patients on how to quit smoking or to eat less fat, this is quite similar to clinic-based primary prevention. Similar messaging may also be provided through social marketing campaigns and other forms of health communication. However, while it is important to educate and counsel people on the benefits of a healthy diet and smoking cessation, these measures, on their own, have been largely ineffective in producing the desired behaviour change. Moreover, there is also an element of "blaming the victim" as well as discouragement and burnout on the part of health care providers and health planners who fail to see any noticeable health gains despite all the time and effort involved. Therefore, developing personal skills should not be used as the only strategy. Rather, it is important to place even greater emphasis on community mobilisation, building healthy public policies and creating supportive environments, which constitute a radical advance in the kinds of strategies that can be used for improving health.

Indeed, decades before the publication of Thaler and Sunstein's popular book *Nudge: Improving Decisions about Health, Wealth and Happiness*,[37] the authors of the Ottawa Charter already recognised that people's behaviours are largely influenced by their physical and social environments, and that restructuring these environments can bring about much more effective change than simply telling people what they should and should not do. Certainly people have some degree of self-determination and responsibility for their actions. Yet the health of an individual is also determined to a great extent by the health of their family, of their community and of the broader society. This interconnectedness is often referred to as the ecological model of disease (Fig. 2.8).

Thus to influence health behaviours, it is necessary to take action on these broader influences. Too often we blame the individual for making unhealthy choices resulting in poor health, when really we need to change the social and physical environment to "make the healthy choices the easy choices" (Fig. 2.9).

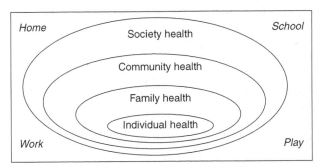

Figure 2.8 Individual health is interconnected with the health of the family, community and society.

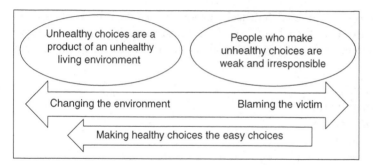

Figure 2.9 Creating supportive environments is needed to make the healthy choices the easy choices.

For instance, imagine you are at the doctor's office. You are found to be in good health but the doctor is nonetheless concerned that you smoke and are overweight – important risk factors for cancer and heart disease. You are once again advised to quit smoking, eat a healthy diet and exercise more. Nothing you did not already know. However, not so easy to put into action, especially as the people around you smoke and, with your busy schedule, it is difficult to eat a balanced diet and fit in time for exercise. In addition to developing the personal skills to change these behaviours, the Ottawa Charter suggests tackling the underlying factors that influence these behaviours. For example, building healthy public policies can range from school and workplace regulations that ban soft-drink machines to laws against smoking in public places and "sin taxes" that increase the cost of cigarettes. Creating supportive environments for health could include installing a workplace gymnasium with fitness classes that employees can attend during their lunch hour or after work, building an extensive network of bicycle paths for recreation and commuting to work, and ensuring that restaurants and cafeterias serve healthy, low-fat meals.

Healthy public policies and supportive environments for health are particularly important strategies since they are "the great equalisers". That is, they do not apply only to certain groups and not to others, but rather, they benefit all members of society and particularly the least well off. For instance, if you advise people to give their children fluoride supplements to protect their teeth, then generally those who are wealthy and well-educated will be more likely to be made aware of these recommendations (i.e. since they are more likely to attend regular dental cleanings, which are generally not covered by publicly funded health insurance and can be quite costly), and they will also have the means to be able to follow these recommendations (i.e. to pay for the fluoride supplements). Thus even well-intentioned recommendations can inadvertently lead to greater health inequities when there are barriers to widespread use. In contrast, by fluoridating the water system, all families, rich and poor, will receive the intervention, and therefore the gap between the rich and the poor will be reduced.

In addition to building healthy public policies and creating supportive environments, it is also important to help communities to mobilise action and support for interventions that reduce risky behaviours and promote health. For instance, changing the social norm from a society that considers smoking as "normal" (and even desirable and sexy) to a society where smoking is regarded as unhealthy and unappealing will make it more likely that people will adhere to no-smoking laws and respect smoke-free zones. Conversely, one can also change the social norm in the opposite direction to promote healthy behaviours, such as breastfeeding, by making it more socially acceptable to breastfeed in public.

The final health promotion strategy involves reorienting health services to provide outreach to vulnerable and marginalised groups that are often at greatest risk and yet have the least access to important resources and services. We cannot wait for patients to appear at our doorstep. Rather, we need to go into the community and reach out to those in need. There are many ways of doing so, from nurse-led home-visitation programmes to community-based self-help groups and so forth.

Therefore, while health promotion is sometimes thought of as a vague and nebulous term, it is actually a powerful combination of strategies that has already had tremendous success, from the reduction of exposure to second-hand smoke to the decline in motor-vehicle injuries. Yet there is still a great deal more to be done. The strategies of the Ottawa Charter that have been most successful are those that focus on building healthy public policies and creating supportive environments. However, as we begin to tackle the upstream social determinants of health, we need to continue to develop new and innovative strategies for improving health.

Addressing the social determinants of health

Indeed, a host of new strategies are being developed to tackle the upstream determinants of health, including intersectoral action and whole-of-government approaches. These strategies – which are not focused on individual patients or specific at-risk groups, but rather on the entire community – require the participation and involvement of partners outside the health sector and of government at all levels. A quarter century after the signing of the Ottawa Charter, our understanding of the opportunities and challenges for improving health has evolved. While the strategies of the Ottawa Charter continue to be highly regarded and valuable tools, the Bangkok Charter places a much greater emphasis on the need to partner with all sectors of government, as well as with civil society and even industry, to improve the health of the population on a global scale.

For instance, tackling the obesity and chronic disease pandemic without the help and cooperation of the food manufacturing industry will be challenging. Social marketing campaigns funded by public health authorities are "drops in the bucket" compared to the global mass marketing of fast food and junk food funded by large multinational corporations. Yet reducing the salt content in pre-prepared foods to reduce blood pressure and the associated risk of stroke is one example of how the food industry can take simple and inexpensive measures that can have a significant and widespread impact on health. Increasingly, low-sodium options are now appearing on grocery store shelves, and fast-food chains are starting to offer low-fat alternatives on their menus, not only because it improves health, but because it is good for business. Building these partnerships and influencing these changes is a challenge, but one that will lead to important health gains.

Even at the local level, there needs to be intersectoral health committees involving many partners such as women's groups, youth groups, schools, urban planners, the police, youth protection, restaurants, stores and so forth, who work together in finding shared solutions to shared health and social problems. There is therefore a need for greater leadership at all levels to ensure that there is "health in all policies" – meaning that we always consider the impact of any decision on health and how to maximise the benefits and minimise harms.

Public health

The continuum of strategies described in this chapter is part of the growing arsenal of approaches used in the field of public health to improve health outcomes and reduce health inequities. In 1920, Charles Edward Amory Winslow, founder of the Yale School of Public Health and an American pioneer in the field, defined public health as follows:

> Public health is the science and the art of preventing disease, prolonging life, and promoting physical health and efficiency through organized community efforts for the sanitation of the environment, the control of community infections, the education of the individual in principles of personal hygiene, the organization of medical and nursing service for the early diagnosis and preventive treatment of disease, and the development of the social machinery which will ensure to every individual in the community a standard of living adequate for the maintenance of health.[38]

More recently, a somewhat shorter definition was proposed by Sir Donald Acheson, former Chief Medical Officer for Health of the United Kingdom and Chairperson of the 1988 report on *Public Health in England*. He describes public health quite simply as "the science and art of preventing disease, prolonging life and promoting health through the organized efforts of society".[39]

Many of the roles described by Winslow almost a century ago are the same core functions[40] and essential services[41] that public health professionals pursue to this day (Table 2.1).[40,41] According to Canada's Advisory Committee on Population Health, the core functions of public health include:

(1) health protection,
(2) disease prevention,
(3) health promotion,
(4) population health assessment, and
(5) surveillance.[42]

Disease prevention and health promotion have been described earlier in this chapter, so I will focus here on health protection, population health assessment and surveillance. Health protection involves addressing imminent and potentially widespread threats to the health

Table 2.1 Core public health functions and essential services.

Assessment
- Monitor health status to identify community health problems
- Diagnose and investigate health problems and health hazards in the community

Policy development
- Inform, educate and empower people about health issues
- Mobilise community partnerships to identify and solve health problems
- Develop policies and plans that support individual and community health efforts

Assurance
- Enforce laws and regulations that protect health and ensure safety
- Link people to health services and assure the provision of health care when unavailable
- Assure a competent public health and personal health care workforce
- Evaluate effectiveness, accessibility and quality of personal and population health services
- Research for new insights and innovative solutions to health problems

Adapted from: Institute of Medicine. *The Future of Public Health*. Washington, DC: National Academy Press, 1988, and Public Health Functions Steering Committee. *Ten Essential Public Health Services*. Atlanta: Centers for Disease Control and Prevention, 1994.

of the population, such as outbreaks of infectious diseases or exposure to contaminants in drinking water. Generally included under the heading of health protection are communicable disease prevention and control, environmental health, occupational health, and emergency preparedness planning. However, to aid public health planning and the optimal use of resources for improving health, a population health assessment is needed. This entails creating a "health portrait" to identify the most pressing health needs of the population and to determine which efforts in prevention, promotion and protection should be prioritised. Finally, surveillance is defined by Teutsch and Churchill as the "ongoing systematic collection, analysis and interpretation of outcome-specific data for use in the planning, implementation and evaluation of public health practice".[43] Surveillance is therefore an important tool for assessing the health of the population and for evaluating the effectiveness of disease prevention and health promotion strategies in improving health. As well, surveillance is also used to rapidly identify and address infectious disease outbreaks or clusters of disease resulting from exposure to contaminants. The five core functions of public health are therefore complementary strategies for improving the health of the population.

While the average life expectancy has more than doubled since the days of John Graunt, the *World Health Report 2008* emphasises that, despite these advances, inequities in health within and between countries have been growing.[44] Yet, according to Geoffrey Rose, "there is no known biological reason why every population should not be as healthy as the best. . . The scale and pattern of disease reflect the way that people live and their social, economic and environmental circumstances".[45] The Institute of Medicine's (IOM's) Committee on Assuring the Health of the Public in the 21st Century recommended that further improving health and reducing health inequities will require adopting a population health approach, strengthening public health capacity, building intersectoral partnerships to address the upstream determinants of health, and ensuring accountability of public authorities. In particular, the IOM highlights the importance of "making evidence the foundation of decision-making for health".[46] The following chapters will examine the intricacies of the decision-making process and how to increase the use of evidence in decision-making.

References

1. International Conference on Primary Health Care. *Declaration of Alma-Ata*. Geneva: World Health Organization, 1978. Available at: http://www.who.int/ publications/almaata_declaration_en.pdf.

2. World Health Organization. *Working for Health: An Introduction to the World Health Organization*. Geneva: World Health Organization, 2007. Available at: http://www.who.int/about/ brochure_en.pdf.

3. World Health Organization. *WHO Constitution*. Geneva: World Health Organization, 1948. Available at: http:// www.who.int/governance/eb/ who_constitution_en.pdf.

4. Royal Commission on Aboriginal Peoples. *Royal Commission Report on Aboriginal Peoples*. Ottawa: Canada Communication Group Publishing, 1996. Available at: http://www.collectionscanada.gc.ca/ webarchives/20071115053257/http:// www.ainc-inac.gc.ca/ch/rcap/sg/sgmm_e. html.

5. Reading J, Kmetic A, Gideon V. *First Nations Wholistic Policy and Planning Model: Discussion Paper for the World Health Organization Commission on the Social Determinants of Health*. Ottawa: Assembly of First Nations, 2007. Available at: http://ahrnets.ca/files/2011/02/ AFN_Paper_2007.pdf.

6. Kleinman A. *The Illness Narratives: Suffering, Healing, and the Human Condition*. New York: Basic Books, 1988.

7. World Health Organization. *International Classification of Functioning, Disability and Health*. Geneva: World Health

Organization, 2003. Available at: http://www.who.int/classifications/icf/en/.

8. Patrick D, Starks H, Cain K, Uhlmann R, Pearlman R. Measuring preferences for health states worse than death. *Med Dec Making* 1994; 14(1): 9–18.

9. Graunt J. *Natural and Political Observations Made Upon the Bills of Mortality*. London: Roycroft Printers, 1662.

10. Organisation for Economic Co-operation and Development. *OECD Factbook 2010*. Paris: Organisation for Economic Co-operation and Development, 2010.

11. World Health Organization. *World Health Statistics Report 2010*. Geneva: World Health Organization, 2010. Available at: http://www.who.int/gho/publications/world_health_statistics/EN_WHS10_Full.pdf.

12. Drummond M, Sculpher M, Torrance G, O'Brien B, Stoddart G. *Methods for the Economic Evaluation of Health Care Programmes*, 3rd edn. Oxford: Oxford University Press, 2005.

13. World Health Organization. *Ottawa Charter for Health Promotion*. Geneva: World Health Organization, 1986. Available at: http://www.phac-aspc.gc.ca/ph-sp/docs/charter-chartre/pdf/charter.pdf.

14. Commission on Macroeconomics and Health. *Investing in Health: A Summary of the Findings of the Commission on Macroeconomics and Health*. Geneva: World Health Organization, 2002. Available at: http://www.who.int/macrohealth/infocentre/advocacy/en/investinginhealth02052003.pdf.

15. Naylor D, Basrur S, Bergeron M *et al*. *Learning from SARS: Renewal of Public Health in Canada*. Ottawa: Health Canada, 2003.

16. Young TK. *Population Health: Concepts and Methods*, 2nd edn. Oxford: Oxford University Press, 2005.

17. The World Bank. *World Development Indicators (WDI) database*. Washington DC: World Bank, Development Research Group, 2012. Available at: http://databank.worldbank.org/ddp/home.do?Step=12&id=4&CNO=2.

18. Australian Bureau of Statistics. *The health and welfare of Australia's Aboriginal and Torres Strait Islander peoples*. Canberra: Australian Bureau of Statistics, 2005. Available at: http://www.ausstats.abs.gov.au/Ausstats/subscriber.nsf/0/DDA14B230A5F3C98CA25715D0019B5BF/$File/4704055002_2005.pdf.

19. Canadian Institute for Health Information. *Improving the Health of Canadians*. Ottawa: Canadian Institute for Health Information, 2004. Available at: https://secure.cihi.ca/free_products/IHC2004rev_e.pdf.

20. Koch R. Die Aetiologie der Tuberkulose. *Mitt Kaiser Gesundh* 1884; 2: 1–88.

21. Heymann D (ed.). *Control of Communicable Diseases Manual*, 19th edn. Atlanta: APHA, 2008.

22. Doll R, Peto R, Boreham J, Sutherland I. Mortality in relation to smoking: 50 years' observations on male British doctors. *BMJ* 2004; 328: 1519–28.

23. Kannel W. The Framingham Study: its 50-year legacy and future promise. *J Atheroscler Thromb* 2000; 6(2): 60–6.

24. Ebrahim S, Beswick A, Burke M, Davey Smith G. Multiple risk factor interventions for primary prevention of coronary heart disease. *Cochrane Database Syst Rev* 2006; (4): CD001561.

25. Federal, Provincial and Territorial Advisory Committee on Population Health. *Toward a Healthy Future: Second Report on the Health of Canadians*. Ottawa: Minister of Public Works and Government Services Canada, 1999. Available at: http://www.phac-aspc.gc.ca/ph-sp/report-rapport/toward/pdf/toward_a_healthy_english.PDF.

26. Evans R, Barer M, Marmor T. *Why Are Some People Healthy and Others Not? The Determinants of Health of Populations*. New York: Walter de Gruyter, 1994.

27. Commission on Social Determinants of Health (CSDH). *Closing the Gap in a Generation: Health Equity through Action on the Social Determinants of Health, Final Report of the Commission on Social Determinants of Health*. Geneva: World Health Organization, 2008. Available at: http://whqlibdoc.who.int/publications/2008/9789241563703_eng.pdf.

28. Lalonde M. *A New Perspective on the Health of Canadians*. Ottawa: Health Canada, 1974. Available at: http://www.phac-aspc.gc.ca/ph-sp/pdf/perspect-eng.pdf.

29. Power M, Faden R. *Social Justice: The Moral Foundations of Public Health and Health*

Policy. Oxford: Oxford University Press, 2006.

30. Hamilton N, Bhatti T. *An Integrated Model of Population Health and Health Promotion.* Ottawa: Health Canada, 1995. Available at: http://www.courseweb.uottawa.ca/pop8910/ Outline/Models/Hamilton-Bhatti.htm.

31. Rose G. Sick individuals and sick populations. *Int J Epidemiol* 1985; 14: 32–8.

32. Andermann A. Screening for abdominal aortic aneurysm: should we lower the intervention cut-off point? [commissioned editorial] *BMJ* 2012; 344:e3111.

33. Last J. *A Dictionary of Epidemiology,* 4th edn. Oxford: Oxford University Press, 2001.

34. Freemantle N, Cleland J, Young P, Mason J, Harrison J. Beta blockade after myocardial infarction: systematic review and meta regression analysis. *BMJ* 1999; 318(7200): 1730–7.

35. Michael Y, Lin J, Whitlock E, *et al. Interventions to Prevent Falls in Older Adults: An Updated Systematic Review.* Rockville, MD: Agency for Healthcare Research and Quality, 2010. Available at: http:// www.uspreventiveservicestaskforce.org/ uspstf11/fallsprevention/fallspreves.pdf.

36. World Health Organization. *Bangkok Charter for Health Promotion in a Globalized World.* Geneva: World Health Organization, 2006. Available at: http://www.who.int/healthpromotion/ conferences/6gchp/hpr_050829_ %20BCHP.pdf.

37. Thaler R, Sunstein C. *Nudge: Improving Decisions about Health, Wealth and Happiness.* New haven: Yale University Press, 2008.

38. Winslow C. The untilled fields of public health. *Science* 1920; 51(1306): 23–33.

39. Acheson D. *Public Health in England: The Report of the Committee of Inquiry into the Future Development of the Public Health Function.* London: HMSO, 1988.

40. Institute of Medicine. *The Future of Public Health.* Washington, DC: National Academy Press, 1988.

41. Public Health Functions Steering Committee. *Ten Essential Public Health Services.* Atlanta: Centers for Disease Control and Prevention, 1994. Available at: http://www.cdc.gov/nphpsp/ essentialServices.html.

42. Advisory Committee on Population Health. *Survey of Public Health Capacity in Canada: Highlights.* Ottawa: Advisory Committee on Population Health, 2002.

43. Teutsch S, Churchill R (eds.). *Principles and Practice of Public Health Surveillance,* 2nd edn. Oxford: Oxford University Press, 2000.

44. Van Lerberghe W, Evans T, Rasanathan K *et al. The World Health Report 2008 – Primary Health Care (Now More than Ever).* Geneva: World Health Organization, 2008. Available at: http://www.who.int/whr/2008/en/index. html.

45. Rose G. *Rose's Strategy of Preventive Medicine.* Oxford: Oxford University Press, 2008.

46. Institute of Medicine (IOM) Committee on Assuring the Health of the Public in the 21st Century. *The Future of the Public's Health in the 21st Century.* Washington DC: Institute of Medicine, 2003. Available at: http://books.nap.edu/openbook.php? record_id=10548.

Available at: http://www.sciencemag.org/ content/51/1306/23.full.pdf.

Understanding how decisions influence health

Decision-making for health is a complex matter. Some decisions are banal everyday choices that we make at the individual level – decisions that are often shaped by many extrinsic forces. Should I buy sweets or a fruit as a snack? Will I drive or cycle to work today? While each individual decision may have relatively little importance, taken together and multiplied across the entire population, the effects can add up. Nonetheless, we are generally very preoccupied with these small decisions, while large-scale decisions made at a population or global level seem entirely beyond our control and tend to go unnoticed, even though they may have even more profound effects on our collective health. For instance, certain countries are attempting to develop nuclear weapons, other countries have a *laissez faire* attitude towards the oversight of financial markets risking worldwide economic crises, and others still continue to produce and export harmful products ranging from asbestos to machine guns and cluster bombs, which could have devastating impacts on the health of large numbers of people worldwide. Who is regulating these decisions? How can we better inform these decisions using the best available evidence? The purpose of this chapter is to provide an overview of decision-making for health from patient choice to global policy as a first step towards better understanding how these decisions are made and how we can intervene to improve health.

Individual health decisions

We all make decisions about our health. Some decisions are rather quick and painless, and others are more important and thought through. Some decisions we make for ourselves, and others are for the health of loved ones. Some decisions, particularly those that deal with questions of life and death, we hope that we never have to face, and, if we do, we would want someone well informed and trustworthy to be there to guide us through it. Thus there are a range of different health decisions made at an individual level, and a wide array of factors that influence these decisions. To illustrate these, and to provide an introduction to the extensive but disparate literature on the subject, I will use three case examples. First, a 55-year-old smoker in Eastern Europe who is considering quitting smoking. Second, a 38-year-old woman in North America with a family history of breast cancer who is considering preventive surgery. And third, a 28-year-old mother in rural Africa who is considering taking her children to be vaccinated. Of course, there are innumerable other examples that could be used, each of which would bring out different subtleties, but these three cases (Box 3.1) will provide an initial basis for understanding the decision-making process at the individual level.

Box 3.1 Individual-level decision-making for health

Case A: Deciding to quit smoking

Mr. X lives in Eastern Europe. He goes to his family doctor for a routine check-up. He is 55 years old and in fairly good health. He has never been hospitalised and takes no medication. He has been feeling well since the last visit but is very concerned about his wife who has recently been diagnosed with lung cancer. In the last few weeks he has been feeling depressed at the thought of losing her and being alone. They have no children. They had tried to have kids for many years but it never happened and they did not want to adopt. Instead, they both focused on their work. Mr. X has worked in the same company for over 30 years as a manual labourer. He is proud that he has never missed a day at work. His wife was a waitress at a local restaurant-bar until she fell ill and had to stop work. After a long day at work, Mr. X enjoys having a drink with friends and smoking a few cigarettes. His wife never smoked or drank alcohol. According to the family doctor, Mr. X has normal blood pressure and blood sugar. His risk for heart disease is however elevated due to his age, his slightly elevated cholesterol and his smoking. As well, smoking is an important risk factor for cancer and lung disease. Therefore the doctor recommends (again) that Mr. X should consider quitting smoking and should also modify his diet and exercise to improve his cholesterol levels. Mr. X is not sure that he is ready to make these changes right now. He needs the cigarettes to calm his nerves and to see him through this difficult time in his life.

Case B: Deciding to undergo surgery

Mrs. Y lives in North America. She just turned 38 years old – the same age that her mother had been when she was diagnosed with breast cancer. Mrs. Y can still recall the day when she was only 14 years old and she came home from school to find her mother waiting for her in the living room with a worried expression on her face. That is when she first learned about the cancer, and she spent the next four years of her adolescence watching her mother suffering through the endless treatments but to no avail. Her mother died 20 years ago, a few days before Mrs. Y's 18th birthday. Mrs. Y has children of her own now – ages 4, 8 and 10 years. She dreads that the same thing will happen to her. What effect will it have on her children? She can't bear to think about it. Her sister, who is two years older than her and lives in Australia, told her about an article in a magazine recommending that women with a family history of breast cancer seek medical advice. Tremendous advances have been made in treatment options over the last few decades. Even effective preventive options are now available. Her sister has already gone to see someone about it and is urging her to get advice as well. Mrs. Y is undecided. She is still so young. Does she want to spend the next 20 or 30 years waiting for the cancer to appear and living under this cloud of uncertainty? What if she is a *BRCA* gene carrier, which predisposes women to develop breast and ovarian cancers at an early age? Would she then require surgery to remove her breasts and ovaries and go into early menopause to avoid repeating her mother's experience? With the kids and her career, Mrs. Y doesn't even know when she could make time to book an appointment even if she did want to explore her options.

Case C: Deciding to vaccinate one's child

Mrs. Z lives in rural Africa. She is 28 years old, recently widowed and has five children. The youngest child is only five months old. Her husband was killed in a road traffic accident and she now has no income and no help at home except for her elderly grandmother who lives with them but is almost blind from cataracts. Mrs. Z no longer has the time to walk one hour each way to go fetch water from the nearest spring and therefore has started to take their water for bathing and cooking from a stream closer to the village where they live. As a result, the family has suffered from multiple bouts of diarrhoea in recent weeks and Mrs. Z once even had to take her three-year-old to the nearest charity hospital, a three-hour walk away, where she had to wait all afternoon for the child's rehydration therapy. Since she was still breast-feeding the youngest child, she brought him along as well. At the hospital, the nurse – a missionary from Europe – asked whether she wanted her children to be vaccinated against life-threatening diseases such as polio, which can be transmitted through unclean water. Mrs. Z was unsure. Her grandmother had always told her that polio was caused by evil spirits that made you fall on the fire. That is how you became paralysed. So how could a vaccine prevent the evil eye? She also once heard from a friend that the colonisers first introduced vaccines to try to sterilise local people to stop them from having children and overpowering the invaders. She already has so many troubles, and although the nurse appeared to be genuine and caring, Mrs. Z wishes that her husband was still alive to help her with these decisions.

Making healthy choices the easy choices

The first case of Mr. X, who is considering whether or not to quit smoking, illustrates an age-old question of why people continue to engage in risky behaviours even though they know it is bad for their health, and what can be done to encourage them to adopt healthier behaviours. Indeed there are many theories that attempt to address this question.

The Health Belief Model, first developed by Hochbaum in the 1950s, suggests that health-related behaviour change depends on whether a person perceives their own health to be at risk (e.g. since I am a smoker it is likely that I could develop lung cancer), the potential severity of the disease (e.g. lung cancer is very often fatal), the advantages and disadvantages of taking action (e.g. I could substantially reduce my risk of cancer by quitting but I would no longer be able to enjoy smoking my cigarettes with friends), and whether there is a trigger to make a change (e.g. my wife was just diagnosed with lung cancer, likely related to second-hand smoke since she herself was never a smoker).[1] However, even though people are often aware that certain behaviours are bad for their health, they continue anyhow. Sometimes it is because these behaviours are pleasurable (e.g. a cigarette after meals), sometimes it is what everyone else is doing (e.g. social pressures), and sometimes there is a physical or psycho-logical dependence (e.g. nicotine addiction).

Therefore, Ajzen and Fishbein developed the Theory of Reasoned Action to explain that a person's knowledge about the risks and their attitudes towards the behaviour are not sufficient to make a change. Rather, this depends on whether they truly have an intention to change.[2] This intention to change depends on beliefs about what people close to you think (e.g. Mr. X's friends have all decided to quit smoking) and what other people around you think (e.g. everyone at Mr. X's workplace thinks that smoking is a dirty habit and almost nobody outside his circle of friends is a smoker). Later, Ajzen made an addition to the theory by adding the notion of Planned Behaviour, explaining that the intention to change also depends on beliefs about one's own capacity to change (e.g. Mr. X has tried quitting before and it never lasted more than a few weeks; as soon as he became stressed out by something he would always start smoking again, and with his wife now ill, he has little confidence that he will be able to quit at this time).[3] Therefore, if Mr. X does not feel ready to make this change now, it is unlikely that he will.

This concept of readiness is described in Prochaska and DiClemente's popular Transtheoretical or Stages of Change model.[4] According to this model, for change to occur, one must balance the pros and cons of changing, consider one's capacity to change (also known as self-efficacy) and, once the change has occurred, resist the temptation to revert back to unhealthy behaviours in times of stress. Therefore, to assist people in making and sustaining a positive change in their behaviour, it is necessary to identify what stage the person is at in the process of change. In the pre-contemplation stage people are not even thinking about making a change in the foreseeable future. In the contemplation stage they have started to think about it. In the preparation stage they have the intention to change and are getting ready to take action. In the action stage they have made a change in their behaviour. In the maintenance stage they are working to prevent a relapse. Finally, in the termination stage, they are no longer tempted by the old behaviour and have made the transition to a healthier way of life. In this example, Mr. X is likely to be in the pre-contemplation or contemplation stage – he may be thinking about quitting but does not yet have the intention to change his behaviour.

While these models can be helpful in assisting us to deconstruct and better understand individual behaviours,[5] critics such as West find that these theories do not always readily translate into policies and programmes that can actually help people to make healthier choices.[6] However, part of the problem is that these theories are mostly focused on the individual, whereas we know that even decisions at an individual level are also largely influenced by external factors in the physical and social environment. Bandura, for instance, describes how behaviours are learned from an early age, thereby emphasising the importance of role modelling and early childhood education both at home and outside the home.[7] What about Mr. X, who grew up in a household where his father was a heavy smoker, and where he himself started smoking when he was still a teenager, resulting in a 40-pack-year smoking history (i.e. smoking 1 pack of cigarettes per day for 40 years). Is it hopeless for him? Certainly not. According to The Task Force on Community Preventive Services, there is strong evidence that population-based measures such as increasing the price of cigarettes (through excise or "sin" taxes) and reducing the cost of smoking-cessation treatments (such as the nicotine-replacement patch or certain antidepressant medications) can assist Mr. X to stop buying cigarettes and adhere to treatments that can help him to quit smoking.[8] Indeed, increasing the cost of cigarettes by 10% results in a 4.1% reduction in tobacco consumption. Reminder systems that prompt Mr. X's family doctor to ask about smoking status at each visit and to provide encouragement and advice about how to quit are also effective, as are multi-component programmes that include individual or group counselling and telephone support to prevent relapse. Smoking bans and restrictions that prohibit tobacco use in certain geographically designated areas as well as smoke-free policies in the workplace are also highly effective. However, in Mr. X's case, there are no laws banning smoking where he lives, cigarettes are still fairly cheap and widely available, and, while some people have started to complain about those who smoke in restaurants or other public places, it is still quite a common and acceptable behaviour. In addition, there are no support groups to help him to quit smoking, and the cost of nicotine replacement treatments is unaffordable to all but the upper classes. Moreover, these treatments are often unavailable in local pharmacies even for those who could afford to pay. Thus, while it is still Mr. X's choice to continue smoking, his choice could be somewhat different if he lived in a country with stricter anti-tobacco laws, higher cigarette taxes, social norms that strongly oppose smoking, and better-developed support systems to assist smokers who want to quit. Many countries are moving in this direction, particularly following the recent ratification in 2005 of the WHO Framework Convention on Tobacco Control (FCTC), one of the very few global treaties negotiated under the auspices of the World Health Organization (WHO),[9] but it is still far from being universal practice.

While Mr. X's case can be used to illustrate the theories of behaviour change for those who engage in "risky" or "unhealthy" behaviours, and how certain population-based measures can help to make the healthy choices the easy choices, influencing decision-making at the individual level is not always so straightforward. Smoking is a fairly clear-cut example of a health risk that one can target and attempt to eliminate. However, what about fatty foods or high-salt content in the diet that can lead to high blood pressure, heart disease and stroke? People need to eat, and it is not possible to ban foods altogether. Therefore the strategies used to promote healthier diets must be more nuanced than simply banning certain products. Instead, it is necessary to partner with industry to lower the sodium content in processed foods and to offer low-fat "healthy options". For instance, a food chain that only sells deep-fried chicken can be encouraged to add to their menu a salad with lettuce, tomatoes, cucumbers and lean, skinless grilled chicken, so that customers can choose to eat healthily if they want to.

Thus, while it is possible to positively or negatively influence decisions, people are not entirely devoid of self-determination and free will. Indeed, Mr. X could choose to quit smoking. After all, what does he really have to lose? If smoking is a stress-relief mechanism or a pleasurable pastime, isn't there something less harmful to one's health that he could use as a replacement? And in any case, is it not the social support from his circle of friends rather than the cigarettes that will see him through the difficult period during his wife's illness? While not downplaying the challenges involved in breaking a nicotine addiction, at least here the answer is clear – smoking kills, and if Mr. X quits smoking he can prolong his life by about five years.[10] If he also adopts other healthy behaviour changes, including increased physical activity and daily consumption of 5 to 10 fruits and vegetables, he could increase his life expectancy even further.[11]

But the case of Mrs. Y is less clear-cut. Her choice is between living with a risk of cancer versus undergoing radical surgery that will artificially put her into early menopause. As well, if she is a carrier of a *BRCA* mutation, this could also have implications for her children and for future generations. Thus the stakes are much higher, and it is also much more difficult to know which is the best choice, since it depends to a greater extent on personal values and contextual considerations. While it may appear counter-intuitive, evidence-informed patient choice is particularly important in cases such as this where there is more of a "grey zone" in identifying the optimal course of action. To get past the uncertainty, whatever evidence is available can be used to help people weigh the benefits and harms of various options and to thereby determine the best way forward in their specific situation.

Promoting patient understanding and informed choice

We may know a lot about what makes people healthy, but there are nonetheless many areas of medicine where there is still tremendous uncertainty, and our understanding can evolve significantly from generation to generation and even from year to year. Indeed, even in situations where there is a great deal of experience, there is no such thing as "zero risk" in medicine. Every medication has potential side effects, every surgery has possible complications, and even test results can be misleading since none are 100% accurate. While in the past it was thought that the physician was in the best position to decide what to do (and even whether to tell the patient at all about their diagnosis and prognosis to save them from any unpleasantness that may be associated with such a disclosure), times have certainly changed. According to Bury, the term *patient* no longer refers to the passive party in the doctor–patient relationship.[12] Patients are now considered as consumers, clients and users of health services. They are partners in shared decision-making, as well as participants (rather than subjects) in medical research.

Tony Hope, Professor of Medical Ethics at Oxford University, was among the first to describe evidence-based patient choice as a process of assisting patients in finding high-quality and relevant information to guide them in making better-informed decisions about their health.[13] However, different individuals want and seek varying types and amounts of information (i.e. some want to know all possible eventualities before deciding and others feel that too many details just cloud the issue and make it even more difficult to make a decision). Benbassat and colleagues similarly found that not all individuals wish to be involved in decision-making in the same way, if at all.[14] Increased patient choice therefore comes with increased uncertainty and responsibility, and some even worry that it may lead to a reduction in physician accountability. Thus the empowerment of patients can at times be a double-edged sword.[15] Nonetheless, while there are pros and cons to shared decision-making, Coulter and others argue that improving access to evidence-informed patient information is important in and of itself, as well as being a pre-requisite to informed patient choice.[16]

Returning to the second case of Mrs. Y, who is considering her preventive options with regard to her family history of breast cancer, there are many different factors at play that influence how she proceeds, and, indeed, there are many decisions, not just one, that she must make on her "medical odyssey". The first decision is whether or not to seek medical advice in the first place. While her sister has encouraged her to do so, Mrs. Y is reluctant, and many reasons can account for this. She is a busy professional and manages the household – who has the time? Depending on which country she lives in, a medical consultation could also cost quite a bit of money – let alone the cost of any further investigations and interventions – which she may not be able to afford and may not be covered by her insurance. There is the distance to the health care provider, the opportunity cost of time off work to go to the appointment, her expectations of whether the visit will be useful, her concerns about whether her husband and children would approve, the logistics of making the arrangements – a long list of potential barriers. But in the case of Mrs. Y, there is probably something else underlying her reluctance to seek medical advice – fear.

Often attempts are made to get people to adopt healthy behaviours to prevent diseases that they have never experienced – directly or indirectly – and know very little about. It would be difficult, for instance, to get an 18-year-old male to avoid smoking cigarettes out of concern about chronic obstructive pulmonary disease. What teenager has ever heard of that? And anyway, even if he did get the disease, he would only likely start to develop bothersome symptoms in his 50s or 60s – a lifetime away. However, tell a young man that excessive alcohol consumption is associated with higher rates of sexual dysfunction,[17] and that is more likely to get his attention. Risk perception – a central component of the health behaviour theories described previously – is therefore an important factor in motivating people's actions. It is also central to the experience of women with a family history of breast cancer, even more so than an understanding of genes and genetics.

There has been a great deal of research on how people understand and make sense of health risks, and much has been written on the difficulties of communicating risks both at the population level and at the individual level. It is also extremely difficult to change a person's perception of risk once established. Women with a family history of breast cancer have often lived through the experience of a loved one with cancer and witnessed the physical and emotional damage that the disease causes. When they reach the age at which their mother was diagnosed with cancer, it is not unusual for women to start thinking about their own risks. As demonstrated by Evans and colleagues, even if detailed investigations indicate that a woman with a family history of breast cancer is not herself at increased risk, it is often very difficult for her to realign her preconceived risk perception with her actual risk.[18] Moreover, an excessive amount of anxiety about one's future health, as in the case of Mrs. Y, can in fact be harmful when people are no longer able to consider their options in a dispassionate way to make free and informed choices.

The classic work of Janis and Feshbach conducted in the 1950s demonstrates how people who are not at all worried about their health are unlikely to change their usual health practices, whereas those who are mildly or moderately concerned are more likely to adopt healthy behaviours and to seek preventive care.[19] On the other hand, evoking high levels of concern can actually be counter-productive and lead to denial and avoidance behaviour, thus creating an inverted U-shaped curve (Fig. 3.1).[19]

While this "fear arousal" theory has been widely debated, it has been shown to hold true in many areas, including breast cancer prevention. In a large, population-based study by Andersen and colleagues, women with higher levels of cancer worries (measured using the validated Lerman Cancer Worries Scale) were less likely to undergo mammography screening, and those with a family history of breast cancer were, understandably, more likely to have stronger cancer worries (Fig. 3.2).[20] Thus the inverted-U curve could explain Mrs. Y's hesitation to seek medical advice. Indeed, Howe has shown that, 20 years ago, most women with a family history of breast cancer did not consider themselves to be at increased risk.[21] However, more recently, and particularly since the discovery of the breast cancer susceptibility genes in the mid 1990s (i.e. *BRCA1* and *BRCA2*), there has been a proliferation of awareness raising and press coverage on the topic. While the multitude of stories in newspapers and women's magazines on breast cancer family history may attempt to encourage women to become more informed and to engage in preventive behaviours, there is a great deal of misinformation,[22] and the shock factor built into these stories (which is often a key selling strategy in the media business) has resulted in unintended consequences. By increasing risk perceptions across the board, women in the general population (i.e. at low risk) are

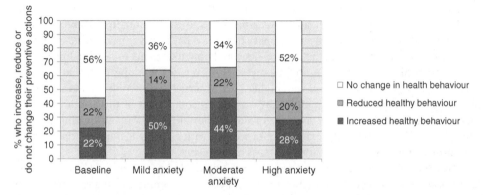

Figure 3.1 Inverted U-shaped curve of preventive action in response to increasing levels of anxiety. Data from Janis I, Feshbach S. Effects of fear-arousing communications. *J Abnorm Soc Psychol* 1953; 48: 78–92.

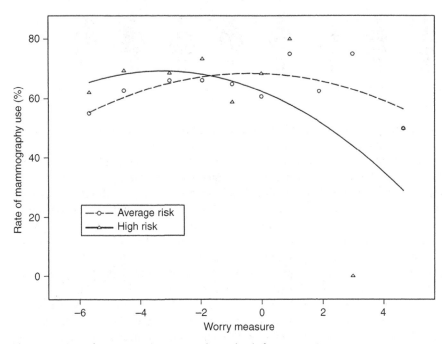

Figure 3.2 Rate of mammography use according to level of cancer worries.
Reprinted from Andersen M, Smith R, Meischke H, Bowen D, Urban N. Breast cancer worry and mammography use by women with and without a family history in a population-based sample. *Cancer Epidemiol Biomarkers Prev* 2003; 12: 314–20, with permission from the American Association for Cancer Research.

now more likely to undergo unnecessary medical consultations and referrals, whereas women with a strong family history (i.e. at high risk) may be too afraid to seek advice, even though they are most in need of attention and care.

Let us imagine that a friend succeeds in allaying Mrs. Y's fears by saying "Even if your mother was a carrier of a *BRCA* mutation, and it is not certain that she was, there would be a 50–50 chance that you did not inherit the gene anyhow, and therefore are not at increased risk – why don't you just find out more about your options from the experts rather than hiding your head in the sand". Thus, while still somewhat reluctant, Mrs. Y decides to seek medical advice. However, even with non-directive counselling that provides patients with all of the information and allows them to make informed choices, there are nonetheless hurdles to be overcome. One issue is the difficulty of understanding risk estimates, another is the issue of framing, and, finally, there is also clinical and scientific uncertainty.

Risk is a complex concept that embodies at least three main dimensions. First, there is the probability of being harmed (i.e. how likely is it that a person will develop the disease – 1 in 10 or 1 in 10,000?). Second, there is the severity of the harm (i.e. how bad is the disease – a mild self-limiting condition or a severe degenerative disease leading to an untimely death?). Third, there is the imminence of being harmed (i.e. when will the person develop the disease – in childhood or late in life?).

When it comes to describing risk, there are many different ways to say the same thing. For instance, women in the general population have about a 10% chance of developing breast cancer by the time they reach the age of 85. Alternatively, 1 in 10 women will develop breast

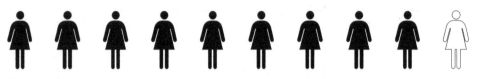

Figure 3.3 Communicating risk estimates using graphic illustrations.

cancer in their lifetime. Or, one could say it using pictures (Fig. 3.3). However, for many people, these population-based risk estimates are difficult to understand. What they really want to know is "Will I get it or not, and, if so, when?" People do not often think of their risk in terms of numbers, but rather they make a more qualitative assessment according to low-risk, average-risk, high-risk and very-high-risk categories. Calman and Royston have suggested developing a standardised language of risk.[23] More often, however, it is considered good practice to present risk information in many different ways to promote understanding.[24] Tennant also considers that it is important to disclose the degree of uncertainty underlying risk estimates to avoid possible misinterpretation and confusion.[25]

Needless to say, it is also important to avoid misrepresenting the risk. A cancer charity advertisement that uses the statistic that one in three people will develop cancer in their lifetime but shows a photograph with three toddlers on it and a caption saying "What do you want to be when you grow up – teacher, doctor, cancer?" is misleading. Perhaps if there was a picture with three octogenarians it would be different. Indeed cancer is very rare among toddlers, and most cancer cases occur after age 50, with the exception of certain childhood leukemias, genetic cancer syndromes and so forth.

Regardless of the actual risk, however, people's perceptions of risk, as described earlier, are not necessarily rational. Generally, people are more afraid of airplane crashes than car crashes, even though car crashes are far more common and can also have very severe outcomes. Yet, people have a sense of control when driving their car and they can see the obstacles. Whereas in a plane crash someone else is at the wheel, and the causes of the crash may sometimes be mysterious and certainly out of the passenger's control, which makes it seem like an unfair tragedy for the innocent passengers who were helpless to do anything about it. Risks and threats are generally more worrisome, anxiety producing and stressful if they are perceived to be involuntary, irreversible, inescapable, invisible, inequitably distributed and poorly understood.[26] When it comes to risk of disease, there is often a greater fear of cancer (i.e. the "C" word), as compared with obesity or heart disease, even though advances in modern medicine have resulted in many types of cancer becoming largely preventable and treatable diseases if identified at an early stage.

Returning again to the case scenario, Mrs. Y finally musters the courage to seek medical advice and her fears are realised. She is evaluated by medical specialists who consider that her family history places her at an elevated risk for developing breast and ovarian cancer. Following genetic counselling, Mrs. Y must face her next decision: whether or not to undergo genetic testing. Mrs. Y is told that if her mother was a *BRCA* mutation carrier, then she has a 50% chance of also being a carrier. If her test results show that she is not a carrier, she will be at the same risk as an average woman in the population. For technical reasons, since genetic testing is far from straightforward, there is also a small chance that she may not have one of the common breast cancer mutations that are included in the panel being tested and therefore test negative, but she may be carrying another mutation that was not tested for and could therefore still be unknowingly at increased risk. If she is a *BRCA* carrier, she will have a 60–80% chance of developing breast cancer in her lifetime (compared to about 10% for the general population – therefore 6 to 8 times higher risk) and also a 20–40% chance of developing ovarian cancer, which is even more difficult to diagnose early.[27] Whether these are good odds or bad odds would depend on whom you ask, since different people have different risk tolerance. For instance, would you choose to undergo surgery with a 15% chance of dying due to complications? What about a surgery with a 5% chance of dying? Or 1%? Not only does it depend on personal preference, but also on how sick the person is, and what they stand to gain or lose from taking that risk. However, Tversky and Kahneman found that even the way you frame the decision affects the choices that are made.[28] A surgery with an 85% chance of survival certainly sounds more appealing than a 15% chance of dying. Therefore framing can pose an important hindrance to rational choice. In a similar vein, Newman shows how stories can be more powerful than statistics.[29] For instance, an emotive description of one person's experience with a preventive mastectomy that resulted in multiple serious complications requiring an extended hospital stay lasting many months and a lengthy recovery over more than a year can greatly affect risk perceptions, even if the data clearly demonstrate that this is a relatively uncommon occurrence and that most people do not share this experience. Thus, while stories can be helpful in conveying risk, it is important that they reflect the "average case" rather than outliers (which one often reads about in the media).

After much agonising over the decision and speaking with many people about what to do, Mrs. Y decides to undergo genetic testing since at least it will provide her with more information to use as a basis for further decisions, and she also feels a responsibility to find out for the sake of her daughters. Once again her fears are confirmed and she is found to be a *BRCA* carrier. While there are many potential preventive options available to her, each has its own risks and inconveniences. As well, it is not a simple "either–or" decision, since she could also choose a combination of these options. But, what should she choose? Should she undergo preventive surgery to remove her breasts and ovaries? Take chemoprophylaxis? Undergo intensive surveillance using mammography or MRI (magnetic resonance imaging) to catch the disease early? Many factors will influence these decisions, but what information does she need to decide? According to Entwistle and colleagues, high-quality patient information is not only written in a way that is easily accessible and understood by the target audience, but also contains key details about the potential risks and benefits of undertaking the intervention, as well as what would be expected to happen if a person chooses to "do nothing".[30] For instance, women who undergo mammography screening may be much less stressed out by abnormal test results or interval cancers (that appear between screenings), if they were aware up front of what to expect. Elmore and colleagues found that the average woman who is screened with routine mammography exams over a period of 10 years has a 23.8% chance of receiving an abnormal test result at some point during this period, but almost 9 times out of 10 this is a false-positive result (i.e. the woman does not actually have cancer upon further examination).[31] There is also a very small chance of having missed a pre-cancerous or cancerous lesion – known as a false-negative test result. Thus even a negative test result is not necessarily an "all clear". Having this information up front before the woman chooses to undergo screening could make a big difference in clarifying expectations and improving her experience of preventive care. Displayed graphically, of 100 women screened for 10 years, 4 will have breast cancer. However, 27 will have a positive test result. But, only 3 of these will actually have cancer, and 1 cancer (or fewer) will be missed (Fig. 3.4).

There is a growing literature on various decision aids to help guide patients through complex decisions to make more evidence-informed choices. Often included in such tools is

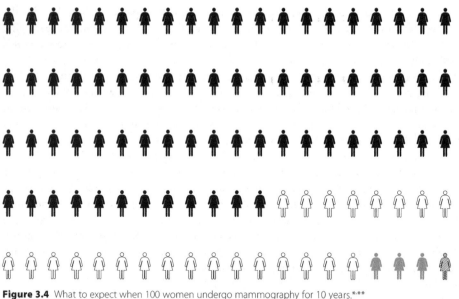

Figure 3.4 What to expect when 100 women undergo mammography for 10 years.*,**
* Black = screened negative, no cancer (true negative); White = screened positive, no cancer (false positive); Grey = screened positive, has cancer (true positive); Diagonal stripes = screened negative, has cancer (false negative).
** In the study by Elmore and colleagues, of 2,227 women who underwent mammography screening over a period of 10 years, 88 women were found to have breast cancer (4%) and 530 (23.8%) had false-positives results.

a decision tree, which illustrates the probabilities that various outcomes will occur if one chooses option A versus option B. Other decision aids are more sophisticated. Some include very elaborate patient information, and others even have computerised calculators to determine a person's individual risk. O'Connor and colleagues have found that "decision aids improve knowledge, reduce decisional conflict, and stimulate patients to be more active in decision-making without increasing their anxiety".[32]

Elwyn and O'Connor are the co-Chairs of the International Patient Decision Aids Standards Collaboration, which has developed quality assurance guidelines for the content and development process of decision aids.[33] With regards to content, options should be explained and compared in sufficient detail to support decision-making, and the probabilities of outcomes should be presented in a balanced and unbiased way. Regarding the development process, the information should be based on the highest quality evidence, and developers should disclose their credentials and any potential conflicts of interest. Nonetheless, even if information is presented in a comprehensive and unbiased manner, and even if it is well understood and integrated by patients, Ubel and Loewenstein have shown that at times decision-making may still proceed in simplified, intuitive ways rather than complex, reasoned ones.[34]

Ultimately, the choice made by Mrs. Y to undergo bilateral mastectomy and oophorectomy (i.e. to remove her breasts and ovaries) was based on many considerations, including the evidence that such surgeries could reduce her risk of developing cancer in future, as well as her own personal values and concerns for the well-being of her young children. Yet she very well could have made a different decision that would have been equally justified and acceptable. It is important to remember that women with a family history of breast cancer are not themselves ill (although they may be labelled as such), and many of them might never develop breast or ovarian cancer during their lifetime. For this reason, it is important that they are made aware of the pros and cons of preventive and early detection options. Regardless of whether or not they actually choose any of these options, at least patients such as Mrs. Y will be able to develop positive coping strategies regarding their risk and feel that they have received sufficient information to allow them to make informed choices about their care. Indeed, Maly and colleagues have shown that the provision of information in itself can increase positive perceptions of health and improve health outcomes.[35]

Improving cultural competency in a globalised world

In our increasingly interconnected world, cross-cultural understandings of health and illness are gradually being recognised as an important factor in determining individual decisions about health. With the recent burgeoning of fields such as transcultural psychiatry and medical anthropology, there is an increasing awareness of cultural factors as key determinants of health, and a growing number of calls for health professionals to become more culturally competent in their day-to-day practice. According to Kirmayer and Minas, "a cultural perspective can help clinicians and researchers become aware of the hidden assumptions and limitations of current psychiatric theory and practice and can identify new approaches appropriate for treating the increasingly diverse populations seen in psychiatric services around the world".[36]

Cultural competency is also receiving a great deal of attention in other fields, from primary health care to nursing, midwifery and dentistry. Indeed the American Academy of Nursing developed their own definition of culturally competent health care almost 20 years ago, describing it as "a complex integration of knowledge, attitudes, and skills that enhances cross-cultural communication and appropriate effective interactions with others".[37] There have been many different definitions proposed since then, as well as alternative terms used to describe similar concepts, including "culture sensitivity", "culturally congruent care" and "intercultural effectiveness". Regardless of the definition or term used, the main idea is that culture matters and needs to be taken into consideration to promote health.

Going back to the case of Mrs. Z, this is not an example of a first- or second-generation immigrant living in a culturally different host society, but rather a health care provider (i.e. the European-born missionary) practising in a foreign country. With the increase of patients, providers and clinical information crossing borders (e.g. diagnostic tests from one country being interpreted by clinicians in another country), cultural competency is becoming a relevant issue no matter where you are. According to Callister, "cultural knowledge can help caregivers avoid cultural imposition and ethnocentrism, or the belief that one's own ways are superior" and can also be used "as a focus for negotiating mutually acceptable solutions to differing cultural perspectives".[38]

Lie and colleagues conducted a review of the literature and found that cultural competency among health care providers has not shown any evidence of harm. Rather, it enhances the patient experience of care and promotes a shared understanding between patient and provider.[39] Willis considers that culturally competent care involves increasing levels of understanding, tolerance, acceptance, appreciation and respect. Even beyond positive patient experiences, cultural competency also provides patients with enhanced feelings of self-worth, a greater sense of control, higher levels of positive coping strategies, increased self-reliance and a greater likelihood of adopting health-promoting behaviours.[40]

Indeed, Mrs. Z faces many challenges that would be important stressors for any person – being a recent widow, lacking financial means, having a sick child. While her decisions about whether or not to vaccinate her children are subject to the same theories of behaviour change and ideas about risk perception and informed choice described previously, there is another layer of complexity that could have an important influence on her choices – her cultural knowledge and beliefs.

A study conducted by Teka and Dagnew in the mid 1990s in the remote town of Gondar in Northern Ethiopia illustrates how mothers are frequently able to identify when their child has an acute respiratory illness. However, the majority believe that the best treatment is a butter and herb mixture applied to the chest, keeping the child's ears clean and dry, and taking the child to the traditional healer.[41] Less than one-third said that they would take their child to the local health clinic, and their decision to do so was not associated with the level of maternal education. From a Western medicine perspective, the behaviour of these mothers would be considered dangerous and unwise, since delays in initiating antibiotic therapy among young children with pneumonia can prove fatal. Indeed, this is an easily treatable condition and even preventable with the more recently available pneumococcal vaccines. However, it is important to understand the prevailing knowledge, beliefs and practices that underlie these health decisions. If Mrs. Z shares her grandmother's views that infectious diseases are caused by evil spirits, then a vaccine or antibiotic therapy will make little sense to her. In contrast, a visit to the traditional healer – someone who is experienced in removing curses and protecting people from evil spirits – would appear to be the rational choice.

All people have certain culturally and socially defined beliefs about health that influence how they understand their illness and the type of care that they seek. According to Hodes, many Ethiopians – both at home and in the diaspora – believe that:

> Health is an equilibrium between the body and the outside. Excess sun is believed to cause mitch ("sunstroke"), leading to skin disease. Blowing winds are thought to cause pain wherever they hit. Sexually transmitted disease is attributed to urinating under a full moon. People with buda, "evil eye," are said to be able to harm others by looking at them. Ethiopians often complain of rasehn, "my head" (often saying it burns); yazorehnyal, "spinning" (not a true vertigo); and libeh, "my heart" (usually indicating dyspepsia rather than a cardiac problem). Most Ethiopians have faith in traditional healers and procedures. In children, uvulectomy (to prevent presumed suffocation during pharyngitis in babies), the extraction of lower incisors (to prevent diarrhoea), and the incision of eyelids (to prevent or cure conjunctivitis) are common. Circumcision is performed on almost all men and 90% of women. Ethiopians do bloodletting for moygnbagegn, a neurological disease that includes fever and syncope. Chest pain is treated by cupping. Ethiopians often prefer injections to tablets. Bad news is usually given to families of patients and not the patients themselves. Zar is a form of spirit possession treated by a traditional healer negotiating with the alien spirit and giving gifts to the possessed patient.[42]

Understanding these culturally specific ideas about health and illness would be important in promoting a greater understanding between the healer and the patient. Lock, however, cautions against oversimplifying and "pigeon-holing" people into ethnic or cultural categories, since often there are many other socio-economic, educational and gender-related explanatory factors that are also intertwined, and not everyone from the same geographic or ethnic origin shares the same belief systems.[43] What is important, however, is to be aware that the healer and the patient may have divergent views with regards to disease causation and appropriate measures for improving health. Therefore it is important to engage in a dialogue to explore these issues, which are often hidden and can lead to great confusion or, even worse, can lead to the medical establishment labelling people as ignorant or non-compliant, breaking down the important bonds of trust and respect between the healer and the patient.[44] A simple way of better understanding what people believe and what are their preferences is to ask them.

Even though vaccines are one of the major public health advances of the last century and have saved the lives of millions of children worldwide each year, there continue to be fears and unfounded myths about vaccines even in Western cultures that are very familiar with the new technologies used by modern medicine. These myths include the fear that "too many vaccines will weaken the immune system" (which is not true, in fact it is just the opposite) or that "vaccines are not effective because people who have been vaccinated nonetheless get the disease" (while no vaccine is 100% effective and therefore a small number of people who have been vaccinated may indeed get the disease, a much smaller percentage of those who have been vaccinated will become symptomatic and suffer complications as compared to those who have not been vaccinated). As a result of vaccine scares in the media and on the Internet, the refusal of parents to vaccinate their children has at times resulted in localised outbreaks of infectious diseases that have largely been absent for decades due to high vaccine coverage rates, which provided "herd immunity", protecting even the small number of children who are not vaccinated. The refusal of parents to vaccinate their children therefore raises ethical concerns that these "free riders" benefit from the participation of others in the vaccination programme without assuming any of the risk themselves. While vaccine safety is highly regulated and the real risks to each child are extremely small, the refusal of parents to vaccinate their children can also place at risk vulnerable members of the community who are unable to be vaccinated, and thereby protect themselves, due to medical reasons (e.g. immune deficiency). Therefore Diekema and the Committee on Bioethics of the American Academy of Pediatrics recommend that health care providers explore and address parental concerns in a respectful way and encourage vaccination of the child without threatening to terminate the patient–provider relationship for repeat refusals.[45] Some jurisdictions go one step further and create laws requiring children to be vaccinated in order to attend school. In more extreme cases, for instance when the child is at greatly increased risk of imminent harm (e.g. due to a deep and contaminated puncture wound and the parents nonetheless refuse the tetanus vaccine), one might go so far as to challenge the refusal and involve the relevant authorities, such as child protective services and even the courts, if necessary.

Returning to the case of Mrs. Z, the nurse could simply dismiss Mrs. Z's reluctance to vaccinate her children and turn her attention to someone else, or she could try to explore further Mrs. Z's reasons as to why she is reluctant. It may turn out that economics and logistics are just as important as cultural beliefs and fears about vaccine safety. Bentley and colleagues found that mothers in a rural village in Peru alter their usual activity patterns only slightly in response to acute diarrhoeal episodes in their children.[46] Unless the episode is considered very severe, mothers generally continue with their usual work and chores (including fetching water, meal preparation, working for wages), although they are more likely to carry the sick child on their back while doing so. Distance to health facilities and lack of infrastructure is another problem. Even if Mrs. Z did consider bringing the children to be vaccinated, there is a large opportunity cost involved in travelling long distances to reach health facilities (and even a real cost if taking transportation). In addition, even if the vaccines are distributed for free, vaccinations generally require multiple booster doses, and therefore it would be necessary for Mrs. Z to return to the clinic with her children at least three of four times, which would be no small task. The nurse may therefore discover that a vaccination outreach programme – perhaps in partnership with local leaders and traditional healers – could be a more effective way of increasing vaccine uptake as compared to the opportunistic counselling of individuals who present to the health centre for other reasons.

The three case examples described above illustrate the tremendous complexity involved in decision-making for health at the individual level, including the interplay of knowledge and beliefs, risk perception and fears; the influences of external economic, social and structural factors; the role of health care providers and health authorities; and the importance of providing balanced and unbiased information in many different formats to promote better-informed choices. Nonetheless, decision-making at a population level involves even more layers of complexity, including the necessity of considering both individual and population-level concerns, as well as balancing the different needs of various groups in society.

Population health decisions

While countless decisions about health are made every day at the individual level, there are also many larger-scale decisions about health that are made at a population level. These include the development and implementation of policies and programmes for promoting health and preventing disease (e.g. the creation of a network of low-cost day care centres to promote early childhood development, or implementing a policy in schools to ban junk food and increase time devoted to physical activity), the enactment and enforcement of laws for health protection (e.g. seat-belt, car-seat and speed-limit laws), the implementation of measures for harm reduction (e.g. opening a safe injection site for injection drug users), and other similar decisions made by health authorities and elected public officials that affect entire segments of the population in a given region or jurisdiction. To illustrate these population-level decisions, and the additional considerations involved in making such decisions as compared to individual-level decisions, I will use the example of developing and implementing a new screening programme for genetic diseases (Box 3.2).

As described in the previous chapter, screening is a form of secondary prevention. In mass screening (Fig. 3.5),[47] a test is offered to all individuals within a defined target population who are recruited through systematic outreach efforts. In opportunistic screening, individuals are recruited when they consult the health system for unrelated medical services. However, genetic screening – whether mass screening or opportunistic screening – should not be confused with genetic testing, which is part of a diagnostic workup within a clinical setting for individuals who present with health-related concerns. Cascade screening, however, which involves the systematic identification and testing of asymptomatic relatives of those affected by a genetic disorder or identified as a carrier, constitutes a grey zone between population-based genetic screening and genetic testing in a clinical setting.[47]

This case example is not focused on whether individual patients with a family history of breast cancer should undergo genetic testing or not (i.e. as in the case example of Mrs. Y from the previous section). Rather, the main decision here is whether or not the government should implement a new screening programme to systematically offer an unsolicited genetic test to the entire population. Thus, when making population-level decisions, instead of focusing on a single person, there are many different groups and viewpoints that need to be taken into account.

Box 3.2 Population-level decision-making for health

Case D: Deciding to screen for genetic disease

For many years, the patient support group for genetic disease X has been lobbying the government to develop a population-based screening programme to detect asymptomatic couples who are both carriers of the disease, who will then have the option of prenatal diagnosis (i.e. detecting during pregnancy whether the unborn fetus is affected) or even pre-implantation diagnosis (i.e. using *in vitro* fertilisation to select an embryo that does not carry the disease to implant into the uterus). The company that has patented the gene is already offering carrier testing direct to consumers at very high prices, and the support group argues that the government should make the test available to all members of society at no cost since health is a human right. The clinical geneticists agree that this can indeed be a devastating disease for patients and their families, even though treatments have greatly improved over the years. While previously most patients with this disease died during childhood and adolescence, some now live well into their 30s and 40s. In addition, the test result is difficult to interpret. The molecular geneticists who first discovered the gene caution that there is a large degree of genotype-phenotype heterogeneity, meaning that not everyone with the same mutation expresses the disease in the same way (i.e. some have milder and others more severe forms of the disease). As well, there are many different mutations that can cause the disease, and each would have to be tested for individually or as part of a panel of tests. However, it is possible that a person who tests negative may still be carrying a mutation that is not included on the panel. Aside from the technical concerns, some ethicists warn that it is important to proceed with caution when it comes to genetic screening, which conjures up ideas of the eugenic legacy in Nazi Germany and elsewhere, where the fervour to improve the human race took precedence over consideration for the autonomy and welfare of individuals and families. Yet proponents of screening argue that there are many genetic screening programmes – ranging from newborn screening for hypothyroidism and phenylketonuria to carrier screening for haemoglobinopathies – that have existed in countries around the world for over 30 years and that are functioning very well with little or no threats to individual autonomy and well-being. These are just a few of the arguments and concerns raised in relation to this screening programme. It is enough to boggle the mind. So, what should the government do now? How to decide whether or not to introduce a new screening pro-gramme? What are the implications of going ahead? Of not acting?

Stakeholders and interest groups competing in the political arena

Perhaps the first thing that is striking about population-level health decisions as compared to individual-level decisions is the very broad range of people involved – often called stake-holders – who tend to have widely divergent opinions about the decision at hand. That is because, like it or not, it is no longer a personal decision, it's political. This is a whole other world with very different rules and modes of operating as compared to the clinical context. This does not mean that the decisions no longer affect individuals – they certainly do. But individual patients no longer have the same degree of direct control over the larger decisions that are made, since these decisions are now being made by policy-makers.

In the case of the patient support group lobbying the government to screen for disease X, it would be important to understand their reasons for wanting this. While not all genetic diseases are the same, and different people with the same disease can have widely varying experiences, very often, being diagnosed with a genetic disorder can be devastating for the

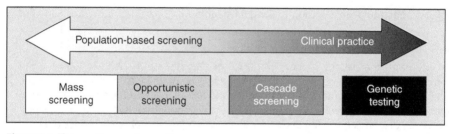

Figure 3.5 The genetic screening continuum.
Reproduced with permission from Andermann A, Blancquaert I. Genetic screening: a primer for primary care. *Can Fam Physician* 2010; 56(4): 333–9.

individual and for their family. Many rare genetic conditions strike very young children and can be severely debilitating. Parents' lives are often derailed as they try to come to terms and cope with the illness. Sometimes one or both parents must stop working to stay home and care for a very ill child. The usual activities of everyday life are often replaced by frequent visits to the doctor and other health care services. Families slide into poverty. Many children die prematurely as a result of the disease. Marriages collapse under the pressure. But what if this could have been prevented? All the pain and suffering caused from not knowing could have been avoided. A simple test could have predicted what would occur and could have provided an opportunity to avert this difficult path. But in most cases these are rare diseases that affect fewer than 1 in 2,000 people. In the case of recessive conditions (i.e. both parents must be gene carriers to have a child affected by the disease), often no one in the family has had this disease before. Parents are unaware that they are silent carriers. The only way that they could have been made aware prior to having an affected child is through screening. And the only way that they would have had access to screening is if the government had developed a screening programme for the entire population (unless they had a family history of the disease, in which case cascade screening is sometimes offered). This is the logic that can lead grieving parents and patient support groups to pressure governments to act-to save others from needlessly experiencing what they lived through.

However, beyond the patients, family members and support groups, there exists an even larger web of stakeholders who are also interested in promoting screening, but for a variety of different reasons (Fig. 3.6).[48] For instance, researchers who have discovered a gene or a new test that could be used for screening are often keen to see the fruits of their labour put into practice. In addition to helping people, this can provide a certain prestige and increase their influence and power in their field. As well, there are often large financial incentives. Whether it is the researchers themselves or biotechnology companies who hold a patent, or whether laboratories will simply be getting a lot of business from processing thousands of samples, there is often money to be made somewhere when developing a population-based pro-gramme. Some genetics conferences now seem more like trade shows, where a respected academic from a top university gives a talk about a new screening test (for which he holds the patent) and explains why it is superior to the other screening tests currently available. This speaker is then followed by someone who left academia to work in a biotechnology company who claims that their screening test is the best. And so forth. With universities now setting up venture capital funds to commercialise research findings, and a growing number of "back door" biotechnology companies emerging each year, the line between science and business is

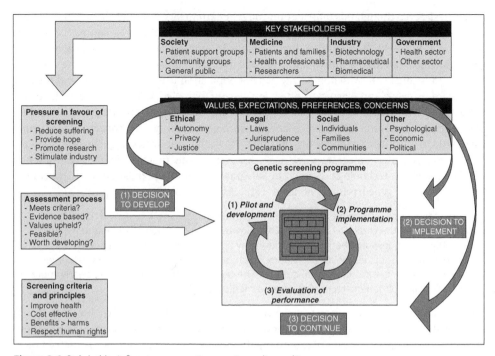

Figure 3.6 Stakeholder influences on genetic-screening policy-making.
Reproduced with permission from Andermann A, Blancquaert I, Déry V. Genetic screening: a conceptual framework for programs and policy-making. *J Health Serv Res Policy* 2010; 15(2): 90–7. Copyright 2010 Royal Society of Medicine Press, UK.

becoming increasingly blurred. Competing interests are now everywhere, to the extent that the mandatory declaration of one's potential conflicts of interest is becoming part of the day-to-day *modus operandi* in medicine, whether as an author of a journal article or as a presenter at a conference. Many blame the US Supreme Court decision of *Diamond v. Chakrabarty* in 1980, which made it possible to patent biological materials.[49] Before that time, living things were not patentable. However, the Supreme Court ruled that "the fact that micro-organisms are alive is without legal significance for purposes of the patent law". At that moment, an entire industry was born. While there are still those who try to challenge the patent laws,[50] and there have been a few small victories,[51] others claim that "the ship has sailed" on this front and we should instead focus our energies on finding new ways to work around it. Knoppers and colleagues are therefore justifiably concerned that strong economic interests, with additional pressures from patient groups, could lead to a market-driven approach to genetic screening policy development before the added value of screening has been demonstrated.[52]

It is one thing to encourage technology transfer of new genetic tests for rare diseases from the research laboratory to the clinical setting (or, as the saying goes, "from the bench to the bedside") so that individuals and families can be tested for specific diseases depending on their family history and individual risk profile (i.e. genetic testing at the individual and family level). Indeed, while many individuals and families at high risk have participated in research studies to help identify new genes, they are often unable to themselves be tested for these diseases since there are no laboratories outside of research settings offering these clinical genetic tests, even though this information could be extremely helpful for them. However, it is quite another thing to systematically offer these tests to the entire population (i.e. genetic screening at the population level). When the focus is on more large-scale applications of new genetic technologies for the entire population, the information has far less immediate relevance for each individual (i.e. by definition the general population is not at high risk), and thus the balance of benefits and harms is often less favourable. Yet, due to the scale involved, population-level applications are more lucrative and therefore more attractive for patent holders. For this reason, there are many dissenting voices who are concerned that rapid technological advances are outpacing the ability of health authorities, regulators and policy-makers to adequately integrate these new discoveries into practice. Some even question whether these new technologies should be integrated at all at a population level and contest the ever-growing "geneticisation" of health care services. According to Lippman:

> [Prenatal] genetic screening is offered as a method of detecting a fetus with defects, thus giving women the choice to abort the fetus. However, another way of looking at the whole situation is to question whether our society may have a defect for not being able to accept people with disabilities or abnormalities. A physical abnormality often only becomes a problem when it is put in a social context. The use of genetic [screening] is clearly more of a social use of genetic technology than a medical use.[53]

Many of these dissenting voices come from academia, and they are often not as active in lobbying the government as those who favour screening. Therefore it is important for decision-makers to have impartial means of examining the arguments both for and against screening to be able to make better-informed decisions at a population level. Is it enough to provide clinical genetic testing and cascade screening to those who have a family history and are therefore at increased risk of transmitting the disease? Should the entire population be offered genetic screening regardless of their *a priori* risk? Should the government listen to the patient groups who only want to prevent further suffering? Should they allow biotechnology companies to make a sales pitch? Should they heed the advice of academic naysayers? How to decide?

Often such population-level decisions involve highly technical issues that require specialised knowledge and expertise. Thus, in recent decades, there has been a burgeoning of health technology assessment (HTA) agencies to fill this need. For instance, there is the National Institute for Health and Clinical Excellence (NICE) in the UK, the Canadian Agency for Drugs and Technologies in Health (CADTH) in Canada, and dozens of other agencies around the world, many of which are members of the International Network of Agencies for Health Technology Assessment (INAHTA). These HTA agencies often work at "arm's length" from governments to examine the technical as well as the social, ethical and contextual implications of introducing new technologies, with the goal of making well-grounded and thoroughly researched recommendations that busy policy-makers can then use in decision-making. In some ways this is analogous to the evidence-based information and decision aids that are developed for patients in a clinical setting, except that, in this case, the patient is the population, and health authorities, bureaucrats or elected government officials are the ones who have the important responsibility of weighing the benefits and harms on behalf of the entire population.

Balancing the benefits and harms of population-level interventions

To be able to balance the benefits and harms, one of course needs to have a good idea of what are the benefits and what are the harms. Population-based genetic screening has been defined as a systematic programme offered to a specified population of asymptomatic individuals whereby a variety of test methods may be used to: (1) detect an inherited disease at an early stage, (2) make a risk estimate regarding an inherited predisposition to disease, or (3) make a risk estimate regarding the possibility of transmitting a disease to offspring, for the purpose of disease prevention, early treatment, or family planning.[54] The benefits of genetic screening have classically involved early diagnosis and treatment, resulting in reductions in morbidity and mortality (e.g. by strictly adhering to a diet that has no phenylalanine – a type of protein – patients with phenylketonuria can avoid developing mental retardation and live a long and healthy life). However, more recently, expanding notions of benefit have emerged. For instance, genetic screening is used to allow couples to make more informed reproductive choices (e.g. having the option of aborting a fetus that has tested positive for a genetic defect or being able to better plan for the delivery of a baby with special needs). Some suggest that screening could even be warranted to shorten the diagnostic odyssey (e.g. newborn screening for cystic fibrosis to avoid the long and drawn-out process of establishing the diagnosis clinically, especially for milder forms of the disease, even if this may not necessarily have an impact on morbidity or mortality in the long term). While some of these benefits are clearly significant reasons to endorse population-based screening programmes (e.g. preventing disease, prolonging life), others are still somewhat controversial (e.g. shortening the diagnostic odyssey).

However, in addition to the benefits of screening, there are also potential harms. Stewart-Brown and Farmer argue that the proponents of screening tend to consider the benefits only from the point of view of those who develop the disease.[55] However, screening is offered to a much larger target population of asymptomatic individuals, most of whom will never develop the disease. Moreover, these individuals can be harmed by screening. Not only can screening cause undue anxiety and concern, for instance from a false-positive test result, it can also lead to unneeded and sometimes invasive diagnostic testing and interventions which can have serious physical consequences. As well, screening can lead to labelling and stigmatisation of those who are discovered to be carriers of a defective gene – even if they themselves will never develop the disease. While certain jurisdictions have passed laws to protect citizens against discrimination, there are quite understandably concerns over the privacy of genetic information and the potential consequences if insurance companies, employers or members of the community were to learn about and misuse this information, for example, by denying insurance coverage, discontinuing employment or ostracising individuals and their families. There are even concerns that knowing one's genetic status may lead people to adopt a fatalistic attitude and engage in harmful, risk-taking behaviours. All of these considerations must therefore be taken into account when balancing the pros and cons of screening.

Austoker cautions that it would be unethical to downplay the potential risks of screening out of concern that screening uptake rates may be low.[56] Even if reduced participation results in compromising the effectiveness of the screening programme (i.e. an intervention cannot improve health if nobody uses it), people should always be given sufficient information to allow them to choose for themselves whether or not they wish to be screened. Of course, many argue that even if people have complete access to information on the benefits and harms it can nonetheless be difficult to make a truly free choice in contexts where one choice is considered far more socially acceptable than another. For example, Woloshin and Schwartz, who oppose what they call "selling screening", cite an old American Cancer Society promotional campaign that says: "If you are a woman over 35, be sure to schedule a mammogram. Unless you're still not convinced of its importance. In which case, you may need more than your breasts examined."[57] Messages such as this certainly made it difficult for women to decline screening even if they wanted to. And while times have changed, even today's promotional materials still have a tendency to use emotional messaging that inflates the risks of disease, overstates the benefits of screening and glosses over the harms, resulting in hidden social pressures that continue to be powerful forces. The mere fact of having a screening programme at all is a sign that this is socially acceptable and judged to be important for the health of the population. Therefore, the decision to introduce any new screening programme needs to be taken with care.

For example, in autosomal dominant conditions such as Huntington's disease where the disease is passed on from one generation to the next even when only one parent is a carrier of the defective gene, it could in theory be possible to wipe out the disease in a single generation if every person in the population is screened before having children and, for those who test positive, they either choose not to have children, to adopt children, to do prenatal testing and abort the fetus if affected, or to select for healthy embryos using *in vitro* fertilisation (IVF), which could then be implanted into the uterus. However, in practice, there are no population-based screening programmes for Huntington's disease outside of a research setting, and only about 15% of people offered testing for Huntington's disease actually decide to take the test.[58] One of the main reasons for this is that the test for Huntington's disease not only informs people of their carrier status for the purpose of making more informed reproductive choices, but also acts as a "crystal ball" that predicts with very high certainty (greater than 90%) whether the person taking the test will themselves develop this terrible degenerative disease during their lifetime. Huntington's disease has no treatment or cure. The average age of symptom onset is at 40 years, followed by a slow decline in functioning over the next two decades involving progressively worsening neuropsychiatric changes such as uncontrolled movements, hostility, and difficulty walking, talking and swallowing, finally ending in premature death at around 60 years of age. Thus, while at first glance it would certainly appear tempting to provide population-based screening services that could relieve future generations of the burden of living with this terrible disease, it is not quite so simple. What about those being screened? For those who test positive, living with the knowledge that one day they will almost certainly become ill and die a slow death as a result of this genetic defect can lead to tremendous psychological distress, resulting in depression, suicide attempts, psychiatric hospitalisation, substance abuse and the breakdown of family relationships.[59] For those who test negative, knowing that they are "saved" but that 50% of their closest loved ones (i.e. parents, siblings) will suffer this terrible fate can result in serious psychological implications all the same. Therefore, one cannot use people living today as a means to an end (i.e. allow those being screened to suffer in the present even if there is a laudable goal of eradicating or even reducing the prevalence of Huntington's disease for the future).

Hubbard and Wald warn that, while eugenics may be a taboo subject since the Second World War, it is important to be vigilant since eugenic thinking persists, albeit in more covert ways.[60] They cite as an example a survey of obstetricians in the 1970s, which found that physicians would be more likely to offer sterilisation as a form of contraception to their patients on welfare than to their wealthier private patients. It is therefore important to proceed with caution when it comes to offering genetic screening services, in order to ensure that patients truly have free and informed consent to choose without being pressured or coerced in any way.[61] Certainly health care providers should not discriminate against nor pressure their patients, but sometimes there are structural factors that limit people's choices indirectly. If, for instance, a woman must choose between aborting an unborn child with a genetic malformation or keeping the child but having to stop working to devote all her time and energy to caring for that child while becoming increasingly impoverished and exhausted due to a lack of publicly funded health and social services for families who have children with disabilities, then it is not really a free choice. Thus, to ensure the real possibility of making free and informed choices, governments need to do more than just provide information on screening. They also need to ensure that they are funding and supporting services for those who are living with the disease (i.e. considering the entire continuum of strategies to improve health and not just focusing on screening as the only approach). Similarly, one could also question whether there are other "upstream" strategies for improving health that could also be used. For instance, in the case of neural tube defects, this could involve fortification of cereals with folic acid and advising all pregnant women to take folic acid supplements during pregnancy (i.e. primary prevention), screening during pregnancy (i.e. secondary prevention) and ensuring adequate services for those who are born with neural tube defects (i.e. treatment and rehabilitation).

Any proposed screening programme (or intervention, more generally) will have various potential benefits as well as potential harms that need to be considered. However, the balance of benefits and harms will very much depend on how decisions are made with respect to the development and implementation of population-level programmes, including how these programmes are organised and what safeguards are in place. Ensuring that screening is conducted in such a way as to minimise risks may entail certain delays in programme development as well as additional costs. Nonetheless, adequate planning, regulations and safeguards are clearly necessary. According to a WHO report entitled *Genomics and World Health*:

> Many countries have yet to establish the regulatory, ethical and policy frameworks that are required to address the economic, legal and social implications of this field, and safeguard against the potential risks and hazards of these technologies in the best interests of their populations.[62]

Therefore, collecting high-quality evidence of the benefits and harms, and putting in place measures that maximise the benefits and minimise the harms, are important aspects when making population-level policy decisions.

Yet another important consideration is the context. Banta, Dobrow and others increasingly emphasise how contextual considerations – such as type of health system, local politics, economic conditions, and so forth – are extremely important when making population-level decisions.[63,64] Indeed, there are a growing number of initiatives to include contextual factors when developing evidence-informed policy recommendations.[65,66] In this way, rather than receiving "generic" advice based on the international literature, decision-makers instead have access to information that is tailored to their specific jurisdiction and/or situation. For instance, HIV prevention in Sub-Saharan Africa would require different approaches as compared to HIV prevention in the Arctic. While the evidence base may be the same, making a positive impact necessitates interventions that make sense and are effective in the local context. Thus, one size does not fit all. Going back over 40 years to Wilson and Jungner's classic report on screening, the authors had already recognised that:

> In theory, screening is an admirable method of combating disease . . . [but] in practice, there are snags. . . The central idea of early disease detection and treatment is essentially simple. However, the path to its successful achievement (on the one hand, bringing to treatment those with previously undetected disease, and, on the other, avoiding harm to those persons not in need of treatment) is far from simple though sometimes it may appear deceptively easy.[67]

Making nuanced decisions about population-level screening therefore requires taking into account all of the different parameters on a case-by-case basis, including the type of disease, the test used, the timing of screening and the target population. For instance, if you offer screening to people in the general population, they are often unaware that they could be affected by this disease and are also more likely to have false-positive test results due to the lower prevalence rates as compared to high-risk groups. Thus greater caution is needed. In contrast, if you offer screening to people at higher risk (i.e. if a certain disease is particularly prevalent in a given sub-population), this group may accept a higher risk of harm due to screening since they also have a greater likelihood of benefit. The Nuffield Council on Bioethics has written an entire report called *Public Health: Ethical Issues* on how to balance individual versus population-level concerns – a recurrent theme in public health.[68] Doing so requires making explicit the many trade-offs that are being made at different levels when decisions are made about population-level interventions.

Considering opportunity costs and making trade-offs

Trade-offs and opportunity costs are inherent to decision-making, although they are generally not made as explicit as they should be. There can be trade-offs regarding the degree to which you minimise harms versus how much you want to spend on implementing a policy or programme. There can be trade-offs in terms of paying for a given programme and therefore having to forego paying for other programmes. There can be trade-offs in terms of doing something for the benefit of a small but marginalised group of individuals, because it is "the right thing to do", even if it is unlikely to benefit the majority of people involved. Making these trade-offs explicit is important since it highlights the kind of value judgements that are being made as part of the decision-making process.

For example, one trade-off is determining how much we as a society should be investing in new genomic technologies versus investments in tackling the social determinants of health. Another trade-off is to determine the extent to which we as a society should be supporting individuals and families suffering from rare and orphan diseases, even if these diseases are not the main causes of death and disability within the population. Before getting into these trade-offs, I want to first clarify the difference between single-gene diseases and common diseases with multifactorial inheritance. Up until now, we have been talking about single-gene diseases (i.e. Huntington's disease, cystic fibrosis, phenylketonuria, etc.). However, in recent years, there has been a growing interest in better understanding the genetic basis of common diseases with multifactorial inheritance (i.e. heart disease, cancer, etc.). Indeed, most diseases result from a combination of genetic and environmental factors. There is, however, an aetiological spectrum, with diseases mostly due to genetic factors at one end, and diseases mostly due to environmental factors at the other. At the "genetic" end of the spectrum, there are more than a thousand single-gene diseases which share certain features: they tend to be rare conditions, they are inherited in a Mendelian fashion (e.g. recessive or dominant transmission), and having the genetic defect is a very strong predictor for developing the disease (i.e. high penetrance). At the "environmental" end of the spectrum, there are common diseases which also share certain features: they tend to affect large proportions of the population, they are caused by the interplay of multiple genes – each of which is a small contributor to the development of the disease – in combination with various behavioural and environmental factors (also known as multifactorial or complex inheritance), and having the genetic defect or genetic marker is only a very small predictor for developing the disease (i.e. low penetrance). For instance, breast cancer is a common disease that is caused by the interplay of a multitude of genetic and environmental factors including age at menarche (first menstruation), age at first live birth, number of previous biopsies and number of first-degree relatives with breast cancer.[69] However, in 5–15% of cases, breast cancer is a single-gene disease with autosomal dominant inheritance (i.e. caused by mutations in the *BRCA1* or *BRCA2* genes that are passed down from generation to generation).

Trade-offs between investing in new technologies versus reducing health inequities

Personalised medicine – a term that is often confused with patient-centred care – proposes to bring the testing of genetic markers for common diseases directly into every doctor's office. Each of these markers (also called genetic variants or low-penetrance genes) would only have a very small role to play in the development of the disease alongside many other genetic and environmental factors. Nonetheless, there are those who believe that this will revolutionise the way that we practise medicine, although this remains highly controversial. Indeed, with the completed sequencing of the entire human genome in the year 2000,[70] the field of genomics has been growing at an exponential rate. There is the oft-repeated promise that new genomic technologies will play a major role in the prevention and treatment of human disease. In particular, population-based screening is being considered as one of the possible vehicles for translating genomic advances into population health gains. However, even John Bell, Regius Professor of Medicine at Oxford and one of the major proponents of personalised medicine, recognises that "very large epidemiological population samples followed prospectively (over a period of years) and characterised for their biomarker and genetic variation will be necessary to demonstrate the clinical utility of these tools".[71] This could take more than a generation, and there is no guarantee that the genomic information will ever prove useful in informing individual health decisions.

For instance, there is great interest in demonstrating that genomic information can be used to create a sufficiently informative risk profile (based on the additive effects of many low-penetrance genes) that would help people to adopt healthier behaviours such as quitting smoking, thereby reducing their risk of cancer and heart disease.[72] However, while there are many evidence-based interventions that have been proven to promote smoking cessation,[73] according to Carlsten and colleagues:

> Empiric data so far provide little or no evidence that knowledge of genetic variants yields long-term benefit in terms of quit rates. For example, a study that incorporated genetic testing for lung cancer susceptibility (genotyping for the glutathione S-transferase M1 gene) in a smoking cessation program found that genetic feedback – regardless of test result – enhanced cessation rates at 6 months, but the effect did not persist at 12 months. Another study examining the impact of genetic testing for alpha-1 antitrypsin on smokers' behavior similarly noted increased attempts to quit but no effect on sustained abstinence. A study of knowledge about L-myc polymorphisms to motivate smoking cessation showed no effect. In contrast, a recent study showed that simply informing a patient of his or her lung age, a low-cost technique requiring only a spirometer, more than doubled the 12-month quitting rate compared with conventional treatment.[74]

Therefore, knowledge of one's genetic variants does not actually help people to change their behaviour and quit smoking. In fact, "considering that the predictive power of genetic testing [for susceptibility to common disease] tends to be underwhelming, perhaps it's no surprise that personalized genetic information induces more shoulder shrugs than lifestyle changes".[75] The one area where there could be some potential for improving health is through pharmacogenomics, where genomic information may help to predict who will be more likely to respond to a given treatment and who should avoid this treatment since they would likely have no benefit or would be at risk for severe side effects. Still, even the widespread use of pharmacogenomics is a long way off, and it remains to be seen whether there will be a substantial added benefit given the significant added costs involved. Therefore, despite all the "genohype", it is no surprise that a recent headline in the *New York Times* reads "A Decade Later, Genetic Map Yields Few New Cures".[76] Yet the "promise" that genomics will yield huge returns continues to drive this research – the question remains whether the real driver is the hope of financial returns or health returns?

Indeed, while genetics is an important determinant of what makes populations healthy or unhealthy, it is only one factor among a long list of determinants of health. As we have seen, the relative contribution of genetics decreases as one moves away from rare, Mendelian single-gene conditions towards more common, multifactorial conditions such as heart disease and cancer. There are therefore growing concerns that these new and costly technologies will fail to improve health at a population level, could draw attention away from other interventions with even greater potential for disease prevention, and may ultimately exacerbate health inequities. According to the *Report of a WHO Meeting on Collaboration in Medical Genetics*:

> All considerations about genetics and genomics... should be placed in the context of the primacy of fundamental overarching strategies to improve health, for example through alleviation of poverty, development of health systems, improved education and classical public health approaches to disease control, prevention and health promotion and states must ensure that genome technology is used to reduce rather than exacerbate global inequalities in health status.[77]

Particularly as the science advances to make it possible to screen for hundreds or even thousands of susceptibility genes that are associated with common diseases (i.e. in contrast with single-gene diseases where a single mutation can be a very high predictor of developing the disease), it will be important to consider the added value of obtaining the genetic profile of individuals as part of the continuum of strategies to improve health, including disease prevention, health promotion and addressing the social determinants of health.

Increasingly, many are starting to question whether it makes sense that budgets for genomics research hugely overshadow spending on other important areas such as global health. When one thinks of the billions of dollars that have been poured into the genomics enterprise with little assurance of making any real impact on population health on a large scale, one wonders whether the money could have been better spent on development aid to build infrastructure for clean water, sanitation, schools, hospitals and so forth in low- and middle-income countries around the world where large segments of the population still live on less than $2 a day and lack access to the most basic necessities. Choosing to spend one's valuable time, money and energy in one way rather than spending it on something else is known as an opportunity cost. On the one hand, governments want to support the growing biotechnology sector, which provides jobs and fuels the economy, while, on the other hand, governments are also responsible for regulating health services and for protecting patients and their families. As well, governments are also part of a global society, and they have pledged to provide financial assistance to poor countries in need.[78] Governments must therefore balance the many different perspectives and needs of society – locally, nationally and globally. In practice, however, some things get more support and other things are left behind.

While it is certainly easy enough to criticise governments for their decisions, it is less obvious what would be the optimal way to balance the various needs of different groups in a fair and rational way. Indeed, governments are not a single entity working as a coherent whole. While one branch of government is funding genomics research and supporting the biotechnology industry, another branch of government is running to catch up with the repercussions that this is causing for the health and well-being of the population, and yet another branch of government is lobbying for social action to reduce health inequities on a global scale. Getting all the branches of government to work together in a coherent way is not always easy. There are, nonetheless, specific interventions involving single-gene diseases where there are real opportunities to make a positive impact on health, as opposed to the hypothetical future opportunities of personalised medicine. In the example of the patient support group lobbying the government to provide a population-based screening programme for disease X, while the decision of whether or not to implement screening depends on many factors, on the whole, supporting those who suffer from rare and orphan diseases is certainly a worthy cause that has been overshadowed by the zealous interest in exploring the genetic causes of common diseases with the hopes of being able to apply these technologies to a much bigger "market", even if people with rare diseases could have a more immediate and obvious benefit.

Trade-offs between improving health overall versus supporting vulnerable groups

Until recently, rare diseases have not been considered a public health concern because, by definition, fewer than 1 in 2,000 people are affected. Approximately 80% of rare diseases are of genetic origin and over 65% are serious and debilitating. According to the European Commission on Public Health, there are between 5,000 and 7,000 distinct rare diseases, which together affect between 6% and 8% of the world's population.[79] Thus, all together, rare diseases are not so rare, affecting an estimated 54 million people in Europe and North America combined, and almost half a billion people worldwide. Nonetheless, it has been very difficult to get rare genetic diseases onto the agendas of policy-makers and pharmaceutical companies. Many rare diseases are therefore orphan diseases for which there is a lack of diagnostic and therapeutic products and services. Individuals and families affected by rare and orphan diseases carry a large social burden and often lack resources and a political voice.[80] Thus, according to Muir Gray, former Programme Director of the UK National Screening Committee:

> From the utilitarian perspective, the case for investing in common diseases is strong, but if a high value is placed on justice or fairness, increased investment may be made in rare diseases, even though the cost per patient treated, and therefore the value assigned to a beneficial outcome for a patient with a rare disease becomes, by this process, higher than the value ascribed to the same outcome for someone with a common condition. These aspects of policy-making are often implicit and unstated.[81]

With a view to promoting greater equity and supporting vulnerable groups, prevention and early treatment of rare diseases, made possible by genetic screening programmes, should be offered when feasible and when the overall benefits outweigh the potential harms. In many countries, babies are screened for congenital hypothyroidism and phenylketonuria using a drop of blood taken from the heel a few days after birth. Modifying the diet or providing hormone replacement before affected infants become symptomatic is crucial in preventing the development of intellectual deficiencies, because if they are diagnosed once they are symptomatic, it would be too late to reverse the effects of the disease.

However, with the advent of new technologies such as tandem mass spectrometry, which makes it possible to greatly expand the number of single-gene diseases that can be screened for by existing population-based programmes,[82] some fear this may lead to a "snowball effect" with important logistical, ethical and cost implications (Fig. 3.7).[83] For instance, different countries, and even different jurisdictions within the same country, are opting to include varying numbers and types of conditions on their newborn screening panels. How can we decide which diseases to add and which diseases not to include on these screening panels? Is it possible to obtain truly informed consent for 30 diseases as compared to 3 diseases? While governments certainly have a role in providing genetic services and screening programmes that aim to improve the health of the population, there is growing concern that the large number of genetic tests that are becoming available may compromise the viability of the health care system overall. Even though the tests themselves may be inexpensive and suitable for large-scale use, the infrastructure and human resources needed to provide appropriate education, counselling, interventions and follow-up are likely to be far more costly. As well, not all genetic diseases are so well suited to population-based screening. And even if screening programmes do not exist, genetic testing or cascade screening could nonetheless be made available in a clinical practice setting for those at increased risk.

Returning to the case of screening for disease X, we are left with more questions than answers. How should the government proceed? In the first instance, screening should not be considered on its own, but rather as part of a continuum of services for the management of these conditions that includes access to health and social services for those affected by the disease. Douste-Blazy and colleagues emphasise the importance of supporting people with rare and orphan disease by developing a comprehensive framework for action. Particularly in publicly funded health care systems where universal access to services is an explicit objective, they consider that:

> Rare diseases present a political problem, in the noblest sense: that of taking into account the needs of the weakest and the fewest in number. If we want to guarantee equal access to treatment, if we are looking for the best quality of care and support, then it is obvious that the problem concerns the entire health and socio-medical system.[84]

Nonetheless, this still leaves the question, what is the role of screening for disease X within the continuum of care? Screening tends to involve large and expensive programmes. Could this money be better used by providing more limited cascade screening to relatives of affected persons, or by providing other forms of support to people with rare diseases, or even by spending the money on programmes for vulnerable groups more broadly to combat poverty and hunger, for instance, which are important determinants of population health? While these are all important questions, at a certain point, one must make a decision and choose – will we offer this screening programme to the specified target population or not? According to Goethe, "Thinking is easy, acting is difficult, and to put one's thoughts into action is the most difficult thing in the world". However, there are tools that can help us to make difficult and complex policy choices, such as the use of criteria.

Criteria for decision-making: sufficient to make good decisions?

Even beyond the field of genetics and genomics, there is a growing understanding that population-level policy decisions – which almost always involve trade-offs and opportunity costs – should be based both on high-quality evidence and on the values of the population. Due to the tremendous complexity involved in genetic screening policy-making, the Nuffield Council on Bioethics recommends that:

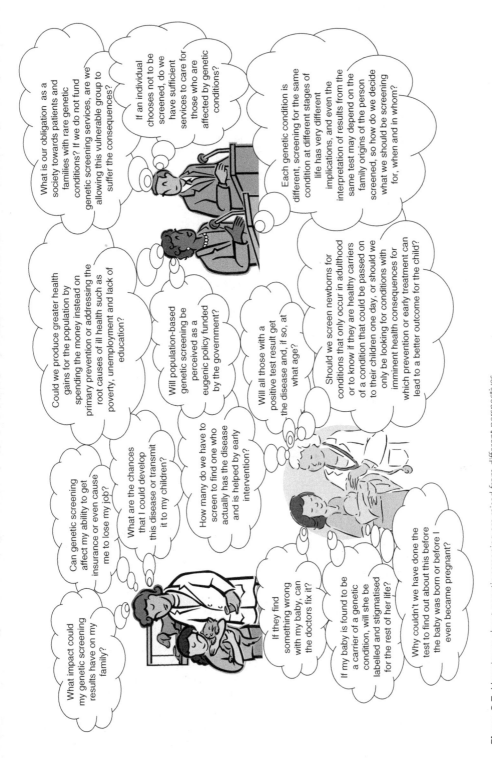

Figure 3.7 Many issues about genetic screening are raised from different perspectives.

Reproduced from Andermann A, Beauchamp S, Costea I, Blancquaert I. *Guiding Decision-Making for Population Based Screening: An Approach Applicable to Genetics* (unpublished report). Montreal: Agence d'évaluation des technologies et des modes d'intervention en santé (AETMIS), 2007.

Table 3.1 The classic Wilson and Jungner screening criteria.

(1) The condition sought should be an important health problem.
(2) There should be an accepted treatment for patients with recognised disease.
(3) Facilites for diagnosis and treatment should be available.
(4) There should be a recognisable latent or early symptomatic stage.
(5) There should be a suitable test or examination.
(6) The test should be acceptable to the population.
(7) The natural history of the condition, including development from latent to declared disease, should be adequately understood.
(8) There should be an agreed policy on whom to treat as patients.
(9) The cost of case-finding (including diagnosis and treatment of patients diagnosed) should be economically balanced in relation to possible expenditure on care as a whole.
(10) Case-finding should be a continuing process and not a "once and for all" project.

Reproduced from Andermann A, Blancquaert I, Beauchamp S, Déry V. Revisiting Wilson and Jungner in the genomic age: a review of screening criteria over the past 40 years. *Bull World Health Organ* 2008; 86(4): 1–3, with permission from the World Health Organization.

Table 3.2 Emerging screening criteria proposed over the past 40 years.

- The screeing programme should respond to a recognised need.
- The objectives of screening should be defined at the outset.
- There should be a defined target population.
- There should be scientific evidence of screening programme effectiveness.
- The programme should intergrate education, testing, clinical services and programme management.
- There should be quality assurance, with mechanisms to minimise potential risks of screening.
- The programme should ensure informed choice, confidentiality and respect for autonomy.
- The programme should promote equity and access to screening for the entire target population.
- Programme evaluation should be planned from the outset.
- The overall benefits of screening should outweigh the harm.

Reproduced from Andermann A, Blancquaert I, Beauchamp S, Déry V. Revisiting Wilson and Jungner in the genomic age: a review of screening criteria over the past 40 years. *Bull World Health Organ* 2008; 86(4): 1–3, with permission from the World Health Organization.

[Governments], in consultation with the appropriate professional bodies, should formulate detailed criteria for the introduction of genetic screening programmes and establish a central coordinating body to review genetic screening programmes and monitor their implementation and outcomes.[85]

Many of the criteria that are generally used are variations on the classic screening criteria developed by Wilson and Jungner for WHO in 1968 (Table 3.1).[86,87]

As well, there are also new criteria that have emerged over the last 40 years in response to broader trends that have shaped both Western medicine and society more generally. These include increased consumerism, the shift away from paternalism towards informed choice, a focus on evidence-based health care, and the rise of managed care models that emphasize cost-effectiveness, quality assurance and accountability of decision-makers (Table 3.2).[87]

Nonetheless, even with criteria, population-level decision-making is far from straightforward. It is beyond the scope of this book to go into all the details that are required to decide whether or not the government should screen for disease X in this specific context. However, what is important is that there is a systematic, transparent and fair process for making such decisions. Involving key stakeholders, through consultations and other means, helps to develop a shared understanding of the issues. Daniels and colleagues emphasise the need for openness and inclusiveness in the decision-making process as a form of procedural justice – since these are, after all, political decisions that can affect the lives of the entire population.[88] The final decision should clearly describe the different options that were examined and make explicit the reasons for choosing one option versus another, so that it would be possible to revisit and revise decisions made as the knowledge base or contextual circumstances evolve.

Although this would be the ideal, Grosse and colleagues find that, in practice, even when the same criteria are being used by different groups, they are not always applied in a consistent manner.[89] According to Pollitt:

> The lack of even broad concordance at the level of national policy is extremely disturbing. Though all discussion is nominally founded on the ten principles laid down by Wilson and Jungner in 1968, there seems no generally accepted way of using these principles, or derived criteria, as objective decision tools.[90]

Thus, while criteria can be helpful tools in providing a more systematic approach to examining the issues, it depends on how they are used. In many instances, criteria are used in a simplistic and instrumental way by proponents to justify screening or by cash-strapped governments to flatly deny screening without really engaging in a broader debate and examination of the issues at stake. In the end, a rational and linear model of policy-making – appealing though it may be – simply does not reflect the reality of how policy-making occurs in practice. Rather, policy-making is more of an "organised anarchy", whereby "a problem is recognized, a solution is available, the political climate makes the time right for change, and the constraints do not prohibit change".[91] It is all about being ready when the "policy window" presents itself to be able to raise the issue higher on the political agenda and generate the support required to push the proposed solution through. Thus policy analysis cannot be disentangled from the political process.[92] Indeed, the complexity is even more pronounced when it comes to decision-making at the global level.

Global health decisions

Global-level decisions for health are a form of population-level decision, but on a much larger scale. The important distinction is that these decisions cross national boundaries. Global health problems have the potential to affect people across many countries or regions, cannot be solved by one country or region alone, and therefore require a transnational response.[93] For this reason, there is much less clarity and far more uncertainty when it comes to making global-level decisions. To illustrate the complexity of decision-making for health at the global level I will use the example of tackling child labour as a means of promoting health equity worldwide (Box 3.3).

At first glance, this may appear to be an unusual example to illustrate global health decision-making. Some would argue that child labour is neither a global issue (i.e. it is a question of domestic policy) nor a health issue (i.e. it is a societal problem). Infectious diseases would be a more traditional global health example. Yet, global health is not limited to infectious diseases. Non-communicable diseases are gaining in importance on the global stage, as are issues relating to the social determinants of health – which include child labour. Affecting an estimated 215 million children worldwide,[94] child labour is an important public health problem that results in numerous physical, psychological and social consequences.

Box 3.3 Global-level decision-making for health

Case E: Deciding to break the entrenched cycle of health inequities

In many low- and middle-income countries, the intergenerational transfer of health inequities can be linked to the problem of child labour. Indeed, when the head of the household suffers from a lack of employment opportunities and poor health, this leads to high rates of child labour – up to 80% and more in some settings – to supplement the family income. Working children are less likely to attend school and are also at increased risk of work-related harms. From child soldiers and rag-pickers to carpet weavers and street vendors, child labour is a key factor in sustaining the cycle of poverty, low educational attainment, social exclusion and poor health from generation to generation. According to one child labourer interviewed as part of a research study, "whenever I see children of my age who are going to school, I get a feeling that... my future would have been better if I had joined in school". Yet the question remains, how to break this vicious cycle, commonly found in South Asia, Africa and Latin America, thereby improving the health of children and adolescents in the short term while also reducing health and social inequities in a more strategic, long-term and sustainable way. What influence do global-level decisions have? Who makes these decisions? What can be done to impact these decisions? How can we tell whether these decisions have made a difference?

Work at an early age is clearly linked to increased rates of injuries, poisonings and even death. Child workers also have higher rates of developmental delay, anaemia, headaches and dizziness (associated with handling toxic products), respiratory problems, cardiovascular problems, cuts and bruises, musculoskeletal problems (such as low back pain), scabies (for instance among rag pickers), motor vehicle injuries (especially among street workers), and neurological symptoms (such as memory loss and poor motor coordination). Child workers are also far more likely to suffer from abuse, including physical abuse, sexual harassment and assault. In one study, up to 77.7% of female child workers had been victims of sexual assault.[95–109] Unsurprisingly, child workers have higher rates of depression, anxiety, substance use and suicidal ideation.[110–113] Moreover, early entry into the labour force results in a lack of schooling and reduced literacy for these children,[114] as well as lower income later in life due to fewer and lower-quality occupational opportunities over time,[115] thus perpetuating the cycle of poverty and poor health when children grow to reach adulthood and start families of their own.[116] With economic pressures, environmental degradation and social unrest leading to increasing migration to find work across borders, as well as the ongoing tragedy of human trafficking, taking action to prevent and mitigate the many different types of harm associated with child labour is indeed a good example of a global health challenge where an intersectoral and transnational response is required.

Who are the global decision-makers?

While the United Nations (UN) was created after the Second World War as a mechanism to promote international cooperation and peace, all 193 member states nonetheless maintain their sovereignty. There is no "global government" that has been elected and has the authority to make decisions at a global level. Just as we have seen with population-level decisions at the national and sub-national levels, there are many different stakeholders and interest groups vying for their concerns to be heard in the political arena – only now the arena is much larger and it is not so clear who has the real authority to decide on behalf of our global society. Ultimately, those who hold the purse strings and the power at the international level are the national governments. Similar to decisions at the individual and population levels, there are many factors that can influence global-level decision-making, from gender and cultural differences among policy-makers to arms races and media effects. According to Mintz and DeRouen, "to survive in a dangerous world with no overarching government, leaders must provide for the security of their states".[117] Thus, while most governments are bound by various bilateral or multilateral agreements and alliances that require them to consult and coordinate their responses,[118] the national governments are nonetheless the primary decision-makers.

Yet when it comes to making decisions at the global level it is important to point out that there is no level playing field. Some national governments clearly wield more power in the global arena and thereby have a greater influence on the decisions that are made. Currently, the G8 governments hold the majority of the global wealth, but with the rise of the middle-income "superpowers" such as China, India and Brazil, this will likely change in the next generation or two. According to Pogge, global institutions "reflect the highly uneven bargaining power of the participating countries and thus tend to reinforce and to aggravate economic inequality".[119] Indeed Manderson and Whiteford consider that global forces are "historical artifacts that derive from Western domination; they reflect Western values of rationality, competition, and progress, in which context there is an implicit assumption that with modernization, local 'traditional' institutions and structures will be replaced by Western systems and patterns".[120] Woods sees little indication that powerful member states have any intention of altering the hierarchical basis upon which order has traditionally been maintained, and while there have been multiple calls for reform over the last few decades, "the most powerful states in the system resist any reform of the institutions they dominate".[121]

Thus, even when global decisions are made with the goal of improving health and social conditions, they are often mere recommendations with no "teeth" to ensure that they are implemented. Sometimes there are conventions, treaties and other forms of international law which hold more sway, but, even so, there is often inaction due to a lack of know-how or political will. For example, Palmer and colleagues have shown that ratification of human rights treaties is poorly correlated with improved population health and social outcomes.[122] Non-governmental organisations such as Amnesty International and others have tried "blaming and shaming" governments to keep to their commitments, often with mixed results. In 2002, the United Nations Commission on Human Rights (now the United Nations Human Rights Council) appointed a Special Rapporteur on the Right to Health. The mandate of the Special Rapporteur is to gather information, develop a dialogue, report on the status of attainment and make recommendations "on appropriate measures to promote and protect the realisation of the right of everyone to the enjoyment of the highest attainable standard of physical and mental health, with a view to supporting States' efforts to enhance public health".[123] While all this looks good on paper, putting it into practice is a different story.

Indeed, taking action on a global level requires the cooperation and action of a large number of players. Importantly, there needs to be the political will and collective action of national governments.[124] Yet, all is not bleak. Countries have been working collectively to tackle common problems such as HIV/AIDS and maternal and child mortality. Moreover, in recent years there have also been some interesting new developments and power shifts whereby the newly emerging economies (i.e. China, India, Brazil, etc.) have begun increasing aid to poorer countries on their own terms.[125] This "silent revolution" of South–South collaboration may soon change the global health landscape and provide even greater opportunities for improving health in more innovative ways.

The politics of recognition rather than denial

Perhaps the first step in addressing a health issue is to ask the question "who knows about this problem and who cares?" In individual-level decisions, there are many people who care very much – namely the patient, their spouse, their children, their extended family members and friends. They all want the very best health outcome since it has such a direct impact on their everyday lives. However, as we move towards population- and global-level decisions, it is far from obvious to discern who knows and who cares. Moreover, those who do care are often least able to actually do something about the problem. Whiteford, Rylko-Bauer and Farmer critique the fact that since the Second World War there have been over 160 wars – a form of socially created violence – that have resulted in over 24 million deaths and millions more suffering disease, disability and displacement. Moreover, "the victims of violence become victimised a second time by being blamed for their suffering and how their experience identifies them as powerless and excluded".[126] Indeed, the existing global power relations are in themselves a form of structural violence against the world's poor who "are not only more likely to suffer; they are also less likely to have their suffering noticed".[127] A century ago, when child labour was still commonplace in North America, most people did not believe that child labour existed or was a problem. Lewis Hine was a sociology professor who was hired in 1908 by the National Child Labour Committee to document how children as young as seven were working in the cotton mills and coal mines.[128] Over a decade he took thousands of photographs that helped convince US lawmakers to introduce new industrial regulations to protect children. Similarly, today, David Parker, an epidemiologist and occupational health physician at the University of Minnesota, has been photographing child labour around the world to raise attention and generate the public outcry and political will needed for large-scale social change.[129] Lee and colleagues argue that, in our increasingly globalised world, the health of the poorest and most vulnerable has direct relevance for all populations due to the increasing "interconnectivities that bring us together".[130] Beck further emphasises that with the advent of globalisation we can no longer focus only on nation states as the main players, since there is a surge of new actors on the global stage, as discussed in greater detail below.[131]

Key players and payers from diplomats to superstars

There is a broad range of stakeholders who try to influence global health decisions.[132] From anti-globalisation protestors wearing black balaclavas and chanting slogans at G8 summit meetings, to rock singers, movie stars and supermodels with a social conscience, a wide variety of people try to have their voices heard. However, only very few people get a seat at the bargaining table, and even fewer still are invited into the high-powered backrooms where the big decisions are made.

Traditionally, the major players in global-level decisions (Table 3.3) have been the national governments (often represented by their various ministries), the UN agencies, other non-UN international fora for government cooperation, the international financial

Table 3.3 Examples of key players in global-level decision-making.

Key players	Examples
National ministries	UK Department of Health, US State Department, Health Canada, Canadian Ministry of Foreign Affairs and International Trade, etc.
UN agencies	World Health Organization (WHO), United Nations Children's Fund (UNICEF), United Nations Development Programme (UNDP), International Labour Organization (ILO), etc.
Other international fora	G8/G20, World Trade Organization (WTO), Organisation for Economic Co-operation and Development (OECD), European Union (EU), Association of Southeast Asian Nations (ASEAN), North Atlantic Treaty Organization (NATO), etc.
International financial institutions (IFIs)	World Bank (WB), International Monetary Fund (IMF), African Development Bank (AFDB), Asian Development Bank (ADB), etc.
International development agencies	Canadian International Development Agency (CIDA), US Agency for International Development (USAID), UK Department for International Development (DFID), etc.
Non-governmental organisations (NGOs)	International Federation of Red Cross and Red Crescent Societies, Save the Children, World Council of Churches, Oxfam, etc.
Professional organisations	World Medical Association, International Council of Nurses, etc.
Lobby groups	International Foodservice Manufacturers Association, International Tobacco Growers' Association, International Association of Heat and Frost Insulators and Asbestos Workers, etc.
Industry	Pharmaceutical companies, biotechnology companies, etc.
Media	CNN, Reuters, etc.

institutions (also known as IFIs), the international development agencies, the secular and faith-based international charities and other non-governmental organisations, as well as various professional organisations, private interest lobby groups, industry and the media.

More recently, private philanthropists are also becoming increasingly active in global politics. However, no one has elected them to represent the views of the world. Therefore, what gives Bono the authority between rock concerts and Louis Vuitton photo shoots to call the Canadian Prime Minister and discuss policy issues? He is not a diplomat or even a Canadian citizen. Why do Bill and Melinda Gates get invited to address the World Health Assembly? Just because they donate more money to global health in a year than the entire annual operating budget of the World Health Organization (WHO), does that give them the right to have a seat at the bargaining table? A recent article in the *New York Times* questions whether billions of dollars spent by the Gates Foundation exploiting new cell phone technologies and developing better bed nets could have had a much greater impact if it had not been so technologically focused and actually tried to implement what is known to work (i.e. clean water, latrines, infrastructure, access to health care, etc.).[133] One might even question whether this is just a veiled form of research and development (also known as R&D) to open up new markets in the developing world, or is this truly philanthropy? Due to these and other similar concerns, there are an increasing number of dissenting voices opposing this new form of "philanthrocapitalism" or "venture philanthropy", which is so dependent upon the whims and wishes of a handful of powerful donors.[134] Indeed, who can oppose these billionaires from doing what they want with their money? What are the mechanisms in place to ensure justice and a fair process at this level? Should these individual superstars and moguls have been taxed more in their countries of origin so that their funds could instead be used in a more democratic forum where there are checks and balances? These are all interesting questions, but, with so many actors and the current piecemeal approach to tackling global health issues, it is unclear who makes the rules, and even if someone does try to set down some rules, the most difficult part is convincing everyone to play by those rules.

Indeed, global health is a burgeoning field with new actors joining each year trying to stake out their claim. This mushrooming industry may in part be due to the fact that much of international development is based on contract work. A wealthy government, for instance, budgets several million dollars to go towards foreign development aid. Channelled through their own international development agency or through one of the development banks, there is often a call for tender for individuals or organisations to provide services that will meet specific objectives – for instance, improving maternal and child health, strengthening school systems, and so forth. Many different organisations ranging from management consulting firms and NGOs to UN agencies apply for funding for specific projects. Selected projects are then funded and implemented, and this process continues until the money runs out.

However, what about those on the receiving end? National ministries in low- and middle-income countries, which are the targets of this development aid, are not always involved or even informed of these projects, and often have far less funding available to be able to coherently plan and implement their own programmes and policies. Even when ministries are consulted, and even when they do have some leverage to influence how aid is spent, either by negotiating directly with donors or via the UN system, donor actions are not always well suited to or coordinated with the needs of recipient countries. Indeed, poor countries are not really in a position to refuse free vaccinations or treatments for their citizens, even if the proposed interventions come with "strings attached" or do not fit with their overall priorities. For instance, mass vaccination against the human papillomavirus (HPV), which is the precursor to developing cervical cancer, is being proposed in many low-income countries. However, many of these countries do not even have adequate coverage of the most basic childhood vaccinations included in the Expanded Programme on Immunization (EPI), which could have a far greater impact on reducing mortality in children under five and throughout the life course. Moreover, most people who develop cervical cancer are over the age of 40 years. In contrast, the average life expectancy in many of the poor countries where they are trying to introduce the HPV vaccine is so low that large segments of the population will never even live to the age when they would be at risk of dying from cervical cancer, since there are many other important causes of mortality that will have already killed them long before (i.e. childhood diseases, injuries, HIV/AIDS, etc.). Nonetheless, drug companies are pulling out all the stops to get the HPV vaccine onto the list of vaccinations funded by the Global Alliance for Vaccines and Immunisation (GAVI), as this would open up a whole new market for their product.[135] As Welsh and Woods point out, "the growing cacophony of donors", each demanding a different set of conditions, meetings and reports, and together eroding rather than strengthening the possibilities for good governance, highlights the need for more predictable and long-term aid flows that empower national and local institutions to be able to develop coherent and sustainable policies and programmes in the best interest of their citizens.[136]

Returning to the example of making an impact on global health and health equity by focusing on the issue of child labour, who are the key players one could partner with? The answer is that there are many. At the global level, there are the UN agencies that work on issues relating to children (e.g. the United Nations Children's Fund, UNICEF), child labour (e.g. the International Labour Organization, ILO) and health equity (e.g. the World Health Organisation, WHO). There are also international NGOs and other organisations which work in the area of child protection (e.g. Save the Children). At the national level there are ministries of health and ministries of labour, as well as national-level NGOs. At the local level, there are municipal governments as well as community groups. All of these knowledge users are involved in making decisions that can affect the health of vulnerable populations where a large proportion of children must work, often under hazardous conditions, to support themselves and their families. Equipped with the evidence on what works, knowledge users at all levels would be better able to make more informed choices and implement more effective interventions for combatting and mitigating hazardous child labour.

Results-based management and greater accountability in global health

In spite of the appearance of a "free for all" at the global level, there has been a push since the early 2000s for greater accountability in global health and international development. In particular, this comes from national governments who are spending public monies and need to have something to show for it, as well as from civil society, which criticises powerful players for the slow progress that has been made in improving global health. This drive to measure the output and impact of the burgeoning development aid for health (which according to World Bank data has exploded from $6 billion per year in 1960 to over $100 billion per year in 2006) is certainly a positive move on the whole.[137] One of the largest and most ambitious global exercises in results-based management is the Millennium Development Goals (or MDGs), which were launched by the United Nations in the year 2000 (Table 3.4).[138]

This "package approach" is akin to having multiple vertical programmes working together simultaneously to address several major diseases and health problems (e.g. HIV/ AIDS, maternal and child mortality), as well as the underlying determinants of health (e.g. poverty, education, access to clean water and improved sanitation). While critics still claim that countries are not doing enough and that the goals will never be reached by the year 2015, at least there are clear objectives, measurable indicators and firm targets, which have focused the world's attention on making a tangible difference. The mere fact of being able to follow the progress that is being made is in itself a positive step forward considering that many countries around the world lack even the most basic vital statistics systems to measure births and deaths.

However, as with many initiatives, there can also be unforeseen perverse effects. For instance, the emphasis on results-based management has led to a tendency to be overly focused on single diseases. Tackling one disease at a time certainly makes it easier to measure success and to attribute that success to specific interventions. Indeed, the Global Fund to Fight AIDS, Tuberculosis and Malaria (commonly referred to as The Global Fund) was established in 2002 to channel contributions from global donors towards concerted action to halt the then growing HIV/AIDS pandemic as well as other major infectious diseases and health problems that continue to kill millions of people each year in countries around the world (i.e. MDGs 4, 5 and 6). One might ask: why did we need a Global Fund? Why wasn't this something that could be done through existing structures? Without getting into rumours about internal power plays and rich donor countries wanting to bypass the UN system to have more control over how their money was being spent, one reason why this new public–private partnership (PPP) between governments, UN agencies, civil society,

Table 3.4 Millennium Development Goals (MDGs).

We resolve by the year 2015 to. . .

(1) **END POVERTY AND HUNGER:**

halve the proportion of the world's people whose income is less than one dollar a day, who suffer from hunger and who are unable to reach or to afford safe drinking water, have achieved a significant improvement in the lives of at least 100 million slum dwellers, develop and implement strategies that give young people everywhere a real chance to find decent and productive work

(2) **UNIVERSAL EDUCATION:**

ensure that children everywhere, boys and girls alike, will be able to complete a full course of primary schooling and that girls and boys will have equal access to all levels of education

(3) **GENDER EQUALITY:**

promote gender equality and the empowerment of women as effective ways to combat poverty, hunger and disease and to stimulate development that is truly sustainable

(4) **CHILD HEALTH:**

have reduced under-five child mortality by two-thirds

(5) **MATERNAL HEALTH:**

have reduced maternal mortality by three-quarters

(6) **COMBAT HIV/AIDS:**

have halted, and begun to reverse, the spread of HIV/AIDS, the scourge of malaria and other major diseases that afflict humanity

(7) **ENVIRONMENTAL SUSTAINABILITY:**

spare no effort to free all of humanity, and above all our children and grandchildren, from the threat of living on a planet irredeemably spoilt by human activities, and whose resources would no longer be sufficient for their needs

(8) **GLOBAL PARTNERSHIP:**

develop strong partnerships with the private sector and with civil society organisations in pursuit of development and poverty eradication

Adapted from: UN General Assembly. *United Nations Millennium Declaration.* New York: United Nations, 2000.

the private sector and affected communities was created is that WHO is largely a normative agency that is mandated to define international standards and to provide technical support to member states. This is unlike UNICEF, which works "on the ground" to provide interventions such as mass vaccination and outreach campaigns. Therefore, The Global Fund, which was affiliated with but distinct from the WHO, has the mandate and capacity to take action and to deploy programmes that could halt or at least slow the progression of the HIV/AIDS pandemic worldwide, and particularly in Sub-Saharan Africa, which was hardest hit.

In 2003, the Joint United Nations Programme on HIV/AIDS (UNAIDS) launched the "3 by 5" initiative, which aimed to treat 3 million people living with HIV by the year 2005 and to ensure that the distribution of this treatment among those in need would be fair[139] – a laudable but challenging task considering the complexity of treatment protocols and the need for strict compliance with medication regimens. While successful at making an impact on prevalence and mortality rates of HIV/AIDS, critics argue that vertical programming, which focuses on single diseases or health conditions, fails to address broader health challenges which require more comprehensive approaches, such as strengthening health systems and, in particular, primary health care. Indeed, while many developing countries saw an influx of clinics devoted to distributing condoms and antiretroviral medications, what happens when a child develops severe dehydration following an episode of diarrhoea or a woman has a post-partum haemorrhage and dies when simple manoeuvres by a skilled birth attendant could have prevented this? Not to worry, there are other maternal, newborn and child health (MNCH) vertical programmes to deal with those issues. But what happens when a health problem falls outside of the scope of these vertical programmes? What about a 15-year-old child labourer who has fallen down a mineshaft? Or a 12-year-old girl working in her cousin's shop who is sexually abused by customers? Or a 10-year-old boy who lives on the street, has to sift through garbage to earn a living and develops an infection from a cut on his hand? Are we going to develop a vertical programme for this too? Where does it end? De Maeseneer and colleagues contend that:

> Vertical disease-oriented programmes for HIV/AIDS, malaria, tuberculosis, and other infectious diseases foster duplication and inefficient use of resources, produce gaps in the care of patients with multiple comorbidities, and reduce government capacity by pulling the best health-care workers out of the public health sector to focus on single diseases. Moreover, vertical programmes cause inequity for patients who do not have the 'right' disease and create an internal brain-drain of health professionals.[140]

Thus vertical programmes – while effective at improving health in specific areas and even contributing to health system strengthening to a certain extent – do not get at the heart of the matter: providing universal access to comprehensive and high-quality health care across the life course, as well as tackling the underlying determinants of health which make these poor countries so vulnerable in the first place. The lack of basic infrastructure, human resources for health, and so forth, cannot be fixed by a simple programme. Much larger issues are at stake, including internal corruption among elite groups within countries, poor governance and financial mismanagement, international loan and trade policies, and the global world order more generally. Until we can find ways to address the fact that masses of people around the world continue to live in substandard conditions and suffer poor health as a consequence of their situation, it will be difficult to make real progress in improving health across the board – rather than for a single disease. While working at WHO someone once said to me "Even if the cure for AIDS was one glass of clean water, we would not be able to cure the world." Therefore there needs to be political will to change the status quo, as well as the "know-how" to be able to make a difference.

While some proponents of vertical programmes claim that horizontal approaches, such as primary health care, are ineffectual, the World Health Assembly's Resolution WHA62.12 advocates for strengthening health systems based on the primary health care approach and urges member states to ensure that any vertical programmes are "implemented in the context of integrated primary health care".[141] The data speaks for itself. Countries with widespread primary health care coverage have improved population health outcomes, even for specific diseases such as HIV/AIDS, as compared to countries which only have vertical programmes and very rudimentary and patchy primary health care systems.[142] Yet, existing health systems will not naturally gravitate towards more equitable, efficient and effective models. This will require strong leadership and accountable governance for health.

Moving towards intersectoral action and a new global health governance

While there have been many exciting developments in the area of global health in recent years, it seems nonetheless that we are still "stuck" in a highly fractioned arena dominated by a disease-based paradigm established over 50 years ago when the world was quite a different place. Indeed, we are having great difficulty breaking free from the previous model to better adapt to new challenges and work in a truly coordinated and intersectoral way. In a recent Lancet commentary, I argue that it is time to make a shift to address the underlying determinants of health in a more integrated way:

> The newly formed Global Task Force on Expanded Access to Cancer Care and Control in Developing Countries proposes to "challenge the public health community's assumption that cancers will remain untreated in poor countries." I strongly support this proactive initiative. Yet I wonder why we continue to tackle health inequities one disease at a time – first HIV, then cancer. What's next? Heart disease? Depression? Will we work our way down the list of the Global Burden of Disease? Even though many vertical programs have become more "diagonal" by incorporating an element of health system strengthening, we are still toiling within the same paradigm as before. To make real progress on global health inequities we must break free from the traditional biomedical model. For instance, child labour does not appear on the list of the Global Burden of Disease, yet 20% of the world's children under the age of 15 years are working, often in hazardous jobs in the informal sector, to help support their vulnerable families. This perpetuates multigenerational health inequities through a cycle of low educational attainment, low income and poor health. Strengthening primary health care and other forms of social protection is crucial, not only to combat HIV and cancer and a host of other diseases, but to impact the shared causes of health inequities. A new paradigm is therefore needed within which we can develop creative and evidence-based solutions to complex and interconnected health and social problems in a more comprehensive way.[143]

Enabling this to happen, however, would require more concerted action. From frontline health workers to high-level policy-makers, the health sector needs to lead the way in advocating for such change by reaffirming that improving health will require more than fancy new technologies and increased expenditures on health care services. Rather, intersectoral action is required at multiple levels, from local communities to the global arena.

There has been a long history of working "in silos" which is only now starting to change. For instance, until recently, the International Labour Organization (ILO) has been largely responsible for tackling the issue of child labour. Indeed, there are multiple conventions and recommendations which aim to protect children from work-related harms, including ILO Convention 138, which prohibits all children from doing hazardous work: "the minimum age for admission to any type of employment or work which by its nature or the circumstances in which it is carried out is likely to jeopardise the health, safety and morals of young persons shall not be less than 18 years".[144] While some forms of child work may be acceptable, or even beneficial, for young people, the real focus is on prioritising action to eliminate "hazardous child labour" including the "worst forms of child labour". ILO Recommendation 190 defines "hazardous work" as: (1) work which exposes children to physical, psychological or sexual abuse, (2) work underground, under water, at dangerous heights or in confined spaces, (3) work with dangerous machinery, equipment and tools or which involves the manual handling or transport of heavy loads, (4) work in an unhealthy environment which may, for example, expose children to hazardous substances, agents or processes, or to temperatures, noise levels or vibrations damaging to their health, and (5) work under particularly difficult conditions such as work for long hours or during the night, or work where the child is unreasonably confined to the premises of the employer.[145] According to ILO Convention 182, the "worst forms of child labour" include: (1) all forms of slavery (including trafficking, bonded labour and forced recruitment of children for use in armed conflict), (2) child sexual exploitation and pornography, (3) illicit activities (e.g. drug trade), and (4) "work which, by its nature or the circumstances in which it is carried out, is likely to harm the health, safety or morals of children".[146]

In the last few years, there have been signs emerging of greater intersectoral action on this issue, but still it is not enough. While the World Health Assembly (WHA) resolutions 62.12 on *Primary Health Care, Including Health System Strengthening* (2009)[147] and 60.26 on *Workers' Health: Global Plan of Action* (2007)[148] call for integrating attention to child injuries into primary health care, including injuries due to hazards at work, the scientific literature on evidence-based interventions to prevent and mitigate the harmful effects of child labour is limited,[149] with relatively few publications on the efficacy of population-level interventions, and even fewer that examine how such interventions impact population health and health equity. Even interventions which at first seem promising, such as microfinance schemes or laws that restrict child labour in the formal sector, sometimes inadvertently increase rates of child labour or shift children from factories to the streets, placing them in even greater danger.[150,151] Conditional-cash transfer programmes, where the condition of payment is that the child attends school, have also been highly regarded, although these too can lead to unintended harms if children are made to attend schools that are so degraded and dangerous that they would have been better off working alongside their parents where at least someone who cares for them is close at hand. Therefore, while some data exists, mostly unpublished or in the grey literature, it is widely recognised that interventions for tackling child labour have been vastly understudied and that there is a need for more intervention research, particularly in low- and middle-income countries.[152,153,154] Developing evidence-based interventions that reduce the prevalence and impact of child labour, particularly in its hazardous and worst forms, and that promote childhood development more generally, is crucial to protect the rights, health and well-being of children as an end in itself and also as a means to redress entrenched multigenerational health inequities in a more long-term and sustainable way. Yet, how to move forward in a more concerted way? It has been said that "given the political will to recognise the problem, children can be removed from hazardous work" although it is more easy to do so by "example than by order".[155] While grassroots action is clearly essential, there also needs to be strong leadership at the very highest levels. Indeed, for many years, there have been multiple calls for strengthening global health governance as a critical first step in addressing global health challenges, including global health inequities. According to Kelley, who describes in detail the complex landscape of global health in its current form, "governance structures for building consensus and for collectively managing public health actions are necessary because the world's inhabitants cannot create societies and economies that are largely self-contained and insulated from outside threats".[156]

A variety of models and forms of what the new global health governance arrangements might look like have been proposed by a variety of authors. The big question is whether these models, which sound nice in theory, can be implemented and made to work in practice amidst all the politics and power plays. For instance, Meier and Fox suggest that "through the development and implementation of collective health rights, states can address interconnected determinants of health within and across countries, obligating the international community to scale-up primary health care systems in the developing world and thereby reduce public health inequities through global health governance".[157] Ruger proposes that there should be "a global health constitution delineating duties and obligations of global health actors and a global institute of health and medicine for holding actors responsible".[158] Kickbusch and colleagues recommend developing a "Committee C" at the World Health Assembly to allow for greater "consensus building and multi-stakeholder decision-making within the unique convening power of the World Health Organization".[159] Gostin has long since advocated for a Framework Convention on Global Health.[160] More recently, there is also a plan to create a Commission on Global Health Governance that will not only focus on the standard global health actors, but will also include partners more broadly from a wide range of sectors to better address the upstream determinants of health:

> Governance challenges in global health have gained attention in recent years. This increased scrutiny is a welcome recognition of the fact that improving health worldwide is not merely a matter of technical intervention or resource mobilisation, but also demands credible, legitimate decision-making processes and effective, efficient, and equitable action. What merits increased attention, however, is a broader consideration of the many actors and forces outside the global health system and the ways in which they influence health.[161]

Some already question whether this new initiative will actually have any teeth since it is being supported by countries that stand to lose a great deal from such an arrangement.[162] So which is the best way forward? According to Pang and colleagues:

> Whether there should be a single global health authority to allocate responsibilities and resources is debatable. Notwithstanding the existence of the 2005 Paris Declaration, in which governments pledged harmonization and alignment of the aid they provide, some would consider the idea of such a global health governance authority an illusion. But there is no doubt that an absence of effective global health governance will exacerbate the current fragmentation of objectives and poor coordination of supported activities, as well as the narrow focus on short-term results, large transaction costs on recipients and the lack of accountability.[163]

Thus, whatever form it takes, effective global health governance is needed to improve the health of our global population and to reduce health inequities. Strengthened global health governance is also a necessary precursor for making more evidence-informed decisions that will be acceptable and applicable on a global scale.

References

1. Hochbaum G. Why people seek diagnostic X-rays. *Public Health Rep* 1956; 71: 377–80.
2. Ajzen I, Fishbein M. *Understanding Attitudes and Predicting Social Behavior.* Englewood Cliffs, NJ: Prentice-Hall, 1980.
3. Ajzen I. The theory of planned behavior. *Organ Behav Hum Decis Processes* 1991: 50: 179–211.
4. Prochaska J, DiClemente C. Stages of change in the modification of problem

behaviors. *Prog Behav Modif* 1992; 28: 183–218.

5. Nutbeam D, Harris E. *Theory in a Nutshell: A Practical Guide to Health Promotion Theories*, 2nd edn. Sydney, Australia: McGraw Hill, 2004.

6. West R. Time for a change: putting the Transtheoretical (Stages of Change) Model to rest. *Addiction* 2005; 100(8): 1036–9.

7. Bandura A. *Social Learning & Personality Development*. NJ: Holt, Rinehart & Winston Inc., 1975.

8. Task Force on Community Preventive Services; Zaza S, Briss P, Harris K (ed.). *The Guide to Community Preventive Services: What Works to Promote Health?* Oxford: Oxford University Press, 2005. Available at: http://www.thecommunityguide.org/library/book/index.html.

9. World Health Organization. *WHO Framework Convention on Tobacco Control*. Geneva: World Health Organization, 2003.

10. Doll R, Peto R, Boreham J, Sutherland I. Mortality in relation to smoking: 50 years' observations on male British doctors. *BMJ* 2004; 328(7455): 1519.

11. Khaw K, Wareham N, Bingham S *et al.* Combined impact of health behaviours and mortality in men and women: the EPIC-Norfolk prospective population study. *PLoS Med* 2008; 5(1): e12.

12. Bury M. *Health and Illness in a Changing Society*. London: Routledge, 1997.

13. Hope T. *Evidence-Based Patient Choice*. London: King's Fund Publishing, 1996.

14. Benbassat J, Pilpel D, Tidhar M. Patients' preferences for participation in clinical decision making: a review of published surveys. *Behav Med* 1998; 24(2): 81–8.

15. Coulter A. Partnership with patients: the pros and cons of shared clinical decision-making. *J Health Serv Res Policy* 1997; 2(2): 112–21.

16. Coulter A. Evidence based patient information is important, so there needs to be a national strategy to ensure it. *BMJ* 1998; 317: 225–6.

17. Peugh J, Belenko S. Alcohol, drugs and sexual function: a review. *J Psychoactive Drugs* 2001; 33(3): 223–32.

18. Evans D, Blair V, Greenhalgh R, Hopwood P, Howell A. The impact of genetic counselling on risk perception in women with a family history of breast cancer. *Br J Cancer* 1994; 70: 934–8.

19. Janis I, Feshbach S. Effects of fear-arousing communications. *J Abnorm Soc Psychol* 1953; 48: 78–92.

20. Andersen M, Smith R, Meischke H, Bowen D, Urban N. Breast cancer worry and mammography use by women with and without a family history in a population-based Sample. *Cancer Epidemiol Biomarkers Prev* 2003; 12: 314–20.

21. Howe H. Social factors associated with breast self-examination among high risk women. *Am J Public Health* 1981; 71: 251–5.

22. Walsh-Childers K, Edwards H, Grobmyer S. Covering women's greatest health fear: breast cancer information in consumer magazines. *Health Commun* 2011; 26(3): 209–20.

23. Calman K, Royston G. Risk language and dialects. *BMJ* 1997; 315: 939–42.

24. Bennett P, Calman K, Curtis S, Fischbacher-Smith D (eds.). *Risk Communication and Public Health*, 2nd edn. Oxford: Oxford University Press, 2010.

25. Tennant D. The communication of risks and the risks of communication. *Risk Dec Pol* 1997; 2(2): 147–53.

26. Hyer R, Covello V. *Effective Media Communication during Public Health Emergencies: A WHO Field Guide*. Geneva: World Health Organization, 2005. Available at: http://www.who.int/csr/resources/publications/WHO%20MEDIA%20FIELD%20GUIDE.pdf.

27. Antoniou A, Pharoah P, Narod S, *et al.* Average risks of breast and ovarian cancer associated with BRCA1 or BRCA2 mutations detected in case series unselected for family history: a combined analysis of 222 studies. *Am J Hum Genet* 2003; 72: 1117–30.

28. Tversky A, Kahneman D. The framing of decisions and the psychology of choice. *Science* 1981; 211: 453–8.

29. Newman T. The power of stories over statistics. *BMJ* 2003; 327: 1424–7.

30. Entwistle V, Sheldon T, Sowden A, Watt I. Supporting consumer involvement in decision-making: what constitutes quality in consumer health information? *Int J Qual Health Care* 1996; 8: 425–37.

31. Elmore J, Barton M, Moceri V, *et al.* Ten year risk of false positive screening mammograms and clinical breast examinations. *N Engl J Med* 1998; 338(16): 1089–96.

32. O'Connor A, Rostom A, Fiset V, *et al.* Decision aids for patients facing health treatment or screening decisions: systematic review. *BMJ* 1999; 319: 731–4.

33. Elwyn G, O'Connor A, Stacey D, *et al.* on behalf of the International Patient Decision Aids Standards (IPDAS) Collaboration. Developing a quality criteria framework for patient decision aids: online international Delphi consensus process. *BMJ*. 2006; 333 (7565): 417.

34. Ubel P, Loewenstein G. The role of decision analysis in informed consent: choosing between intuition and systematicity. *Soc Sci Med* 1997; 44(5): 647–56.

35. Maly R, Bourque L, Engelhardt R. A randomized controlled trial of facilitating information giving to patients with chronic medical conditions: effects on outcomes of care. *J Fam Pract* 1999; 48(5): 356–63.

36. Kirmayer L, Minas H. The future of cultural psychiatry: an international perspective. *Can J Psychiatry* 2000; 45: 438–46.

37. American Academy of Nursing Expert Panel on Culturally Competent Nursing Care. Culturally competent health care. *Nurs Outlook* 1992; 40(6): 277–83.

38. Callister C. What Has the literature taught us about culturally competent care of women and children. *MCN Am J Matern Child Nurs* 2005; 30(6): 380–8.

39. Lie D, Lee-Rey E, Gomez A, Bereknyei S, Braddock C. Does cultural competency training of health professionals improve patient outcomes? A systematic review and proposed algorithm for future research. *J Gen Intern Med* 2011; 26(3): 317–25.

40. Willis W. Culturally competent nursing care during the perinatal period. *J Perinat Neonatal Nurs* 1999; 23(3): 45–59.

41. Teka T, Dagnew M. Health behaviour of rural mothers to acute respiratory infections in children in Gondar, Ethiopia. *East Afr Med J* 1995; 72(10): 623–5.

42. Hodes R. Cross-cultural medicine and diverse health beliefs: Ethiopians abroad. *West J Med* 1997; 166(1): 29–36.

43. Lock M. On being ethnic: the politics of identity breaking and making in Canada, or, nevra on Sunday. *Cult Med Psychiatry* 1990; 14(2): 237–54.

44. Fadiman A. *The Spirit Catches You and You Fall Down: A Hmong Child, Her American Doctors, and the Collision of Two Cultures.* New York: Farrar, Strauss and Giroux, 1997.

45. Diekema D and the Committee on Bioethics of the American Academy of Pediatrics. Responding to parental refusals of immunization of children. *Pediatrics* 2005; 115(5): 1428–31.

46. Bentley M, Elder J, Fukumoto M *et al.* Acute childhood diarrhoea and maternal time allocation in the northern central Sierra of Peru. *Health Policy Plan* 1995; 10(1): 60–70.

47. Andermann A, Blancquaert I. Genetic screening: a primer for primary care. *Can Fam Physician* 2010; 56(4): 333–9.

48. Andermann A, Blancquaert I, Déry V. Genetic screening: a conceptual framework for programs and policy-making. *J Health Serv Res Policy* 2010; 15(2): 90–7.

49. Diamond, Commissioner of Patents and Trademarks, v. Chakrabarty 447 U.S. 303 100 S. Ct. 2204 65 L. Ed. 2d 144, 1980.

50. Benowitz S. French challenge to BRCA1 patent underlies European discontent. *J Natl Cancer Inst* 2002; 94(2): 80–1.

51. Brice P. Latest twist in gene patent saga as BRCA patent revoked. *PHGfoundation: making science work for health*, March 30, 2010. Available at: http://www.phgfoundation.org/news/5324/.

52. Knoppers B, Hirtle M, Glass K. Commercialization of genetic research and public policy. *Science* 1999; 286(5448): 2277–8.

53. Lippman A. Prenatal genetic testing and screening: constructing needs and reinforcing inequities. *Am J Law Med* 1991; 17(1–2): 15–50.

54. Andermann A, Blancquaert I, Beauchamp S, Costea I. Guiding policy decisions for genetic screening: developing a systematic and transparent approach. *Public Health Genomics* 2011; 14 (1): 9–16.

55. Stewart-Brown S and Farmer A. Screening could seriously damage your health: Decisions to screen must take account of the social and psychological costs. *BMJ* 1997; 314(7080): 533–4.

56. Austoker J. Gaining informed consent for screening is difficult – but many misconceptions need to be undone. *BMJ* 1999; 319(7212): 722–3.

57. Woloshin S, Schwartz L. Numbers needed to decide. *J Natl Cancer Inst* 2009; 101 (17): 1163–5.

58. Langbehn D, Brinkman R, Falush D, Paulsen J, Hayden M. A new model for prediction of the age of onset and penetrance for Huntington's disease based on CAG length. *Clin Genet* 2004; 65: 267–77.

59. Lawson K, Wiggins S, Green T *et al.* Adverse psychological events occurring in the first year after predictive testing for Huntington's disease. The Canadian Collaborative Study Predictive Testing. *J Med Genet* 1996; 33(10): 856–62.

60. Hubbard R, Wald E. *Exploding the Gene Myth: How Genetic Information is Produced and Manipulated by Scientists, Physicians, Employers, Insurance Companies, Educators and Law Enforcers*. Boston: Beacon Press, 1993.

61. Holtzman N. *Proceed with Caution: Predicting Genetic Risks in the Recombinant DNA Era*. Baltimore: John Hopkins University Press, 1989.

62. World Health Organization. *Genomics and World Health: Report of the Advisory Committee on Health Research*. Geneva: World Health Organization, 2002.

63. Banta H. Considerations in defining evidence for public health. *Int J Technol Assess Health Care* 2003; 19(3): 559–72.

64. Dobrow M, Goel V, Lemieux-Charles L, Black N. The impact of context on evidence utilization: a framework for expert groups developing health policy recommendations. *Soc Sci Med* 2006; 63(7): 1811–24.

65. Morestin F, Gauvin F-P, Hogue M-C, Benoit F. *Method for Synthesizing Knowledge about Public Policies*. Quebec: National Collaborating Centre for Healthy Public Policy, Institut national de santé publique du Québec (INSPQ), 2011. Available at: http://www.ncchpp.ca/docs/MethodPP_EN.pdf.

66. Pawson R, Greenhalgh T, Harvey G, Walshe K. Realist review – a new method of systematic review designed for complex policy interventions. *J Health Serv Res Policy* 2005; 10(Suppl 1): 21–34.

67. Wilson J, Jungner G. *Principles and Practice of Screening for Disease*. Geneva: World Health Organization, 1968. Available at: http://whqlibdoc.who.int/php/WHO_PHP_34.pdf.

68. Nuffield Council on Bioethics. *Public Health: Ethical Issues*. London: Nuffield Council on Bioethics, 2007.

69. Gail M, Brinton L, Byar D *et al.* Projecting individualized probabilities of developing breast cancer for white females who are being examined annually. *J Natl Cancer Inst* 1989; 81(24): 1879–86.

70. Lander E, Linton L, Birren B *et al.*. Initial sequencing and analysis of the human genome. *Nature* 2001; 409(6822): 860–921.

71. Bell J. Predicting disease using genomics. *Nature* 2004; 429(6990): 453–6.

72. Collins F. Shattuck lecture – medical and societal consequences of the Human Genome Project. *N Engl J Med* 1999; 341(1): 28–37.

73. Task Force on Community Preventive Services; Zaza S, Briss P, Harris K (ed.). *The Guide to Community Preventive Services: What Works to Promote Health*? Oxford: Oxford University Press, 2005. Available at: http://www.thecommunityguide.org/library/book/index.html.

74. Carlsten C, Halperin A, Crouch J, Burke W. Personalized medicine and tobacco-related health disparities: is there a role for genetics? *Ann Fam Med* 2011; 9(4): 366–71.

75. Collier R. Predisposed to risk but not change. *CMAJ* 2012; 184: E407–8.

76. Wade N. A Decade Later, Genetic Map Yields Few New Cures. *The New York Times*. June 12, 2010. Available at: http://www.nytimes.com/2010/06/13/health/research/13genome.html.

77. World Health Organization. *Report of a WHO Meeting on Collaboration in Medical Genetics*. Geneva: World Health Organization, 2002.

78. Organisation for Economic Co-operation and Development. *The Paris Declaration on Aid Effectiveness*. Paris: Organisation for Economic Co-operation and Development.

Available at: http://www.oecd.org/
dataoecd/11/41/34428351.pdf.

79. European Commission on Public Health.
    What are Rare Diseases? Brussels, Belgium:
    European Commission on Public Health,
    2006.

80. MacDonald N. Aboriginal children suffer
    while governments ignore Jordan's
    Principle *CMAJ* 2012; 184: 853.

81. Gray J. Evidence based policy making. *BMJ*
    2004; 329(7473): 988–9.

82. Makni H, St-Hilaire C, Robb L, Larouche K,
    Blancquaert I. *La spectrométrie de mass en
    tandem et le dépistage néonatale sanguine au
    Québec: rapport sommaire.* Montréal:
    Agence d'évaluation des technologies et des
    modes d'intervention en santé, 2007.

83. Andermann A, Beauchamp S, Costea I,
    Blancquaert I. *Guiding Decision-Making for
    Population Based Screening: An Approach
    Applicable to Genetics* [unpublished report].
    Montreal: Agence d'évaluation des
    technologies et des modes d'intervention en
    santé (AETMIS), 2007.

84. Douste-Blazy P, Monchamp MA, d'Aubert
    F. *French National Plan for Rare Diseases
    2005–2008: Ensuring Equity in Access to
    Diagnosis, Treatment and Provision of Care.*
    Paris, France: Ministère de la santé et de la
    protection sociale and Secrétariat d'État aux
    personnes handicapées, 2004.

85. Nuffield Council on Bioethics. *Genetic
    Screening: A Supplement to the 1993 Report
    by the Nuffield Council on Bioethics.* London,
    UK: Nuffield Council on Bioethics, 2006.

86. Wilson J, Jungner G. *Principles and Practice
    of Screening for Disease.* Geneva: World
    Health Organization, 1968. Available at:
    http://whqlibdoc.who.int/php/
    WHO_PHP_34.pdf.

87. Andermann A, Blancquaert I, Beauchamp S,
    Déry V. Revisiting Wilson and Jungner in the
    genomic age: A review of screening criteria
    over the past 40 years. *Bull World Health
    Organ* 2008; 86(4): 1–3.

88. Daniels N, Kennedy B, Kawachi I. Justice,
    health and health policy. In: Danis M,
    Clancy C, Churchill L (eds.). *Ethical
    Dimensions of Health Policy.* Oxford:
    Oxford University Press, 2002,
    pp. 19–50.

89. Grosse S, Boyle C, Botkin J *et al.* Newborn
    screening for cystic fibrosis: evaluation of

benefits and risks and recommendations for
state newborn screening programs. *MMWR
Recomm Rep* 2004; 53(RR13): 1–36.

90. Pollitt R. International perspectives on
    newborn screening. *J Inherit Metab Dis*
    2006; 29(2–3): 390–6.

91. Kingdon J. *Agendas, Alternatives and Public
    Policies*, 2nd edn. New York, NY: Longman
    Press, 2003.

92. Stone D. *Policy Paradox: The Art of Political
    Decision Making.* New York, NY: WW
    Norton & Company, 2002.

93. Manciaux M, Fliedner T. World health: a
    mobilizing utopia? In: Gunn S, Mansourian P,
    Davies A, Piel A, Sayers B, (eds.).
    *Understanding the Global Dimensions of
    Health.* New York, NY: Springer, 2005,
    pp. 69–82.

94. International Labour Organization.
    Accelerating Action against Child Labour.
    Geneva: International Labour Organization,
    2010. Available at: http://www.ilo.org/
    wcmsp5/groups/public/—dgreports/—
    dcomm/documents/publication/
    wcms_126752.pdf.

95. Roggero P, Mangiaterra V, Bustreo F,
    Rosati F. The health impact of child labor in
    developing countries: evidence from cross-
    country data. *Am J Public Health* 2007; 97
    (2): 271–5.

96. Dantas R, Santana V. Child and adolescent
    labor, socioeconomic status, and reduced
    adult height. *Int J Occup Environ Health*
    2010; 16(2): 153–9.

97. Asogwa S. Sociomedical aspects of child
    labor in Nigeria. *J Occup Med* 1986;
    28(1): 46–8.

98. Mathews R, Reis C, Iacopino V. Child
    labor. A matter of health and human
    rights. *J Ambul Care Manage* 2003; 26(2):
    181–2.

99. Esin M, Bulduk S, Ince H. Workrelated risks
    and health problems of working children in
    urban Istanbul, Turkey. *J Occup Health*
    2005; 47(5): 431–6.

100. Noweir M, Osman H, Abbas F, Abou-Taleb
     A, Mansour T. Child labour in Egypt. II.
     Impact of work environment on health.
     J Egypt Public Health Assoc 1993; 68(3-4):
     443–67.

101. Mull L, Kirkhorn S. Child labor in Ghana
     cocoa production: focus upon agricultural
     tasks, ergonomic exposures, and associated

injuries and illnesses. *Public Health Rep* 2005; 120(6): 649–55.

102. Awan S, Nasrullah M, Cummings K. Health hazards, injury problems, and workplace conditions of carpet-weaving children in three districts of Punjab, Pakistan. *Int J Occup Environ Health* 2010; 16(2): 115–21.

103. Mallik S, Chaudhuri R, Biswas R, Biswas B. A study on morbidity pattern of child labourers engaged in different occupations in a slum area of Calcutta. *J Indian Med Assoc* 2004; 102(4): 198–200.

104. Pinzon-Rondon A, Koblinsky S, Hofferth S, Pinzon-Florez C, Briceno L. Work-related injuries among child street-laborers in Latin America: prevalence and predictors. *Rev Panam Salud Publica* 2009; 26(3): 235–43.

105. Saddik B, Williamson A, Nuwayhid I, Black D. The effects of solvent exposure on memory and motor dexterity in working children. *Public Health Rep* 2005; 120(6): 657–63.

106. Feingold E, Wasser J. Walk-through surveys for child labor. *Am J Ind Med* 1994; 26(6): 803–7.

107. Fineran S, Gruber J. Youth at work: adolescent employment and sexual harassment. *Child Abuse Negl* 2009; 33(8): 550–9.

108. Doocy S, Crawford B, Boudreaux C, Wall E. The risks and impacts of portering on the well-being of children in Nepal. *J Trop Pediatr* 2007; 53(3): 165–70.

109. Audu B, Geidam A, Jarma H. Child labor and sexual assault among girls in Maiduguri, Nigeria. *Int J Gynaecol Obstet* 2009; 104(1): 64–7.

110. Fekadu D, Alem A, Hagglof B. The prevalence of mental health problems in Ethiopian child laborers. *J Child Psychol Psychiatry* 2006; 47(9): 954–9.

111. Largie S, Field T, Hernandez-Reif M, Sanders C, Diego M. Employment during adolescence is associated with depression, inferior relationships, lower grades, and smoking. *Adolescence* 2001; 36(142): 395–401.

112. Chen C, Chen W, Lew-Ting C *et al.* Employment experience in relation to alcohol, tobacco, and betel nut use among youth in Taiwan. *Drug Alcohol Depend* 2006; 84(3): 273–80.

113. Tandon S, Marshall B, Templeman A, Sonestein F. Health access and status of adolescents and young adults using youth employment and training programs in an urban environment. *J Adolesc Health* 2008; 43(1): 30–7.

114. Santana V, Cooper S, Roberts R, Araujo-Filho J. Adolescent students who work: gender differences in school performance and self-perceived health. *Int J Occup Environ Health* 2005; 11: 294–301.

115. Kassouf A, McKee M, Mossialos E. Early entrance to the job market and its effect on adult health: evidence from Brazil. *Health Policy Plan.* 2001; 16: 21–8.

116. Leinberger-Jabari A, Parker D, Oberg C. Child labor, gender and health. *Public Health Rep* 2005; 120: 642–7.

117. Mintz A, DeRouen Jr. K. *Understanding Foreign Policy Decision Making.* Cambridge: Cambridge University Press, 2010.

118. Walt G. *Health Policy: An Introduction to Process and Power.* London: Zed Books, 1994.

119. Pogge T. Relational conceptions of justice: Responsibilities for health outcomes. In: Anand S, Peter F, Sen A, (eds.). *Public Health, Ethics and Equity.* Oxford: Oxford University Press, 2004. pp. 135–62.

120. Manderson L, Whiteford L. Health, globalization and the fallacy of the level playing field. In: Whiteford L, Manderson L (eds.). *Global Health Policy, Local Realities: The Fallacy of the Level Playing Field.* Boulder, CO: Lynne Rienner Publishers, 2000, pp. 1–19.

121. Woods N. Order, globalization and inequality in world politics. In: Hurrell A, Woods N eds. *Inequality, Globalization and World Politics.* Oxford: Oxford University Press, 1999, pp. 8–35.

122. Palmer A, Tomkinson J, Phung C, *et al.* Does ratification of human-rights treaties have effects on population health? *Lancet* 2009; 373(9679): 1987–92.

123. Commission on Human Rights. *The Right of Everyone to the Enjoyment of the Highest attainable standard of physical and mental health* [Resolution 2002/31: E/2002/23-E/CN.4/2002/200]. Geneva: Commission on Human Rights, 2002.

124. Sandler T. *Global Collective Action.* Cambridge: Cambridge University Press, 2004.

125. Woods N. Whose aid? Whose influence? China, emerging donors and the silent revolution in development assistance. *Int Aff* 2008; 84(6): 1205–21.

126. Whiteford L, Rylko-Bauer B, Farmer P. Global Health in times of violence: finding hope. In: Rylko-Bauer B, Whiteford L, Farmer P, (eds.). *Global Health in Times of Violence*. Santa Fe: School for Advanced Research Press, 2009, pp. 223–32.

127. Farmer P. *Pathologies of Power: Health, Human Rights and the New War on the Poor*. Berkley, CA: University of California Press, 2005.

128. Sutherland T. Lewis Hine: The Child Labour Photos That Shamed America. *BBC News* April 11, 2012. Available at: http://www.bbc.co.uk/news/magazine-17673213.

129. Parker D. *Before their Time: The World of Child Labour*. New York: Quantuck Lane Press, 2007. Available at: http://www.childlaborphotographs.com/.

130. Lee K, Buse K, Fustukian S (eds.). *Health Policy in a Globalising World*. Cambridge: Cambridge University Press, 2002.

131. Beck U. *Power in the Global Age*. Cambridge: Polity Press, 2005.

132. Jacobsen K. *Introduction to Global Public Health*. Sudbury MA: Jones and Bartlett Publishers, 2008.

133. McNeill Jr. D. Five Years In, Gauging Impact of Gates Grants. *The New York Times* December 20, 2010. Available at: http://www.nytimes.com/2010/12/21/health/21gates.html?pagewanted=all.

134. Bowman A. The flip side to Bill Gates' charity billions. *New Internationalist Magazine*. April 1, 2012. Available at: http://www.newint.org/features/2012/04/01/bill-gates-charitable-giving-ethics/.

135. Kane M. Preventing cancer with vaccines: progress in the global control of cancer. *Cancer Prev Res* 2012; 5(1): 24–9.

136. Welsh J, Woods N (eds.) *Exporting Good Governance: Temptations and Challenges in Canada's Aid Program*. Waterloo, ON: The Centre for International Governance Innovation and Wilfrid Laurier University Press, 2007.

137. World Bank. *World Development Indicators Online*. Washington, DC: World Bank, 2008.

138. UN General Assembly. *United Nations Millennium Declaration: Resolution Adopted by the General Assembly (A/55/L.2)*. New York: United Nations, 2000. Available at: http://www.un.org/millennium/.

139. Macklin R. *Ethics and Equity in Access to HIV Treatment – 3 by 5 initiative*. Geneva: World Health Organization, 2004. Available at: http://www.who.int/ethics/en/background-macklin.pdf.

140. De Maeseneer J, Roberts R, Demarzo M et al. Tackling NCDs: a different approach is needed. *Lancet* 2012; 379(9829): 1860–1.

141. Sixty-Second World Health Assembly. Resolution WHA62.12: Primary health care, including health system strengthening. Geneva: World Health Organization, 2009. Available at: http://www.who.int/hrh/resources/A62_12_EN.pdf.

142. Van Lerberghe W, Evans T, Rasanathan K et al. World Health Report 2008. *Primary Health Care: Now More than Ever*. Geneva: World Health Organization, 2008. Available at: http://www.who.int/whr/2008/en/index.html.

143. Andermann A. Breaking away from the disease-focused paradigm. *Lancet* 2010; 376(9758): 2073–4.

144. International Labour Organization. *Minimum Age Convention (C138): Convention Concerning Minimum Age for Admission to Employment (Entry into Force: 19 Jun 1976)*. Geneva: International Labour Organization, 1973. Available at: http://www.ilo.org/ipec/Action/Time-BoundProgrammes/Legal/Conventions/lang–en/index.htm.

145. International Labour Organization. *Worst Forms of Child Labour Recommendation (R190): Recommendation Concerning the Prohibition and Immediate Action for the Elimination of the Worst Forms of Child Labour*. Geneva: International Labour Organization, 1999. Available at: http://www.ilo.org/ipec/Action/Time-BoundProgrammes/Legal/Conventions/lang–en/index.htm.

146. International Labour Organization. *Worst Forms of Child Labour Convention (C182): Convention Concerning the Prohibition and Immediate Action for the Elimination of the Worst Forms of Child Labour (Entry into*

Force: 19 Nov 2000). Geneva: International Labour Organization, 1999. Available at: http://www.ilo.org/ipec/Action/Time-BoundProgrammes/Legal/Conventions/lang–en/index.htm.

147. Sixty-Second World Health Assembly. *Resolution WHA62.12, May 2009. Primary Health Care, Including Health System Strengthening*. Geneva: World Health Organization. Available at: http://apps.who.int/gb/ebwha/pdf_files/A62/A62_8-en.pdf.

148. Sixtieth World Health Assembly. *Resolution WHA60.26, May 2007. Workers' Health: Global Plan of Action*. Geneva: World Health Organization. Available at: http://apps.who.int/gb/ebwha/pdf_files/WHA60/A60_R26-en.pdf.

149. Hesketh T, Gamlin J, Woodhead M. Policy in child labour. *Arch Dis Child* 2006; 91(9): 721–3.

150. Carothers R, Breslin C, Denomy J, Foad M. Promoting occupational safety and health for working children through microfinance programming. *Int J Occup Environ Health* 2010; 16(2): 180–90.

151. Parker D. Street children and child labour around the world. *Lancet* 2002; 360(9350): 2067–71.

152. Horton R. The continuing invisibility of women and children. *Lancet* 2010; 375: 1942–3.

153. Scanlon T, Prior V, Lamarao M, Lynch M, Scanlon F. Child labour. *BMJ* 2002; 325(7361): 401–3.

154. National Institute for Occupational Safety and Health. *Child Labour Research Needs: Recommendations from the NIOSH Child Labor Working Team* (NIOSH Publication No. 97-143). Atlanta: US Centers for Disease Control and Prevention, 1997.

155. Gunn S, Ostos Z. Dilemmas in tackling child labour: the case of scavenger children in the Philippines. *Int Labour Rev* 1992; 131(6): 629–46.

156. Kelley P. Global health: governance and policy development. *Infect Dis Clin North Am* 2011; 25(2): 435–53.

157. Meier B, Fox A. International obligations through collective rights: moving from foreign health assistance to global health governance. *Health Hum Rights* 2010; 12(1): 61–72.

158. Ruger J. Global health governance as shared health governance. *J Epidemiol Community Health* 2012; 66(7): 653–61.

159. Kickbusch I, Hein W, Silberschmidt G. Addressing global health governance challenges through a new mechanism: the proposal for a Committee C of the World Health Assembly. *J Law Med Ethics* 2010; 38(3): 550–63.

160. Gostin L. Meeting the survival needs of the world's least healthy people: a proposed model for global health governance. *JAMA* 2007; 298(2): 225–8.

161. Ottersen O, Frenk J, Horton R. The Lancet-University of Oslo Commission on Global Governance for Health, in collaboration with the Harvard Global Health Institute. *Lancet* 2011; 378(9803): 1612–3.

162. Braillon A. Who will fear the Commission on Global Governance for Health? *Lancet* 2012; 379(9818): 803–4.

163. Pang T, Daulaire N, Keusch G, *et al.* The new age of global health governance holds promise. *Nat Med* 2010; 16(11): 1181.

Producing evidence to inform health decisions

4

Since the purpose of this book is to help people make better-informed decisions about improving health and reducing health inequities, an important question is what counts as evidence in supporting these decisions? Often, if a person has a health problem, they might ask a family member or a friend for advice. If they are sufficiently concerned that this health problem could be serious, they may make an appointment to go see their family doctor or a local lay health worker and ask them what to do. In this technological age, many people learn about health issues from the media or go on the Internet and use Google to find guidance. In government, high-level officials – who may not have any health training even though they are responsible for important decisions that affect the health of thousands or even millions of people – often turn to their scientific and technical advisors for assistance. Friends, family, newspapers, television, blogs and so on, are all sources of health information. But, will this information lead to better-informed decisions? Doctors and technical advisors may have greater knowledge about what makes individuals and populations healthy, but what evidence do they use as a basis when they provide advice? When a friend recommends chicken soup for a cold because that is what he learned from his grandmother, does this count as evidence? What if the friend says that the chicken soup helped someone else to feel better when they had a cold – now is this evidence? What if the friend says that they read in the newspaper that a randomised controlled trial of chicken soup versus placebo reduced the average length of a cold from seven to five days – now is this evidence? What about when it comes to social policies – what would be the optimal length of parental leave to promote health? Is 3 months enough? What about 12 months? How could one investigate this? The purpose of this chapter is to explore further what counts as evidence, how evidence is produced and how it can be used to make better-informed decisions to improve health.

What counts as evidence?

According to the *Oxford English Dictionary*, evidence is "the available body of facts or information indicating whether a belief or proposition is true or valid".[1] Evidence is used in many different contexts. In a court of law, evidence can help to build up a case in an attempt to prove whether a person is innocent or guilty of having committed a crime. Similarly, in the health field, evidence is used to build up the knowledge base about the distribution and extent of a given health problem (often called the epidemiology of the disease), the various causes of the health problem, and what works to prevent or reduce the burden related to the health problem. However, unlike in the court of law, the type of evidence used is very different. There are no photographs of fingerprints, testimonials by eyewitnesses or handguns sealed in numbered plastic bags. Instead, much of the evidence is based on various types of research and clinical observation.

Indeed, for many centuries, determining the causes of disease and whether different treatments were effective was generally conducted in an empirical way – through trial and error. While there were standard medical texts by authors such as Galen and Avicenna that students studied, physicians largely learned through experience what worked well and what didn't work, and passed on their knowledge through apprenticeship. On the whole, their success rate in terms of improving health outcomes was not too impressive, with some notable exceptions, such as the treatment of scurvy with plants and fruits containing high levels of vitamin C. Indeed, long before Dr. James Lind of the British Royal Navy recommended the "citrus cure" for scurvy in the mid eighteenth century,[2] the French explorer Jacques Cartier published an account of his second voyage to what is now Canada, where he describes how most of his crew suffered from scurvy during the particularly harsh winter of 1535. While many died, Cartier explained how those who survived had used local indigenous knowledge to brew teas from the bark of the white spruce tree, which proved highly effective in warding off the disease.[3] However, pre-globalisation, with limited means of incorporating new information into the corpus of medical knowledge, many advances were lost over time and some later rediscovered. That being said, in hindsight, not all of the advances were worthy of being included as they may well have done more harm than good. For instance, Dr. Lind also recommended fumigating the sailors' quarters below deck with sulfur and arsenic – now known to be highly toxic poisons.[4] Nonetheless, even in 1762, the quest was to identify "the most effectual means of preserving health" – a quest which continues to this day. But how can we know if a proposed treatment or intervention is really beneficial or whether it is harmful? Where does the truth lie? What are the different methods that we can use to determine what is true and what is not? Which of these methods is more reliable than the others?

Different approaches to uncovering the truth

To better understand why certain methods used for uncovering the truth and acquiring knowledge (e.g. a randomised controlled trial) are considered in many scientific and medical circles to be more reliable and effective than other methods (e.g. personal experience), it is helpful to look back in history to examine how knowledge is created in different periods and what is considered to be the truth.

Since biblical times, for many, the truth is taken to be the word of God, which has been handed down through holy writings such as the Bible and the Koran. That being said, how to interpret the word of God has been the subject of a great deal of debate across the centuries. For instance, devout Creationists fiercely oppose Darwinian evolutionists with regard to the origins of humankind.[5] Indeed, Darwin himself almost became a priest earlier in his career and was married to a very pious woman. He therefore waited decades before publishing *On the Origin of Species by Means of Natural Selection* out of concern for how this would be received and the potential social unrest that could be provoked by his new theory.[6] Darwin was not the first to face opposition from religious leaders in relation to theories of the world that are not coherent with the teachings of the holy books. Already in the early seventeenth century, Galileo was persecuted as a heretic – even Socrates was put on trial and condemned to death in 399 BC for corrupting the minds of youth and for impiety. Interestingly, many ancient and medieval philosophers did not hold God as being in opposition to reason, but, rather, conceived God as pure intellect (*Nous*). By using reason to understand the world around them, they claimed to be coming closer to God.[7] Although, many of their theories – such as Aristotle's cosmology and Ptolemy's geocentric worldview – were later overturned from the early modern period onwards, one can hardly accuse ancient and medieval philosophers of not being concerned with reason and knowledge.

Indeed, one of Plato's dialogues, *Theaetetus*,[8] is among the earliest writings in epistemology, the philosophical discipline that investigates the nature of knowledge and how one arrives at the truth (i.e. through perception, through inferences, etc.). At its core, epistemology attempts to distinguish between "justified belief and opinion".[9] So how is it that such learned men, so preoccupied with reason and knowledge, who were even engaged in scientific experimentation,[10] developed theories that were widely accepted as true for almost two millennia, and yet these theories were still able to be overturned? Part of the answer is simply that new evidence showed a competing theory to be superior – i.e. a better explanation of the phenomena – and therefore is considered closer to the truth.

Starting in the seventeenth century, the scientific method, which consists of "systematic observation, measurement, and experiment, and the formulation, testing, and modification of hypotheses",[11] was increasingly used as a means of ascertaining knowledge. Many scholars, from Copernicus to Newton, were involved in making the systematic astronomical observations and mathematical calculations that built up the body of evidence in support of a heliocentric model (i.e. that the planets revolve around the sun) that eventually overturned the deeply entrenched geocentric model (i.e. that the earth is the centre of the universe and that all other objects revolve around it). Although the process of refuting the geocentric theory took over 200 years,[12] the scientific method nonetheless gained in popularity during this time. Many believed that because this approach was so effective at uncovering the laws governing the physical world (e.g. Newton's laws of motion),[13] the scientific method should form the basis for unveiling the truth in all areas of human inquiry – "from the man of business to the bookworm"[14] (i.e. from industry to academia).

In the mid nineteenth century, John Stuart Mill published *A System of Logic: Ratiocinative and Inductive being a Connected View of the Principles of Evidence and the Methods of Scientific Investigation*, which attempted to coherently describe "the modes of investigating truth and estimating evidence, by which so many important and recondite laws of nature have, in the various sciences, been aggregated to the stock of human knowledge".[15] In essence, by describing the scientific method, Mill wanted to better understand the steps used in the sciences for determining what is true. In so doing, he was hoping to "rescue from empiricism" the study of mankind and explore "how far the methods, by which so many of the laws of the physical world have been numbered among truths irrevocably acquired and universally assented to, can be made instrumental to the gradual formation of a similar body of received doctrine in moral and political science". Mill claimed that, at first, people making these scientific discoveries (e.g. Newton) did not realise that they were following the "scientific method" – it was just a logical way of working through a problem and arriving at the truth. However, by analysing how these scientists came to the truth, Mill's intention was to use the same methods to better understand how to tackle even more complex moral and political problems. His hope was that, one day, the decisions governing society (e.g. the laws and policies enacted by government) would also derive from a solid evidence base, rather than popular opinion:

> Principles of evidence and theories of method are not to be constructed *a priori*. The laws of our rational faculty, like those of every other natural agency, are only learnt by seeing the agent at work. The earlier achievements of science were made without the conscious

observance of any scientific method; and we should never have known by what process truth is to be ascertained, if we had not previously ascertained many truths. But it was only the easier problems which could be thus resolved: natural sagacity, when it tried its strength against the more difficult ones, either failed altogether, or it succeeded here and there in obtaining a solution, had no sure means of convincing others that its solution was correct. In scientific investigation, as in all other works of human skill, the way of attaining the end is seen as it were instinctively by superior minds in some comparatively simple case, and is then, by judicious generalization, adapted to the variety of complex cases. We learn to do a thing in difficult circumstances, by attending to the manner in which we have spontaneously done the same thing in easy ones. This truth is exemplified by the history of the various branches of knowledge which have successively, in the ascending order of their complication, assumed the character of sciences; and will doubtless receive fresh confirmation from those, of which the final scientific constitution is yet to come, and which are still abandoned to the uncertainties of vague and popular discussion.

However, even if the scientific method can be used as a reliable means of building up the evidence in support of a certain hypothesis or theory, not everyone views this approach as enthusiastically as Mill.

Scientific facts are socially constructed

Scientists today (myself included) are often criticised by certain people in the humanities as being "positivists" and "reductionists" who naively believe that "all things are measurable" and that the use of the scientific method leads to "an objective progression toward the truth". Bruno Latour, a prominent French sociologist, is one of many who argue that scientific facts are socially constructed and therefore cannot be wholly objective.[16] Even the choice of what to study and what research gets funded is socially determined. Indeed, historians and philosophers of science have long been interested in better understanding how it is that a set of facts become generally recognised as the truth.

Ludwig Fleck, a Polish doctor and scientist, was interested in epistemology as it pertains to the medical sciences. He therefore examined the process by which a fact emerges as the truth using the discovery of the Wassermann reaction for the diagnosis of syphilis as a case study. Fleck contends that discoveries are not made by individuals in isolation, but, rather, people work within a certain context or field which he coined the "thought collective" (Denkkollektiv).[17] Making a discovery or unveiling a scientific fact requires a change in the way of thinking which is initially greeted with resistance by the thought collective. Indeed, at the centre of the thought collective, there is often a heated debate among the experts and a great deal of uncertainty over the facts. This is quite understandable since those who are involved in conducting the research are aware of all the minutiae in terms of what elements fit and what elements do not fit with the original hypothesis. However, as the research findings permeate to the outer boundaries of the thought collective, and the details are lost in the process, the uncertainty is glossed over and the facts become accepted more easily as truths. Once there is a critical mass of approval that a given fact is indeed true, even those who are somewhat more sceptical eventually come around.

Thomas Kuhn refers to this as a "paradigm shift", whereby a scientific revolution occurs and one belief system is replaced by another, after which there is a point of no return.[18] Although Kuhn questions the idea of linear "scientific progress", once it was generally agreed that the planets revolve around the sun, there was no going back to the old geocentric worldview. Similarly, once the germ theory of disease was accepted, there was no going back to miasmas. Of course, that is the Western scientific worldview, and many cultures see things very differently. For instance, even if all Westerners (and those who share Western beliefs) believe that epilepsy is a disease caused by bursts of uncontrolled electrical activity in the brain, there are those who believe that it is a falling sickness due to evil spirits or curses. Therefore, prescribing anticonvulsant medications, which prevent the excessive firing of neurons, may be the "gold standard" treatment in Western medicine, but it would not make much sense to people in a different context, who may prefer a shaman or traditional healer. Some would argue that the evidence-based Western worldview should prevail and those who do not share this worldview need to be educated on how their bodies work and how to improve their health. However, as discussed in the previous chapter, understanding and respecting alternative worldviews is increasingly recognised as being important in promoting health across cultures. So, whether or not everyone believes in the same realities, if the goal is improving health and reducing inequities, then more than indoctrination matters. While we needn't fall into the trap of cultural relativism, greater cultural competency is nonetheless required so that we can create an ongoing dialogue and discuss our differences in a respectful way when confronted with alternative concepts of reality and truth.

So, where does all this leave us? First, the quest for truth and the appeal to evidence have been around for many millennia. However, the way that people build up the evidence base has evolved. In particular, the scientific method, which has been used increasingly over the last several centuries, has become the dominant mode of generating evidence in the health field – to elucidate the nature and causes of poor health as well as the cures. Even more recently, many of the specific study designs commonly used in generating the evidence (i.e. randomised controlled trials, qualitative research studies, etc.) have been developed in the past 50–100 years, and the methods for synthesising the evidence base (i.e. systematic reviews) have only been developed in the past few decades. Thus, while critics are correct when they point out that even scientific evidence is not wholly objective, the results of research studies are clearly valuable in better understanding health and disease, and, to date, there have been no better alternatives proposed for coming closer to the truth.

To make better-informed decisions about health, we must therefore rely upon the best available research evidence while recognising that all research has certain biases and flaws, and that these need to be critically reflected upon and made explicit as part of the decision-making process. It is also important to recognise, as discussed in earlier chapters, that, in addition to the research evidence, context and values are also important in decision-making for health – whether at the patient level or at the population and global levels. Once again, these considerations also need to be made explicit. Thus it is neither a question of whether we should use evidence (yes, we should), nor whether the use of evidence means that we are avoiding important issues relating to context and values (indeed, all of these elements are important ingredients in decision-making). Rather, the real question is how best to use evidence as part of the decision-making process. This requires a nuanced understanding of how evidence is produced and what are the various shortcomings of research studies, which is described in greater detail in the remainder of this chapter.

The evidence-based medicine (EBM) movement

Although the evidence-based medicine (EBM) movement has been subjected to its fair share of criticism (see Table 4.1),[19] a core feature of EBM involves teaching people how to

Table 4.1 A summary of the criticisms of evidence-based medicine (EBM).

Limitations

- Universal to the practice of medicine
- Shortage of coherent, consistent scientific evidence
- Difficulties in applying evidence to the care of individual patients
- Barriers to the practice of high-quality medicine
- Unique to the practice of evidence-based medicine
- The need to develop new skills
- Limited time and resources
- Paucity of evidence that evidence-based medicine "works"

Misperceptions

- Evidence-based medicine denigrates clinical expertise
- It ignores patients' values and preferences
- It promotes a cookbook approach to medicine
- It is simply a cost-cutting tool
- It is an ivory-tower concept
- It is limited to clinical research
- It leads to therapeutic nihilism in the absence of evidence from randomised trials

Reproduced with permission from Straus SE, McAlister FA. Evidence-based medicine: a commentary on common criticisms. *CMAJ* 2000; 163: 837–41.

be critical thinkers, to judge for themselves the quality and utility of research studies so that they can base decisions on the best available evidence, with the overall aim of improving health.

Indeed, evidence-based medicine has been defined as the conscientious, explicit and judicious use of current best evidence in making decisions about the care of individual patients (or populations).[20] The classic EBM cycle starts with a clinical (or policy) question. It is therefore rooted in the local context. For instance, a 59-year-old, post-menopausal woman has been taking hormone replacement pills for 9 years. At first, the pills were prescribed to relieve symptoms relating to menopause such as hot flashes and vaginal dryness. However, even though she hasn't experienced these symptoms in years, she continues to take the medication and is reluctant to stop. Repeatedly she has been told that extended use of these pills could lead to an increased risk of developing breast cancer and heart disease. Nonetheless she asks "Must I stop doctor? I feel well when I take these pills. Are the risks really so high?" The first step in the EBM approach would be to formulate the clinical (or policy) question in a way that can be answered more easily. For instance, among post-menopausal women aged 50 to 70 years old, what is the 10-year risk of developing heart disease related to hormone replacement therapy (HRT) as compared to placebo? The next steps are to search for the evidence and to critically appraise the research findings to be sure that the advice is based on high-quality research. The final step is to return to the local context to see whether the evidence applies. Here is where the decision-making process comes in. Even if there is an increased risk of harm from extended use of HRT (which there is), what is most important is that the patient is well informed about the potential risks and benefits and is actively involved in the decision-making process. The patient's values and preferences are thereby taken into consideration when negotiating the treatment plan. Perhaps rather than stopping the hormones altogether, since she has no family history of heart disease or other risk factors such as high blood pressure or diabetes, she could consider switching from the oral formulation of the HRT medication to a vaginal cream, which could provide similar benefits at a lower dose. Alternatively, she may be willing to have a one-month trial off the hormones to see whether they are still providing a true benefit or whether she may feel just as well without them. Similarly, for population-level questions, evidence should not supersede societal values and a fair process, but rather the evidence should be used to support the decision-making process.[21] In the policy world, the term "evidence informed" rather than "evidence based" has been adopted to further emphasise that evidence is just one of many factors taken into account when making decisions about population health.

While not dismissing the criticisms, much of the controversy over the EBM movement has been raised by physicians working within the medical establishment who are either disgruntled by the new approach and what this change entails for their medical practice, or who are annoyed by the implication that what they were doing previously was not rigorous and even ineffective. There have also been multiple critiques from social scientists who complain that EBM is just a handmaid for rationing health care[22] or that EBM attempts to shy away from making difficult, value-based decisions by providing a "technocratic fix".[23] As with any large movement, EBM can mean different things to different people,[24] and therefore risks being misunderstood and misused. While acknowledging that the EBM movement has certain limitations, as does any scientific research study which is used as evidence, trying to make decisions for health without using this evidence at all would be like trying to sail the seas without a map (even if at times this map can be quite tricky and difficult to read). Indeed, a major reason for writing this book is to expose the many nuances underlying the evidence so that decisions are made which take these shortcomings into account. But rather than denounce the EBM movement altogether and "throw out the baby with the bathwater", it is helpful to instead look back to the origins of the EBM movement, and to some of the key players involved, to better appreciate why and how it was created.

The founders of EBM

In 1972, Dr. Archie Cochrane, a Scottish physician, published a seminal work called *Effectiveness and Efficiency: Random Reflections on Health Services.*[25] In this book, he called for a better understanding of which medical treatments work. He believed that effective treatments should be provided free of charge to all citizens through the publicly funded universal health care system with the aim of improving the health of the population. At the same time, he also believed that it was important for physicians (and policy-makers) to know which treatments do not work, not only to save taxpayers from spending money on useless or potentially harmful interventions, but also to ensure that universal access to health care services would be sustainable.[26] Dr. David Sackett, the founding director of the Department of Clinical Epidemiology and Biostatistics at McMaster University in Canada, was concerned with these same issues. In an article published in 1973 questioning the utility of periodic health exams, he cites Cochrane's newly released book and argues for more and better quality research that can be used as a basis for rational decision-making:

At the present growth rate, health expenditures in Canada would absorb almost the gross national product by the year 2000, and pressures are increasing to develop some rational method of allocating limited funds. In the health sector, there are various methods of evaluating the allocation of resources, economists and physicians tending to use different criteria. The economists view is reflected through studies such as cost-benefit analysis... The other view is found in the medical literature, where the measure of benefits has mainly been in terms of changes in mortality rates... Unless we, as academic clinicians, rapidly expand our randomized clinical trials of screening, diagnostic and treatment manoeuvres so that we can free resources spent on worthless clinical procedures and reinvest them in valid clinical innovations, we will have only ourselves to blame when we are faced with government edicts which restrict hospital beds and physician incomes.[27]

Both Cochrane and Sackett devoted their careers to building up that evidence base. Cochrane's main focus was on conducting systematic reviews of controlled trials in perinatal medicine. In 1978, he became the founding director of the National Perinatal Epidemiology Unit (NPEU) at Oxford University. The mission of the unit, which is still going strong to this day, is "to produce high quality research evidence that can improve the care provided to women and their families during pregnancy, childbirth, the newborn period and early childhood as well as promoting the effective use of resources by perinatal health services". Cochrane was involved in collecting, reviewing and synthesising the findings from over 3,500 controlled trials, which contributed to the creation of *A Guide to Effective Care in Pregnancy and Childhood*. This work spawned an international collaboration to assist in preparing systematic reviews of controlled trials in pregnancy and childbirth and the neonatal period,[28] and this model was later expanded to include other areas of medicine and population health.

In 1993, the Cochrane Collaboration was formally established to produce systematic and up-to-date reviews of all relevant randomised controlled trials of health care, with the first Cochrane Centre located in Oxford. By the year 2010, there were more than 28,000 people working within the Cochrane Collaboration in over 100 countries. The collaboration has over 50 review groups focusing on a wide variety of disciplines in medicine and public health, and together they have published over 5,500 reviews. There is also a sister organisation, the Campbell Collaboration, which was established in 2000 and focuses on systematic reviews in areas such as education, justice and social policy.

Unlike Cochrane, the focus of Sackett's early career was somewhat different. Rather than writing reviews based on syntheses of the evidence from randomised controlled trials that had already been conducted, Sackett instead attempted to fill existing knowledge gaps by becoming an expert in conducting randomised controlled trials. The results of these trials demonstrated that patients cared for by nurse practitioners had similar outcomes and satisfaction as compared to those who were cared for by a physician,[29] defined which strategies were effective in encouraging patient compliance with anti-hypertensive medications,[30] suggested that deep vein thrombosis could be diagnosed just as accurately using a less invasive ultrasound procedure,[31] concluded that physicians should not screen for carotid artery stenosis by listening for bruits,[32] and proposed that aspirin could be used to prevent stroke.[33] Sackett strongly believed that there were three ways to answer clinical questions: "1) induction from our own individual prior experiences, 2) abdication to the authority of our teachers and those who write review articles, and 3) deduction from the reports of randomized clinical trials".[34] The first two, he argues, are fallible. The third can also have its disadvantages and involves more work on the part of the knowledge user, but it is less prone to serious errors in judgement. Sackett was therefore actively involved in promoting evidence-based medicine and developed materials for continuing medical education to encourage physicians to become better acquainted with the evidence.[35] As well, he was also very active in training junior doctors to use evidence in their day-to-day clinical decision-making, which was greatly assisted by the advent of personal computers, handheld devices and the Internet.[36] In 1994, Sackett moved to Oxford University, where he was the founding director of the Centre for Evidence Based Medicine and the founding co-editor of the journal *Evidence Based Medicine*, as well as the founding chair of the Cochrane Collaboration Steering Group.

The conventional hierarchy of evidence

By the late 1990s, there was growing consensus that the double-blind randomised controlled trial (RCT) is the gold standard for producing unbiased, relevant and reliable evidence for health. Nonetheless, even RCTs can be poorly designed and subject to flaws. Ian Chalmers, then Director of the UK Cochrane Group, wrote that:

> Randomised trials conducted over the past half century have helped to bring about a situation in which health care has been credited with three of the seven years of increased life expectancy over that time and an average of five additional years of partial or complete relief from the poor quality of life associated with chronic disease. But we should not be complacent. Systematic reviews of some of the hundreds of thousands of reports of trials published since 1948 are beginning to make painfully clear that, in most of these studies, inadequate steps were taken to control biases, many questions and outcomes of interest to patients were ignored, and insufficient numbers of participants were studied to yield reliable estimates of treatment effects. In brief, a massive amount of research effort, the goodwill of hundreds of thousands of patients, and millions of pounds have been wasted.[37]

Therefore, when making evidence-informed recommendations, it is not just a matter of collating all of the existing research on a given topic, but also ensuring that the studies included as a basis for these decisions are valid and reliable. As early as 1976, the Canadian Task Force on the Periodic Health Exam (now the Canadian Task Force on Preventive Health Care) attempted to base their recommendations on the strength and quality of the evidence, followed in 1984 by the US Preventive Services Task Force. While frameworks depicting the hierarchy of evidence may vary (Fig. 4.1), well-conducted RCTs are generally considered as the most reliable form of evidence, with systematic reviews of RCTs (with or without meta-analyses) as the only other studies higher on the pyramid.[38]

The reason why "randomised controlled trials (RCTs) yield stronger evidence than other study designs"[39] is because randomisation safeguards against bias due to known and unknown factors. Randomised controlled trials are not only useful in the clinical arena, but have also been widely used to assess the impact of education and social policies.[40] Yet RCTs are not always feasible or ethical depending on the context. Some argue that well-conducted observational studies are just as valid as RCTs.[41] Others argue that too much attention has been focused on RCTs, downplaying the value of alternative forms of research, such as qualitative studies, which are useful in answering different types of research questions (for example, rather than comparing the number of people who exercise more than 30 minutes per day in group A versus group B, a qualitative study might ask people why

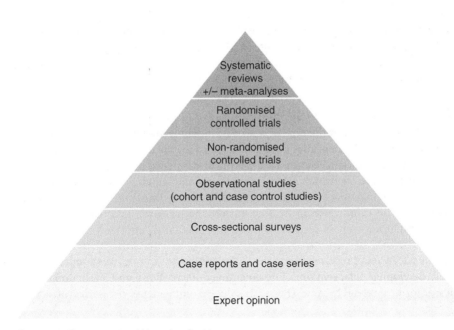

Figure 4.1 The conventional hierarchy of evidence.

they exercise and what are the facilitators and barriers to making time for exercise). Therefore, rather than being too dogmatic regarding the hierarchy of evidence, it is important to recognise that the most appropriate study design depends on the type of question that is asked.

Indeed, when it comes to determining what constitutes evidence, the medical establishment is showing greater openness as to the types of research that are considered valuable. Scientific or medical facts are not limited to laboratory science or even to clinical and epidemiological studies (including RCTs). Increasingly, the utility of mixed-methods research is being recognised, which includes qualitative research (e.g. interviews and focus groups with key informants) as well as quantitative research (e.g. surveys and experimental trials). Economic evaluations are also being included as part of the evidence base for improving health. Even econometric modelling – although at times quite hypothetical and very much dependent on the underlying assumptions that are presupposed from the outset – can also be considered as evidence. With the increasing emphasis on developing healthy public policies and promoting intersectoral action to tackle the upstream determinants of health, a better understanding of political and social science is of growing importance. As well, ethnographic research to better understand cultural values and beliefs, and participatory research that involves communities in taking control over their health and its determinants are playing increasingly important roles.

Therefore there is a wide range of possible types of research that can assist us in better understanding the magnitude of a health problem, the causes of poor health, what works to improve health, and how to evaluate whether progress has been made. In contrast to the fingerprints, testimonials and smoking gun from the courtroom example above, it is safe to say that the type of evidence generally used in the health field is research evidence. While initially research evidence was predominantly generated to answer clinical questions, increasingly, there is a growing evidence base which also attempts to address population-level questions[42] to promote more evidence-informed programmes and policy.[43, 44, 45, 46] The remainder of this chapter will examine in greater detail how such evidence is produced, as well as illustrating the various shortcomings that are inherent to research evidence.

How research evidence is produced

It may appear self-evident, but the type of research studies needed to build up the evidence base depends on the research questions being asked. For instance, if you want to know how to improve health outcomes in relation to a specific disease, then an RCT would be a good choice of study design to test which interventions work and which do not work. However, if instead you want to know which are the most pressing health priorities in a given population, then you cannot use an RCT to answer that research question. Rather than an RCT, you might use a cross-sectional survey or a qualitative interview study with key informants.

The main categories of research questions – i.e. defining health priorities, understanding the causes, developing interventions, implementing interventions and evaluating health outcomes – form a research cycle (Fig. 4.2) which complements the series of actions

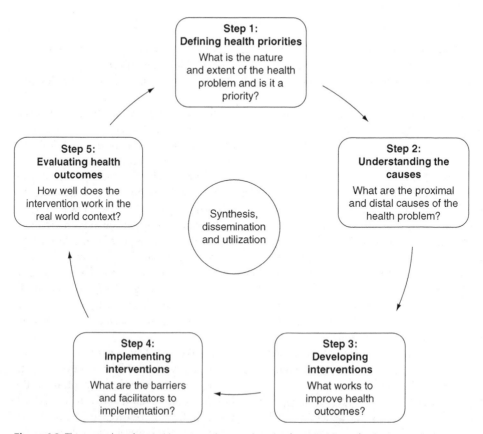

Figure 4.2 The research cycle: priorities, causes, interventions, implementation, evaluation.

Box 4.1 Tackling non-communicable diseases through global tobacco control

In September 2011, the United Nations held a high-level meeting on non-communicable diseases (NCDs), including heart disease, stroke, cancer, diabetes and obesity, which constitute an increasing global crisis. The most urgent priority identified to reduce premature mortality worldwide is tobacco control. The NCD Action Group and the NCD Alliance "propose as a goal for 2040, a world essentially free from tobacco where less than 5% of people use tobacco".[47] You are the Minister of Health in your country, which also happens to be a major producer of tobacco for export. You know that you will need to have very strong evidence to build a local movement in support of this "world free from tobacco" goal. You are concerned that in your country there will be a great deal of opposition from farmers and from industry, from transport companies and from advertisers – not to mention from smokers. Anticipating this, you want to be well prepared to answer the tough questions that you will face from the many critics. Conceding to the authority of the United Nations or to the opinion of medical experts will not be enough. To get people on board, it will be necessary to go back to basics and to explain the logic behind this recommendation. Of course, it will also be important to ensure that people will not lose their livelihoods and will be able to find work that is not related to tobacco manufacture or export. The transformation of the economy and people's way of life will be a massive undertaking and it will not be easy unless everyone has a shared understanding and commitment as to why this change is important.

---

that are likewise required to improve the health of individuals and populations as described in the health planning cycle in Chapter 2. The case example in Box 4.1 will be used to illustrate the different types of research studies that can be used to answer different research questions at each step in the research cycle.

Step 1: Defining health priorities

The first step in improving the health of individuals and populations is better understanding what are the main health problems and, of these, which are the most urgent priorities and why. In the absence of reliable and comparable surveillance data, different types of research studies can also be used to make this assessment. Table 4.2 illustrates a number of possible research questions relating to the first step in the research cycle, as well as examples of research study designs that can be used to answer these questions and thereby help to build up the evidence base. This is the first of a series of tables – one for each step in the research cycle. It is important to note that these tables are not intended to be exhaustive. Rather, they provide examples of the types of research that are possible at each step.

The nature of the health problem

Using the case above of the Minister of Health, to better understand what are non-communicable diseases and how they develop we can first turn to laboratory research to provide some of the evidence. For instance, pathological studies can show how heart disease and certain types of stroke result from atherosclerosis (i.e. the build-up of fatty deposits in the arteries) that can already begin to accumulate in adolescence and early adulthood,[48] even if symptoms only appear much later in life (i.e. when the fatty plaques partially or completely block off the blood vessel thereby compromising blood flow and the transport of oxygen to the tissues resulting in cell death). Similarly, research in molecular biology can help us to

Table 4.2 Research evidence on defining health priorities.

Question	Research	Study type	Evidence
The nature of the health problem			
What is the nature of the health problem?	Laboratory research	Molecular biology, genetics, anatomy, physiology, pathology, etc.	Pathophysiology of the health problem
The frequency of the health problem			
What proportion of the population is affected?	Epidemiological research	Cross-sectional surveys, secondary analysis of medico-administrative databases, etc.	Prevalence
How many new cases are there each year?	Epidemiological research	Serial surveys, cohort study	Incidence
The severity of the health problem			
How many people die as a result of this health problem each year?	Epidemiological research	Secondary analysis of vital statistics, verbal autopsy surveys	Cause-specific mortality
What proportion of people die from this health problem as compared to the total number of deaths?	Epidemiological research	Secondary analysis of vital statistics, verbal autopsy surveys	Proportional mortality
What is the extent of premature deaths due to this health problem?	Epidemiological research	Secondary analysis of vital statistics, verbal autopsy surveys	Potential years of life lost (PYLL)
What is the burden of suffering due to this health problem?	Epidemiological research / economic evaluations	Secondary analysis of vital statistics combined with assessments of values and preferences	Disability-adjusted life years (DALYs)
How does this health problem affect people's lives?	Qualitative research	Interviews, focus groups, etc.	Personal experience
What is the economic burden of the health problem?	Economic evaluations	Cost analysis	Cost
Is this health problem a priority?			
Is this health problem perceived to be an important priority?	Qualitative research	Interviews, focus groups	Perceived or subjective health needs

understand the step-wise process that leads to cancer formation. This involves exposure to carcinogens resulting in a series of mutations that overwhelm the DNA repair mechanisms such that certain cancer-promoting genes are activated more than they should be, whereas other protective genes (e.g. tumour suppressor genes) are inactivated. This then leads to unregulated cell growth and the formation of tumours that can invade local tissues as well as metastasise to more distant parts of the body.[49] Indeed, there is a huge literature and thousands of researchers working on better understanding the pathophysiology and molecular basis of heart disease and cancer.

The frequency of the health problem

To estimate what proportion of the population is affected by non-communicable diseases, we turn to epidemiological research. One of the most basic epidemiological study designs is the cross-sectional survey (sometimes also referred to as a household survey). Surveys are classified as descriptive studies since they do not attempt to test any hypothesis. They are simply used to measure the frequency of a specific health problem (or risk factor or attitude or belief or behaviour), as well as its distribution in a given population (i.e. is it more common in men versus women, at different ages, in specific ethnic groups, in certain geographic areas, etc.). Conducting a survey is like taking a "snapshot" of the population at a single point in time. It involves selecting a random sample of the population and using a standardised questionnaire (either self-completion or completed with the help of a data collector) to ask people questions about their health. For instance, a cross-sectional survey can be used to determine how many people have diabetes by asking them "Have you ever had a diagnosis of diabetes?" If 3 out of 100 people answer "yes", then the prevalence of diabetes in the population would be estimated to be 3%. It is important to qualify this finding as an estimate since all research has certain limitations. For instance, a person may have diabetes, but they may not want to disclose this information or they may not be aware that they have the disease. For those who are unaware, either they were never tested for diabetes, or they may not have understood that they were diagnosed with diabetes, or they simply might not remember. Therefore, people may respond "no" to the survey question for various reasons, even if they do have the disease. For this reason, some surveys, such as the US National Health and Nutrition Examination Survey (NHANES), and similar surveys in other countries, also include direct assessments of the health condition (e.g. by doing blood sugar tests).[50] Thus, while the prevalence of people diagnosed with diabetes may be 3% in a given population according to people's subjective assessment, laboratory findings could demonstrate that 5% actually have the disease and an additional 10% have a precursor of the disease (e.g. impaired fasting glucose, also known as pre-diabetes), which would certainly make diabetes a much bigger priority.

In addition to knowing how many people are living with the disease (i.e. the prevalence), it is also worthwhile to understand how many new cases of the disease appear each year (i.e. the incidence). This helps to distinguish whether the disease is truly on the rise because more people are becoming affected each year or whether people are just living with the disease for a longer period of time (since prevalence equals incidence times duration: $P = I \times D$). A single cross-sectional study can give an indication of incidence depending on how you ask the question. If you ask "Have you ever been diagnosed with diabetes?" this gives you the prevalence. However, if instead you ask "In the last 12 months, were you diagnosed with diabetes?" this gives you an estimate of the incidence in the last year.

To be able to determine the trend over time, you would need to conduct serial surveys each year or every few years. Alternatively, a cohort study, which follows a specific group of people (or cohort) over time, can also provide data on incidence. Other potential sources of data on prevalence and incidence include medical records (i.e. a patient's chart), disease registries (e.g. tumour registry), medico-administrative databases (which contain data on prescriptions filled, doctor visits, hospitalisations, etc.), and so forth. Whereas, in most research studies, researchers collect the data themselves (i.e. primary research), in this case, the data from these other sources were already collected for another purpose (e.g. to care for the patient or to monitor the use of public funds). The researchers are therefore analysing data that they did not collect (i.e. secondary analysis of primary data), and therefore what they can do with the data is limited to what already exists in the data set. Nonetheless, if the data has been collected in a reliable way, it can also be used to determine what proportion of the population has the disease (i.e. prevalence), although it will only capture the subset of people who presented for medical care and were diagnosed, rather than a true population-based estimate.

The severity of the health problem

In addition to knowing about how many people have the health problem and how many new cases develop each year, it is also important to assess the severity of the health problem. Often, this is taken to mean how many people die or suffer prolonged disability as a result of this health problem. Vital statistics records (e.g. death certificates), where available, can be used to provide evidence on cause-specific mortality rates (i.e. the number of deaths due to the health problem in a given time period divided by the total population) and proportional mortality (i.e. the number of deaths due to the health problem in a given time period divided by the total number of deaths in the same time period). Once again, this kind of research often involves secondary analysis of data with the various limitations that this entails (e.g. quality and availability of death certificates, which are the main sources of data). In countries where vital statistics are unavailable or not routinely collected, alternative sources of data may be used such as verbal autopsies (i.e. a method for determining cause of death using a trained interviewer).[51] However, while mortality rates are certainly an important measure of the severity of a health problem, they are not the only measure.

Some health problems which predominantly affect children are given more weight by calculating the potential years of life lost (PYLL), which factors in the age at which the death occurred. Other health problems, particularly mental health conditions and certain disabilities, may not lead to premature death, but can cause extended periods of suffering. Thus, other measures, such as disability-adjusted life years (DALYs) are used to take this into consideration. Ultimately, to better understand in what ways health problems actually affect people, it is necessary to ask people directly. Therefore, qualitative research using in-depth interviews and focus groups (i.e. a group interview often with 6–12 people), can help to tease out how a health problem impacts people's lives and what kind of support would be most helpful. For instance, one study identified that male cancer survivors are concerned about their changing role in relation to their family and friends, financial issues and body image.[52] This type of evidence would be impossible to elicit from a survey, which can count how many people share these concerns, but not what are the concerns and why. DIPEx is an online database of patient experiences which repertories how various diseases can impact people's wellbeing and social functioning. Another type of impact would be to look at the economic burden of the disease, from an individual as well as a societal standpoint. Economic evaluations such as costing studies can be used to calculate the direct, indirect and intangible costs related to a particular health problem. Direct costs include the amount paid for medical treatments, indirect costs include time off from work and lost productivity, and intangible costs include other factors such as pain and suffering.

Is this health problem a priority?

Whether a certain disease or health problem is an important priority depends not only on how common it is in the population (i.e. the prevalence and incidence) but also the severity and impact on those affected, their families and society. Therefore, when prioritising which health problems should be the focus of further research (i.e. moving to Step 2 in the research cycle), it is not sufficient to simply make a ranking of the health conditions which result in the largest number of deaths or DALYs, or which cost the most money. According to Lawrence Green and Marshall Kreuter's "Precede-Proceed" model for health planning, in addition to the "objective needs assessment" there should also be a "subjective needs assessment".[53] People want to be involved,[54] and their voices should be heard to ensure a fair process,[55] since these decisions will ultimately affect them. Qualitative research is an important way of involving various populations or target groups in providing their own viewpoints and empowering them in determining their own health priorities and identifying their preferred solutions.[56]

Returning to the case example of the Minister of Health who is building up the knowledge base to rally support for the "world free from tobacco", what evidence can he use? Some of the evidence, such as the pathophysiology of disease, can be taken from the international literature. The Minister can also use global health data on the incidence, prevalence and mortality associated with common non-communicable diseases such as heart disease, stroke, diabetes and obesity. However, it would certainly be even more powerful if it is possible to demonstrate that these diseases are also a major problem in the local population. In the absence of vital statistics or other research in this area, the Minister could partner with researchers at the local universities to conduct verbal autopsy studies and/or prevalence surveys to see whether these conditions really are common in the national context. As well, when it comes to understanding how these diseases impact people's day-to-day lives, and what people think should be the major health priorities, qualitative studies can be conducted which will produce powerful narratives and guidance for whether and how this global priority fits with the national and local priorities. Costing studies can also be used to determine how much the government and individuals spend out of pocket on health care expenses related to non-communicable diseases, and the degree to which these diseases lead to catastrophic illness resulting in already fragile families sliding deeper into poverty. It is important though that research evidence is not taken out of context or used as a political tool. The research can be used to answer questions. But it is important to avoid bias in analysis, interpretation and use of the evidence.

What if the research shows that only a very small proportion of the population smokes and that the rates of heart disease and cancer are relatively low? What if instead the research shows that the main causes of death nationwide are poverty-related diseases among children under five years of age and injuries among young people, especially in relation to child work? It is important not to disregard this. Even if globally non-communicable diseases and tobacco control are an urgent priority, this country may have different problems to contend with. Of course, increasingly health problems transcend national borders and require a concerted international effort to be overcome. Allowing the country to continue producing and exporting tobacco is an important barrier to achieving the global targets and goals. Nonetheless, the Minister cannot use people as a means to an end, and the local health needs must be the primary focus for health planning. Yet, there may still be creative solutions. For instance, multilateral agreements can be arranged such that if the Minister can co-opt his colleagues in the Ministry of Finance and the Ministry of Labour to reorient the economy to one that is less reliant on tobacco production, then additional funds will be made available to help address the more pressing health and economic development needs identified by the local people. That being said, non-communicable diseases are becoming so pervasive that most countries around the world are facing sharp increases in adult mortality resulting from these conditions. For the purpose of this example, we will therefore continue to focus on tobacco control and non-communicable diseases. Although, on the basis of the initial research findings, the Minister may reasonably decide to reorient the focus of the research conducted nationally. In Step 2 of the research cycle a greater emphasis could thus be placed on better understanding the causes of infant mortality and injuries among working children and adolescents to develop better-adapted solutions for these problems, which could have an even greater impact on the health of the local population.

Step 2:   Understanding the causes of the health problem

Once the first step of the research cycle identifies the major health priorities, the next step is to better understand the causes of the health problem as a basis for developing effective interventions. Once again, there are several different types of research that can be used to accomplish this task (Table 4.3).

Basic science

Basic science or laboratory research can help us to better understand which factors promote the development of the disease, which factors protect against the disease, the biological mechanisms that lead to poor health (e.g. how does stress lead to chronic health problems such as heart disease), and the natural history of disease (i.e. what are the different stages in the development of the disease from pre-clinical changes to disability and death), so that we are then better able to prevent, diagnose and treat the disease. For instance, laboratory research has shown that tobacco smoke contains hundreds of chemicals, and it has long been known that many of these compounds are carcinogenic, meaning that they can cause genetic mutations to occur in cells which can lead to these cells growing out of control.[57] Further research in the laboratory has shown that other compounds found in tobacco smoke, such as nicotine, which is not in itself carcinogenic, can nonetheless promote the growth of cancers through other cellular mechanisms.[58] Therefore, basic science is very helpful in determining the factors that lead to disease and how disease develops. However, laboratory research alone is not sufficient. Indeed, there is often a complex interplay between basic science, clinical research and population-level studies, to more fully tease out the causes of health problems.

Clinical research

In hindsight, it may seem obvious that smoking causes cancer. However, a century ago, smoking was extremely popular. In the UK, many doctors were also smokers. So, back in those days, who would even think of examining tobacco smoke for the presence of harmful chemicals that could lead to premature death from cancer and heart disease? Yet, already in 1604, King James I of England wrote a treatise condemning the use of tobacco as an unpleasant and harmful substance. He claimed that men "smoke themselves to death",[59] and therefore levied a high tax as a disincentive to its use – incidentally, raising taxes is used today as one of the main strategies in the World Health Organization (WHO) Framework Convention on Tobacco Control. While not himself a physician, King James I was making a clinical observation linking smoking and mortality. Therefore to provide us with clues as to what the causes of health problems might be, there are many different types of research that we could use which do not look at cells or molecules in a laboratory, but rather involve people, especially in a clinical setting.

Notwithstanding the historical anecdote above, clinical research in a previously unexplored and poorly understood area of medicine generally begins with the publication of case

Table 4.3 Research evidence on the proximal and distal causes of the health problem.

Question	Research	Study type	Evidence
Basic science			
How does the health problem develop and what are the contributing factors involved?	Laboratory research	Molecular biology, genetics, anatomy, physiology, pathology, etc.	Natural history of the health problem, contributing factors in a laboratory setting
Clinical research			
What are the different factors that tend to accompany the health problem in practice?	Clinical research	Case reports, case series, etc.	Potential causal factors
What do patients believe are the underlying causes of their own health problem?	Qualitative research	Interviews, focus groups, etc.	Potential causal factors
What do people think are the causes of the health problem in other cultures?	Qualitative research	Ethnographic studies, etc.	Potential causal factors
What does the body of scientific literature suggest as the potential causes of this health problem?	Secondary research	Reviews of the literature, etc.	Potential causal factors
Population-based studies			
Is this potential cause (whether a proximal risk factor or an upstream determinant) associated with the health problem?	Epidemiological research	Cross-sectional surveys, case-control studies, cohort studies, randomised controlled trials, etc.	Presence or absence of an association
Is this potential cause harmful or protective with respect to the health problem?	Epidemiological research	Cross-sectional surveys, case-control studies, cohort studies, randomised controlled trials, etc.	Positive association is harmful, negative association is protective
What is the strength of association between the potential cause and the health problem?	Epidemiological research	Cross-sectional surveys, case-control studies, cohort studies, randomised controlled trials, etc.	Correlation Odds ratio Relative risk Hazard ratio
Does the potential causal factor or exposure fulfil the criteria for causality?	Secondary research	Systematic reviews +/− meta-analyses, etc.	Strength of association Dose-response Temporal relationship Biological plausibility Experimental evidence Consistency Coherence, etc.

reports and case series to provide an initial indication of what might be causing the disease. For instance, a hundred years ago, before the link between smoking and mortality was widely recognised, if a physician saw a patient with a lung tumour who happens to be a smoker he might not think much of it. But, if he then sees another lung cancer patient who is also a smoker, and then another, and another, it begs the question of whether there may be an association. Physicians use their clinical observations to write up a case report or, if there are many cases, a case series, to describe findings that are new and have not been described before. By publishing these case reports or case series in widely read medical journals, thereby drawing attention to the possible connection between smoking and cancer, other physicians may also become more attuned to whether there are similar cases in their clinical practice. We can also ask the patients themselves what they think are the causes of their health problem by using qualitative research methods, since patients may have important insights that others may not be aware of (e.g. a specific hobby or type of work that leads to the exposure to a certain chemical, or a special type of diet). Similarly, cross-cultural research can provide an understanding of how health problems are viewed in different parts of the world. These insights, whether from physicians, from patients or from other cultures – and, of course, from the existing research literature – can be very helpful in developing hypotheses about the causes of health problems. However, how do we know for certain whether this is just coincidence based on a few observations and anecdotes or whether there is truly an association? This is where population-based research comes in, building on existing basic science and clinical research to further elucidate the causes of disease.

Population-based studies

In 1950, Richard Doll and Austin Bradford Hill sought to test the hypothesis of whether smoking could be a cause of lung cancer.[60] They were prompted to do so in response to the remarkable rise in lung cancer mortality in the UK during the first half of the twentieth century. The number of lung cancer deaths jumped from 612 in 1922 to 9,287 in 1947. What could be the cause of this tremendous 15-fold rise? Well, perhaps it has something to do with data collection. If, for instance, in 1922 physicians had difficulty diagnosing lung cancer and wrote "unknown cause" on the death certificate and in 1947 were better at diagnosing this health problem (whether due to improvements in education, greater awareness or new diagnostic tools) and therefore wrote "lung cancer" on the death certificates, this could result in an artefactual increase. Yet, this is unlikely to have been the case since the rise in lung cancer deaths was similar in the cities – with the best diagnostic equipment – and in the countryside. As well, there was no similar increase in diagnosing other respiratory diseases. So, what else could explain it? Well, it could have something to do with the population growth. If there was a wave of immigration or simply the maturing of the population such that in the 1940s many more people in the UK were above the age of 50 when cancer is more common, then that could also be an explanation. Yet, Doll and Hill calculated the age-standardised, cause-specific mortality rates, which were 1.1 for males and 0.7 for females per 100,000 population between 1901 and 1920 and 10.6 for males and 2.5 for females per 100,000 population between 1936 and 1939. They also noted that many other countries had similar increases in lung cancer cases. Doll and Hill therefore proposed two possible causes for this increase: pollution or smoking. Some studies had been done in the past exploring these associations, but it was difficult to draw any conclusions since the number of partic-ipants was generally too small for the results to be statistically significant. Therefore, they decided to conduct further research studies that would be large enough so as to be sufficiently powered to determine whether there truly is an association between the potential causes (i.e. smoking and/or pollution) and the health problem (i.e. lung cancer).

In the first instance, to determine which of these hypotheses is most likely, Doll and Hill conducted a case-control study. Then to test the most likely hypothesis, they conducted a cohort study. Case-control and cohort studies are a form of epidemiological research. Unlike cross-sectional surveys described above, which are purely descriptive (i.e. how many people have a particular health problem, of those with the health problem how many have a specific risk factor, etc.), case-control and cohort studies are classified as analytical studies that are able to test a hypothesis since they use a control group as a basis for comparison. These studies are also sometimes called observational studies since, unlike experimental trials, there is no intervention, but rather, they simply compare two different groups. As the name suggests, in a case-control study the two groups consist of the cases (e.g. patients with lung cancer) and the controls (e.g. patients of similar age, gender, social class, place of residence, and other background), who ideally only differ from the cases in that they do not have the disease under study (i.e. lung cancer). By asking the cases and the controls about their history of exposure to various potential causal factors, it is possible to determine which exposures are associated with the health problem, as well as the direction of the association. If an exposure is positively associated with the health problem, then it is harmful and can lead to the development of poor health. If an exposure is negatively associated with the health problem, then it is protective and can prevent disease.

What Doll and Hill found was that 647 out 649 male lung cancer patients (99.7%) were smokers, as compared to 622 out of 649 male controls (95.8%). The numbers appear to be quite similar when looking at the simple proportions – 99.7 / 100 versus 95.8 / 100 – because the prevalence of smoking among males was extremely high at the time (i.e. almost all men were smokers). However, statistically, the fact that 25 fewer men were smokers in the non-lung cancer group as compared to the lung cancer group is a highly significant difference ($p < 0.0001$). This indicates that there is indeed an association between smoking and lung cancer. As well, because lung cancer patients are more likely to be smokers, there is a positive association between lung cancer and smoking. This indicates that smoking is likely harmful and is a potential causal factor in the development of lung cancer. To get a better idea of the strength of the association, one can use the results of the case-control study to draw a two-by-two table and to calculate an odds ratio (Table 4.4).[60] Using the following formula to calculate the odds ratio: OR = ad / bc, this study shows that men with lung cancer are 14 times more likely to be smokers than male controls who do not have lung cancer. This is an absolutely huge association, since many associations that are published nowadays linking other types of exposures to other types of health problems are in the range of two to three times higher among cases as compared to controls.

Table 4.4 Drawing a two-by-two table and calculating an odds ratio based on a case-control study.

	Cases (males with lung cancer)	Controls (males with no lung cancer)	Total
Potential cause present (smokers)	647	622	1269
	a b		
	c d		
Potential cause present (non-smokers)	2	27	29
Total	649	649	1298

Adapted from data in Doll R, Hill AB. Smoking and carcinoma of the lung. Preliminary report. *BMJ* 1950; ii: 739–48.

Case-control studies are relatively inexpensive and quick to complete since they are retrospective, meaning that you are starting with people who already have the disease (e.g. lung cancer), and all you have to do is ask them about their past exposures to various potential causes. However, case-control studies can be subject to potential bias. The results depend on how people answer the questions, and, as we have seen for surveys, this can sometimes be problematic. For instance, if someone has a disease, they may remember many more exposures that in their mind could have caused their current predicament as compared to someone who does not have the disease. This is called recall bias. Indeed, there are many different types of bias that can affect the validity of the research results. These occur when one group systematically responds differently or is treated differently as compared to the other group. This results in apparent associations appearing which do not really exist but result from these biases.

To get around this, in 1951 Doll went on to conduct one of the first large-scale cohort studies.[61] Rather than starting with people who already had lung cancer, he started instead with 34,439 healthy men – all of whom were doctors and therefore shared similar socio-economic and other backgrounds. These British male doctors were then divided into two groups according to whether or not they were smokers. Doll then followed this cohort for over 50 years and measured the rates of disease that developed in each group. He was able to demonstrate many things through this study. One important finding is that smoking was not only associated with increased rates of lung cancer, but also with heart disease, stroke and many other types of cancers (especially mouth and throat cancer), as well as overall mortality from all causes. Indeed, being a smoker reduces one's life expectancy on average by 10 years. The good news is that the earlier people quit smoking, the longer they live. If a person quits smoking at age 30, they could lower their risk sufficiently so as to gain back the 10 years that would otherwise have been lost and end up with the same life expectancy on average as a non-smoker. Even if a person quits at age 60, they could still gain 3 years of life over someone who continues to smoke.

Using a cohort study, more than just demonstrating whether there is an association between the exposure and the health problem (i.e. harmful association versus protective association versus no effect), it is possible to determine the strength of the association. This is done by calculating the relative risk (RR) of developing the health problem among people with the exposure as compared to those without (Table 4.5).[61] Indeed, the odds ratio calculated using data from case-control studies is just an approximation of the relative risk. Ideally, when one actually has data from a cohort study, then it is preferable to calculate the relative risk directly. To do this, once again, the results of the study can be plugged into a two-by-two table and the relative risk can be calculated using the following formula: $RR = [a / (a + b)] / [c / (c + d)]$. The data shows that, over the 50-year follow-up, 86% of smokers had died from all causes $[a / (a + b)]$ as compared to only 55% of life-long non-smokers $[c / (c + d)]$. The relative risk of death is therefore 1.6 times higher (86% / 55%) among smokers (including former and current smokers, cigarette and other smokers) than non-smokers. Going back to the lung cancer data more specifically, the rate of death due to lung cancer is 2.49 per 1,000 man-years among current smokers and 0.17 per 1,000 man-years among life-long non-smokers. Therefore, the relative risk of lung cancer death among smokers is 15 times higher (2.49 / 0.17), which is similar to the odds ratio calculated from Doll and Hill's original case-control study.

However, is the strength of association based on these studies enough to prove that smoking causes lung cancer (and heart disease, and stroke, and other cancers, and premature

Table 4.5 Drawing a two-by-two table and calculating a relative risk based on a cohort study.

	Disease (death from all causes)	No disease (still alive in 2001)	Total
Exposure group (smokers)	22,429	3,507	25,936
Control group (lifelong non-smokers)	2,917	2,395	5,312
Total	25,349	5,902	31,248

Adapted from data in Doll R, Peto R, Boreham J, Sutherland I. Mortality in relation to smoking: 50 years' observations on male British doctors. *BMJ* 2004; 328: 1519–28. Note: the paper reports that 17% of the original cohort of 34,439 male British doctors were lifelong non-smokers. However, the proportion of lifelong non-smokers among the 31,248 who were successfully followed up until 2001 (i.e. 50 years later) is not reported. For the purposes of this illustration, I have retained the proportion of 17% although this may not exactly reflect the data (i.e. if more smokers were lost to follow-up as compared to non-smokers, for instance).

death in general)? In 1965, Austin Bradford Hill, who co-authored the original case-control study with Richard Doll, wrote another influential paper entitled "The environment and disease: association or causation?"[62] In this article he argues that strength of association is only one criterion for causality. It is important but not sufficient to prove causation. He then describes eight more criteria which are now known collectively as the Bradford Hill criteria for causality. But before we look at these criteria in more detail, why isn't strength of association sufficient to determine causality?

Threats to internal validity: chance, bias and confounding

While external validity refers to the extent to which we can generalise research findings, internal validity refers to whether the research findings are an accurate and reliable reflection of the truth. As any basic epidemiology text will explain, there are three main factors that can influence the internal validity of research findings: chance, bias and confounding.

Chance

Sometimes researchers find that there is an association between a potential causal factor and a health problem just by chance. Indeed, researchers are aware of this possibility from the outset and, by convention, set the level of uncertainty that is permissible to 5% (i.e. alpha = 0.05). Therefore, if a researcher attempts to determine whether 20 factors are linked with a given health problem, then, by chance, one of the associations is likely to appear positive, even if it is not truly a cause. If the researcher tests 100 factors, then, on average, 5 would appear positive, even if they are not truly causes either. And so forth. Thus while most people are uncomfortable with uncertainty, and despite the use of the scientific method, none of these estimates are 100% reliable. For this reason, it is important to guard against "fishing expeditions" in research where the researchers test all possible permutations and combinations hoping to get a publishable positive result. Rather, the main research questions and hypotheses should be stated from the outset as part of the research protocol. As well, more recently, the use of the 95% confidence interval is favoured over the binary *p*-value (i.e. statistically significant versus not statistically significant) because it illustrates more clearly the likely range where the truth lies.[63] In very large studies which include thousands of research participants, the uncertainty is much smaller and therefore the confidence intervals (CIs) will also be small (e.g. RR = 1.5; 95% CI: 1.3 to 1.7). In contrast, in very small studies with only a few dozen people, there is far more uncertainty and the confidence intervals may be very wide (e.g. RR = 1.5; 95% CI: 0.8 to 2.4). Similar to the function of the *p*-value, when the confidence intervals cross 1 (the point at which both the exposure group and the control group have the same rates of the health problem under investigation), it is not possible to tell whether there is an association at all and therefore the results of the study are not statistically significant. Intuitively, this makes sense. If you ask two people for their opinion about whether smoking causes premature death, one may say "yes" and the other says "no". If you ask 10 people, 8 may say "yes" and 2 say "no". If you ask 100 people, 83 may say "yes" and 17 say "no". And so forth. Thus, with increasing sample size of the study, you have greater power to detect a difference and greater precision of the estimate.

Bias

Even if the association did not occur by chance, there is also concern about potential bias. Bias has been defined as "deviation of results or inferences from the truth, or processes leading to such deviation".[64] However, "the term bias does not necessarily carry an imputation of prejudice or other subjective factor, such as the experimenter's desire for a particular outcome. This differs from the conventional usage in which bias refers to a partisan point of view". Therefore bias is used here as a technical term whereby there is a systematic difference that arises between the two comparison groups that leads us to believe there is an association when in fact there is not. There are many different types of bias, and they generally fall into two main categories: information bias and selection bias. Recall bias, which was raised earlier in the context of the case-control study, is a form of information bias. However, this is not a problem in a cohort study where the study prospectively follows people over time. Nonetheless, there could still be other forms of information bias. For instance, observer bias occurs when the researchers recording the rates of disease pay closer attention to collecting all new cases of disease in the exposure group while missing new diagnoses in the control group. Selection bias occurs when the people in the exposure group differ from those in the control group in more ways than just the presence of the exposure. This was the case in the recent uproar over hormone replacement therapy, which called into question the utility of observational studies (i.e. case-control and cohort studies) altogether. Which brings us to the third reason for being cautious: confounding.

Confounding

At times, there can appear to be an association between an exposure and a health problem when in fact there is no such association but, rather, there is a confounding factor that makes it appear so. A confounder is both associated with the exposure and also associated with the health problem, but does not lie along the causal pathway between the two (Fig. 4.3). To provide a simple example to start off with, one might conduct a study and find an association between living in nursing homes and being diagnosed with cancer. This might lead you to wonder whether all nursing homes are built from some toxic carcinogenic substance. However, most people in nursing homes are relatively old, and most people who get cancer are also relatively old, therefore age could be a confounding factor which could explain this

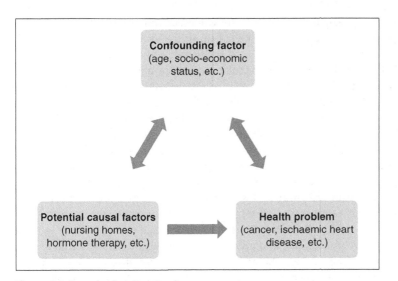

Figure 4.3 Example of confounding factors.

spurious association (i.e. advanced age is associated with living in nursing homes and is also associated with cancer). If you control for age (i.e. using different statistical techniques such as matching or stratification), you would likely find that the number of new cancer cases diagnosed each year among people who are over age 75 and living in nursing homes is the same as for those of the same age who are not living in nursing homes.

However, it is only possible to control for confounding if you can predict in advance what the confounders are likely to be (i.e. generally factors such as age, gender, etc.) or if you realise that there is a confounder that needs to be controlled for in the final analysis (e.g. if the association somehow does not make sense). This was a major problem in the observational studies on hormone replacement therapy (HRT), which neglected to control for an important and very common confounding factor, namely socio-economic status (SES). While there was quite a bit of discordance in the HRT literature and many HRT studies were quite small and therefore had wide confidence intervals that crossed 1 (i.e. difficult to conclude whether there is an association at all – positive or negative), several observational studies, including some larger ones, showed that women on hormone replacement therapy had a reduced risk of heart disease.[65] However, women in the exposure group who were already on HRT when recruited into the study tended to be wealthier and more educated than those in the control group who did not use HRT. Socio-economic status was therefore associated with the exposure (i.e. HRT) and was also associated with the outcome (i.e. heart disease). However, none of this really became apparent until a large randomised controlled trial was conducted of HRT versus placebo, called the Women's Health Initiative (WHI) study.[66]

Contradicting the conventional wisdom, which was even based on a systematic review of dozens of observational studies, the WHI study, which included over 16,000 women, showed that HRT was associated with an increased risk of heart disease (Hazard ratio = 1.29; 95% CI 1.02–1.63), breast cancer (1.26; 1.00–1.59), stroke (1.41; 1.07–1.85) and pulmonary embolus (2.13; 1.39–3.25). This was an important finding because pharmaceutical companies were seeing dollar signs flashing before their eyes with the prospect of being able to sell HRT to every woman on earth as soon as she turned 50 for the primary prevention of heart disease.

While HRT nonetheless appears to be protective for colorectal cancer (0.63; 0.43–0.92) and hip fractures (0.66; 0.45–0.98), there are other medications to prevent and treat osteoporosis (a condition associated with an increased risk of fractures), and the benefit–risk balance makes it unlikely that HRT will ever be used for colon cancer prevention. Indeed, it was a sad day for the pharmaceutical industry when the WHI results were announced, and it certainly put the scientific community into a tailspin – making them question what they can truly believe.[67] Later, when researchers went back and controlled for the confounding relating to socio-economic status, the findings of the observational studies were similar to the trial.[68] This illustrates a major benefit of randomisation, which can control for both known and unknown confounding factors. Rather than allowing research participants to self-select which study group they will be in, as occurs in observational studies (i.e. women already on HRT are placed in the exposure group and women not on HRT are placed in the control group), a randomised study recruits participants and then randomly assigns them to be in one "arm" or the other "arm" (e.g. to be in the intervention arm and receive HRT or to be in the control arm and receive placebo or standard of care). This obviates any selection bias or "healthy-woman effect" among women who are HRT users. As well, through double-blinding (i.e. when neither the researcher nor the research participant knows who has been assigned to which group), information bias is also less likely. Nonetheless, when entering the realm of experimental studies, there are other issues to consider such as precautions to safeguard against potential breaches of ethical conduct. But this is a whole other topic that I will save for a later section. The main point here is that even when there is evidence of an association, and even if it is a strong association, it is important to retain a certain sense of scepticism and to consider whether the other criteria for causality have also been met, often requiring further research.

Criteria for causality: association is necessary but not sufficient

Returning to the case example of a "world free from tobacco", the Minister of Health needn't reinvent the wheel and redo any of the research that has already been done to link cigarette smoking with poor health outcomes such as lung cancer, heart disease and premature death (unless there are very different types of exposures locally and questions as to whether these are also just as harmful as cigarette smoke). Rather, gathering the evidence that has already been produced by the international community is likely sufficient. Yet, the criteria for causality are helpful in gaining a better overview of the big picture (Table 4.6)[62] and can help in making the argument for the link between smoking and disease.

Table 4.6 The Bradford Hill criteria for causality.

(1) Strength of association
(2) Consistency
(3) Specificity
(4) Temporal relationship
(5) Dose-response relationship or biological gradient
(6) Biological plausibility
(7) Coherence
(8) Experimental evidence
(9) Analogy

Adapted from Hill AB. The environment and disease: association or causation? *Proc R Soc Med* 1965; 58: 295–300.

Beyond the impressive 14-fold strength of association (i.e. from the odds ratio and relative risk calculated based on Doll and Hill's observational studies), another important indicator that smoking is truly the cause of lung cancer, other types of cancer, heart disease and premature death is the dose-response relationship. A dose-response relationship exists when higher levels of exposure lead to higher levels of disease. In the case-control study there was already an indication of this relationship (Table 4.7).[60] There were twice as many heavy smokers and fewer light smokers among patients with lung cancer as compared with controls. The trend is even more apparent in the cohort study. Here we have prospective data on the rates of death (number of deaths per 1,000 man-years) according to whether a person was a light, moderate or heavy smoker. The risk of death due to these diseases was shown to increase with the average number of cigarettes smoked per day (Table 4.8).[61] This gradient is therefore strong additional evidence in support of causality.

Table 4.7 Example of the dose-response gradient from the case-control study.

	Light smoker: 1–14 cigarettes/day	Moderate smoker: 15–25 cigarettes/day	Heavy smoker: over 25 cigarettes/day
Lung cancer (n=647)	283 (43.7%)	196 (30.3%)	168 (26.0%)
Controls (n=622)	348 (56.0%)	190 (30.5%)	84 (13.5%)

Adapted from data in Doll R, Hill AB. Smoking and carcinoma of the lung. Preliminary report. *BMJ* 1950; ii: 739–48.

Table 4.8 Example of the dose-response gradient from a cohort study.

Health problem	Lifelong non-smokers	Light smoker: 1–14 cigarettes/day	Moderate smoker: 15–25 cigarettes/day	Heavy smoker: Over 25 cigarettes/day	Relative risk (heavy vs. light smoker)
Lung cancer	0.17	1.31	2.33	4.17	3.18
Mouth cancer	0.09	0.36	0.47	1.06	2.94
Other cancer	3.34	4.21	4.67	5.38	1.28
Heart disease	6.19	9.10	10.07	11.11	1.22
All-cause death	19.38	29.34	34.79	45.34	1.55

Adapted from data in Doll R, Peto R, Boreham J, Sutherland I. Mortality in relation to smoking: 50 years' observations on male British doctors. *BMJ* 2004; 328: 1519–28. Data is expressed as age-adjusted mortality rates per 1,000 man-years, except for the last column, which is a ratio.

Using a cohort study also satisfies the criteria for a temporal relationship. For an association between an exposure and an outcome to be truly causal, the exposure must occur before the outcome. In 1951, all of the doctors who entered the study were healthy. Smoking (i.e. the exposure) clearly occurred before the doctors developed the disease and died (i.e. the outcome). In contrast, in a case-control study, people are selected as cases when they already have the disease. Therefore, even if they report historical exposures, it is not as clear whether the exposure truly occurred before the disease. If the exposure occurred after the disease already developed, then it could not be a cause.

Even though observational studies (i.e. case-control and cohort studies) can provide valuable information on many of the criteria for causality, the addition of experimental evidence is quite powerful. Indeed, in the conventional hierarchy of evidence, experimental evidence is at the very top. The trouble with experimental evidence, however, is that it raises a wide range of ethical issues. Even though it is possible to conduct experiments in the laboratory on cell cultures, exposing them to chemicals found in cigarette smoke and determining the toxicity and carcinogenicity of these substances, it would certainly be highly unethical to conduct a randomised controlled trial where one group is randomly assigned to a potentially harmful exposure (i.e. tobacco smoke). Such trials are only possible when there is real doubt as to whether an exposure is harmful or beneficial. This is often referred to as "clinical equipoise", although it can be difficult to determine in practice.[69] Nonetheless, one could turn things around and instead conduct a randomised controlled trial that removes the harmful exposure to see whether people's health is improved. This is what Geoffrey Rose and Linda Colwell did. They conducted a randomised controlled trial (RCT) of anti-smoking advice. Out of over 16,000 civil servants enrolled in the UK Whitehall study, they selected 1,445 male smokers aged 40–59 years who were randomly assigned to two groups. After 20 years of follow-up, they found that the intervention group who received the anti-smoking advice had a 7% reduction in total mortality, a 13% reduction in heart disease mortality and an 11% reduction in lung cancer mortality as compared to the control group who did not receive the intervention.[70] Thus the data from the case-control study, the cohort study and the RCT all lead us to the same conclusion: that smoking is very likely a cause of lung cancer, as well as heart disease and premature mortality.

However, these are only three studies. True, they are classic studies which were well conducted and adequately powered to demonstrate an effect. But we rarely base our conclusions on such a small number of studies when there is a huge literature on the topic. This is where the value of systematic reviews and meta-analyses comes in – to give us a sense of the overall body of literature. Indeed, consistency and coherence are additional factors that help to determine whether an association is truly causal. According to researchers at the International Agency for Research on Cancer (IARC), "a meta-analysis of over 50 studies on involuntary smoking among never smokers showed a consistent and statistically significant association between exposure to environmental tobacco smoke and lung cancer risk".[71] Unlike in the HRT example above, the consistency of the findings among different research groups, using different types of epidemiological research studies, in different countries, with different study populations, further supports the link between smoking and cancer. Coherence exists when the epidemiological data are also in agreement with the basic and clinical science data. For instance, when lung cells are removed from the body and exposed to tobacco smoke in the laboratory, they exhibit signs of inflammation, which is a precursor to the initiation and progression of tumours.[72] As well, in a review of autopsy studies, "almost all studies indicate a significant association between cigarette smoking and degree of aortic atherosclerosis",[73] a precursor to heart disease. These are just a couple of examples of the numerous studies that illustrate the coherence between basic science research and the clinical and population-based research, which brings us to the next criterion on biological plausibility.

If an association is biologically plausible, there exists a logical biological explanation that explains how the exposure can cause the disease. For instance, the chemicals in tobacco smoke cause inflammation of the lung cells as well as genetic mutations within these cells, which leads to uncontrolled cell growth and tumour formation. This makes sense and is supported by the evidence. However, one should nonetheless be cautious. As noted previously, 5% of associations are found by chance alone, and if there is no basic explanation for the link, then this should raise some degree of scepticism. That being said, just because there is a good explanation, it does not automatically lead to the conclusion that the association is causal. Indeed, this was deceptively misleading in the case of HRT and the prevention of heart disease.[74] According to Bradford Hill, there can be no absolute certainty. Rather, the criteria are helpful in supporting or refuting whether a certain exposure causes a certain health outcome:

> Here then are nine different viewpoints from all of which we should study association before we cry causation. What I do not believe – and this has been suggested – that we can usefully lay down some hard-and-fast rules of evidence that must be obeyed before we can accept cause and effect. None of my nine viewpoints can bring indisputable evidence for or against the cause-and-effect hypothesis and none can be required as a *sine qua non*. What they can do, with greater or less strength, is to help us to make up our minds on the fundamental question – is there any other way of explaining the set of facts before us, is there any other answer equally, or more, likely than cause and effect?

Certainly, when it comes to smoking, the body of evidence is so large, and there is such strong support of almost all of the criteria for causality (except specificity, since tobacco smoke is associated with many different outcomes, not just one), that even sceptics could reasonably conclude that smoking is indeed an important cause of lung cancer, other types of cancers, heart disease and premature death.

Logic models: mapping out the causes and opportunities for intervention

Often the causes of health problems are complex and involve a number of proximal risk factors as well as upstream determinants of health. For instance, smoking (i.e. a risk factor) causes lung cancer, but what causes people to start smoking in the first place, and to continue smoking for decades? Indeed, there is a whole literature on the various factors, such as peer pressure, marketing and social norms, which influence young people to start smoking. Then, because nicotine is an addictive substance, once smokers develop a dependence to tobacco it is much more difficult to quit smoking. Even non-smokers are at risk of disease and therefore need to be protected from environmental tobacco smoke (ETS). A "logic model" can explain the complex relationship between the various causal factors and the health problem as a starting point for developing interventions to target these causes. For instance, the Task Force on Community Preventive Services developed a logic model for interventions to prevent the initiation of smoking, to promote smoking cessation, and to reduce exposure to ETS, as a means of reducing disease incidence and mortality (Fig. 4.4).[75]

The next step in the research cycle is determining what works to improve health. This involves developing new interventions or identifying existing interventions that act on the causes of poor health, and then conducting further research to assess which of these interventions actually makes a difference in improving health outcomes.

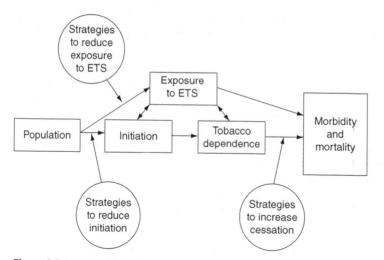

Figure 4.4 Logic model to reduce tobacco use and exposure to environmental tobacco smoke. Adapted from Hopkins DP, Briss PA, Ricard CJ *et al.* on behalf of the Task Force on Community Preventive Services. Reviews of evidence regarding interventions to reduce tobacco use and exposure to environmental tobacco smoke. *Am J Prev Med* 2001; 20(2 Suppl): 16–66.

Step 3: Developing interventions to improve health

As with the previous steps in the cycle, there are many different types of research needed in developing, piloting and testing interventions for improving health outcomes (Table 4.9). While intervention research in a clinical context has long been an important fixture (e.g. does drug X work to treat disease Y? Does screening for early signs of disease Z reduce mortality?), the field of intervention research in a community and population context is just beginning to take off.[76] Interventions can range from clinical preventive services to national and global-level policies and programmes such as anti-smoking laws, "sin taxes" and the WHO Framework Convention on Tobacco Control. Since population health has two main goals – to improve the health of the population and to reduce health inequities – there can therefore be two types of population-level health interventions: those that aim to improve the health of the population overall and those that aim to reduce health inequities. Increasingly, the focus is on the latter – i.e. interventions which promote greater health equity.

In 2004, the Canadian Institutes of Health Research created the Population Health Intervention Research Centre (PHIRC) based in Calgary, Alberta and directed by Professor Penny Hawe. According to Hawe and colleague Louise Potvin from the Léa-Roback Research Centre on Social Inequalities and Health at the University of Montreal:

> Population-level health interventions are policies or programs that shift the distribution of health risk by addressing the underlying social, economic and environmental conditions... [and] population health intervention research involves the use of scientific methods to produce knowledge about policy and program interventions that operate within or outside of the health sector and have the potential to impact health at the population level.[77]

Hawe and Potvin argue that population intervention research can also incorporate aspects of implementation and evaluation research, which occur further along in the research cycle.

Table 4.9 Research evidence on interventions that can improve health.

Question	Research	Study type	Evidence
The potential impact of an intervention			
How much disease is caused by this particular exposure?	Epidemiological research	Cohort studies, etc.	Attributable risk (AR) Attributable risk proportion (AR%)
How much disease would remain even if you had an intervention that could eliminate this exposure entirely?	Epidemiological research	Cohort studies, etc.	Baseline risk
In a population with a given incidence of disease, by how much could the incidence be reduced if you had an intervention that could eliminate the exposure entirely?	Epidemiological research	Cohort studies, population-level data, etc.	Population attributable risk (PAR) Population attributable risk proportion (PAR%)
Considering that not everyone in the population will receive the intervention, and that the intervention will not have 100% efficacy, what will be the likely impact on the population?	Epidemiological research	Randomised controlled trials (RCTs), population-level data, etc.	Population impact number (PIN)
Developing the intervention			
What is likely to be a useful intervention and what would be the important health outcomes to measure?	Qualitative research / historical research	Interviews, focus groups, historical analysis, etc.	Potential interventions Patient/population-informed outcomes
What are the mechanisms by which the intervention could eliminate or prevent the exposure?	Laboratory research /social science research	Laboratory studies, social science studies, etc.	Biological and social mechanisms
Efficacy, harms and costs of the intervention			
What is the efficacy of the intervention in preventing or treating disease?	Epidemiological research / secondary research	Randomised controlled trials, quasi-experimental studies, systematic reviews, etc.	Attributable risk reduction (ARR) Relative risk reduction (RRR)
How many people would need to receive the intervention to prevent one person from developing the disease or to result in one person suffering harm due to the intervention?	Epidemiological research	Randomised controlled trials (RCTs), etc.	Number needed to treat (NNT) Number needed to harm (NNH)
What is the overall cost of the intervention and what is the incremental cost per incremental improvement in health?	Economic evaluations	Cost analysis, cost–benefit analysis, cost-effectiveness analysis, cost–utility analysis, etc.	Cost Cost–benefit ratio Cost-effectiveness ratio Cost–utility ratio

Indeed, at the population level, given the size of these interventions and the complexity involved, it is not always feasible to consider these as three distinct steps in the research cycle (i.e. intervention development, implementation and evaluation occur simultaneously). However, for the sake of simplicity and a clearer understanding, the latter two will be described separately in the following section.

The potential impact of an intervention

Before developing interventions for a specific health problem, let alone testing whether the interventions work, it is important to think about which of the causes to prioritise and where to intervene to have the greatest impact on improving health (something that is not always done in an explicit way). Until now, we have been more interested in *whether* an exposure causes a disease. Once we are satisfied that there is sufficient evidence to support a causal link, we still need to know *how much* disease is caused by the exposure, and therefore how much disease can be prevented by eliminating, reducing or in some way modifying the exposure. This can be achieved using the same data as previously from Doll's cohort study plugged into a two-by-two table (Table 4.5). But instead of calculating the relative risk, we can calculate the attributable risk (also known as the absolute risk or risk difference) using the following formula: $AR = [a / (a + b)] - [c / (c + d)]$ (Table 4.10).[61]

Over the 50-year follow-up of the British male doctors, we saw that 86% of smokers had died from all causes $[a / (a + b)]$ as compared to only 55% of life-long non-smokers $[c / (c + d)]$. The attributable risk (i.e. the percentage of deaths due to smoking) is 86% − 55%, which comes to 31%. Therefore, out of every 100 deaths, 31 can be attributed to smoking, and the remainder are due to other causes (i.e. unhealthy diet, lack of exercise, injuries, etc.).

Going back to the lung cancer data more specifically, the rate of death due to lung cancer was 2.49 per 1,000 man-years among current smokers $[a / (a + b)]$ and 0.17 per 1,000 man-years among life-long non-smokers $[c / (c + d)]$. The attributable risk (AR) is therefore 2.49 − 0.17, which comes to 2.32 per 1,000 man-years. The number of deaths that remain (i.e. in this example, 0.17 deaths per 1,000 man-years) is the baseline rate of lung cancer deaths

Table 4.10 Drawing a two-by-two table and calculating attributable risk based on a cohort study.

	Disease (death from all causes)	No disease (still alive in 2001)	Total
Exposure group (smokers)	22,429	3,507	25,936
Control group (lifelong non-smokers)	2,917	2,395	5,312
Total	25,346	5,902	31,248

Adapted from data in Doll R, Peto R, Boreham J, Sutherland I. Mortality in relation to smoking: 50 years' observations on male British doctors. *BMJ* 2004; 328: 1519–28. Note: the paper reports that 17% of the original cohort of 34,439 male British doctors were lifelong non-smokers. However, the proportion of lifelong non-smokers among the 31,248 who were successfully followed up until 2001 (i.e. 50 years later) is not reported. For the purposes of this illustration, I have retained the proportion of 17% although this may not exactly reflect the data (i.e. if more smokers were lost to follow-up as compared to non-smokers, for instance).

due to other causes (i.e. asbestos exposure, occupational causes, etc.). We can also calculate the attributable risk proportion (AR%). This is essentially the attributable risk divided by the incidence in the exposed group: AR / $[a / (a + b)]$. From the same example, this comes to 2.32 / 2.49, which is 93%. Therefore, if an intervention is 100% effective in getting people to quit smoking, then 93% of lung cancer deaths could be eliminated.

However, not everyone in the population will be a smoker. Before spending money on an intervention, policy-makers will want to know the impact that it will have on the population. This can be calculated using the population attributable risk (PAR), which is the incidence of death or disease in the total population minus the baseline risk (i.e. the incidence in lifelong non-smokers). If you do not know the population incidence, then you can use the following formula:

(Incidence exposed × Percentage exposed in population)
+ (Incidence unexposed × Percentage unexposed in population)
− (Incidence unexposed).

Among the entire cohort, 83% were smokers and 17% were life-long non-smokers. Therefore the PAR for the cohort overall is $(2.49 \times 0.83) + (0.17 \times 0.17) - (0.17)$, which comes to 1.93 per 1,000 person-years. Similarly, the population attributable risk proportion (PAR%) is PAR / Incidence in the total population. So what does all this mean? In the cohort of British doctors, had they all received an intervention that was 100% effective at helping people to quit smoking, and since not all of them were smokers, then 1.93 lung cancer deaths per 1,000 person-years could have been prevented (rather than 2.32 per 1,000 person-years). Since, nowadays, the prevalence of smoking in many countries is already greatly reduced (e.g. 20–30%, rather than over 80%), the added value of anti-smoking interventions could be calculated using the above formulas, but would be considerably less as compared to the historical cohort, where there was a very high prevalence of smoking. That being said, many low- and middle-income countries have very high smoking rates, and therefore anti-smoking interventions could potentially have an even greater impact in these contexts.

Until now, we have been assuming that the intervention would be 100% effective and that everyone who is exposed will actually receive the intervention. In real life, however, this is rarely the case. Heller has therefore proposed a population impact number (PIN) which takes into consideration the proportion of people in the population who have the exposure, the proportion of those with exposure who will realistically receive the intervention, and the efficacy of the intervention, defined as the number needed to treat to prevent one negative health outcome. The number needed to treat is a measure that has emerged from the evidence-based medicine (EBM) movement and can be derived from RCT data. To do so, you first need to calculate the attributable risk reduction (ARR), which is the rate of negative outcomes (e.g. lung cancer deaths) in the control group minus the rate of negative outcomes in the intervention group. The ARR is therefore the absolute reduction of negative outcomes that can be attributed to the intervention. The number needed to treat (NNT) is then calculated as 1 / ARR. It is the number of people who would have to receive the intervention to avoid one person with a negative outcome. For instance, in the RCT of an anti-smoking intervention reported by Rose and Colwell, there was an 11% reduction in lung cancer mortality in the intervention group as compared to the control group (i.e. ARR = 11%).[70] The number needed to treat is 1 / 0.11, which is 9. One would therefore have to offer the anti-smoking intervention to 9 people for 1 person to benefit from an averted lung cancer death. The other 8 people receiving the intervention would have no benefit. Indeed, since no intervention is without some risk of adverse effects, there is also the possibility that the intervention may cause unintended harm. One can, in a similar way, calculate the number needed to harm (NNH), to help in assessing the balance of benefits and harms.

Thus the population impact number (PIN) provides a more nuanced estimate of what kind of effect can be expected as a result of developing and implementing an intervention. Starting out already thinking about the final impact that an intervention could potentially have on the health of the population is helpful in prioritising which types of interventions should be developed, which outcomes are likely to be affected and what one might reasonably expect as a result of widespread implementation.

Developing the intervention

With a better sense of which causes are the greatest contributors to the health problem, and what could be the potential impact on the health of the population if these causes were addressed, the next step is to actually develop the intervention. This is a whole process in and of itself which can also be informed by research. One can conduct historical research or ethnographic research to see what has been done across different periods or what has been successful in different cultures around the world to get ideas for potential interventions. One can conduct basic science research or social science research to better understand the bio-logical and social mechanisms and targets for interventions. One can conduct secondary research to know what interventions have already been tested and how well they work. One can ask people affected by the health problem using participatory research and qualitative research methods to better understand what they consider would be good solutions and what they think would be the most important health outcomes that should be used to measure success. One can use theoretical frameworks based on previous research findings as a basis for developing the intervention. Interventions can be single component or multi-component. They can be aimed at a clinical level or a population level. The common theme here is that an intervention is intended to improve the health of the individual and the population, and that the benefits in terms of improved health outcomes should outweigh any potential harms, ranging from the side effects of a medication to stigmatisation and discrimination from genetic screening.

Efficacy, harms and costs of the intervention

Once the intervention has been developed, we would want to know whether it works, how well it works, whether there are any unwanted negative consequences, whether the benefits of the intervention outweigh the harms, and how much this will cost per incremental improve-ment in health. Often, when we speak about whether an intervention works in a research setting where there is generally a more controlled environment and greater attention to ensuring that the intervention is well delivered, we call this "efficacy". In contrast, once an intervention has been proven efficacious and is scaled-up in practice, the effect may become diluted since not everyone may know the intervention exists, it may not be used exactly as intended, and so forth. Therefore, how well the intervention works in a real-life setting is generally called "effectiveness". For now, our focus is on efficacy.

As mentioned previously, the "gold standard" for determining the efficacy of an inter-vention is the double-blind randomised controlled trial (RCT). Essentially, an RCT is an experimental study whereby participants are recruited to the study, and, if they consent to participate, they are randomly assigned to one of two groups. In the first group, the participants receive the intervention (i.e. intervention arm) and, in the second group, the participants do not receive the intervention (i.e. control arm). Thus, the study is controlled by the researchers who provide the intervention to one group but not the other group and then measure the outcomes. This is in contrast to observational studies such as case-control and cohort studies described previously, where there is no intervention and researchers simply observe groups with different outcomes to determine whether there was any difference in exposures between the two groups (i.e. case-control studies) or observe groups with different exposures to determine whether there was any difference in outcomes between the two groups (i.e. cohort studies). Rather, in RCTs, randomisation ensures that both groups (i.e. the intervention arm and the control arm) are identical in all respects with the exception that one group receives the intervention and the other group does not. Indeed, randomisation is a powerful tool to reduce selection bias and control for confounding (as described earlier) by ensuring that factors such as age, gender and so forth are equally distributed among both groups. Randomisation can even equally distribute factors that one may not have thought about in advance of the study. In double-blinded RCTs, neither the researchers nor the participants are aware of who is in the intervention arm and who is in the control arm. This further reduces possible observation bias and placebo effect.

However, even though RCTs are the gold standard, not all such studies have been carried out with the same rigour, thus affecting the internal validity and hence the usefulness of the results. In 1993, 30 experts, comprised of medical journal editors, clinical trialists, epidemiologists and methodologists, met in Ottawa, Canada with the aim of developing a new scale to assess the quality of randomised controlled trials. However, they found that many of the suggested scale items were irrelevant because they were not routinely reported by authors. The CONSORT statement was therefore developed to standardise the reporting of RCTs so that it would be possible to better judge the quality of such trials.[78]

According to the recently updated CONSORT 2010 statement, all RCTs must be reported in a systematic way. For instance, the authors should use the word "randomised" in the title so that it will be possible to identify the study as being an RCT when searching in Medline or other online databases. The abstract should include a structured summary of the trial design, methods, results and conclusions. The introduction should clearly state the scientific background, the rationale for the study, the study objectives and the hypothesis being tested (e.g. the intervention will improve outcomes A and B without causing harm C). The methods section should describe in detail the main features of the study, which are given the acronym "PICO". These features include: (1) the population (i.e. recruitment procedures, inclusion criteria, exclusion criteria), (2) the intervention (i.e. who receives what, when and how), (3) the control or "routine care" (i.e. who receives what, when and how), and (4) the outcomes (e.g. primary outcome death, secondary outcomes quality of life, cost, etc.). The methods should also specify the trial design, the analysis used (i.e. subgroup analyses, etc.), the sample size calculations (i.e. the number of people needed in each group to detect a difference between the intervention arm and the control arm), how randomisation and blinding were carried out (i.e. computer-generated tables, etc.) and the stopping rules (i.e. allowing the study to be terminated early if the interim analysis shows a significant difference or excessive harm from the intervention). The results section should begin with a flow chart describing the number of participants enrolled in the study, the number who were then excluded for various reasons, the number randomly assigned to each group, the number allocated to each group who actually received the intervention/control, losses to follow-up, and the number included in the analysis. Next, in Table 1, the intervention arm and the control arm are compared at baseline for important demographic and clinical characteristics so that readers can assess how comparable the groups were before receiving the intervention or control (i.e. placebo or standard of care). Finally, the outcomes are reported (both positive outcomes and adverse events) including the number and percentage with each outcome in the intervention arm and in the control arm, as well as the difference between the intervention and control arm, the 95% confidence interval (CI) of the difference and whether this difference is significant (e.g. p-value < 0.05 or 95% CI that does not cross 1). The discussion section then wraps up with a summary of the limitations of the study, the generalisability of the findings and the interpretation in light of other relevant evidence.

Even though in an ideal world all interventions would be tested using an RCT or a variation thereof (i.e. cross-over study, factorial design, cluster RCT, etc.), in practice this is not always possible. RCTs are extremely expensive and are also subject to important ethical considerations. Therefore, alternative study designs can also be used, such as quasi-experimental studies (which will be described in greater detail in the next section).

Ethical considerations in research

While all types of research raise various ethical questions, experimental research – including RCTs – is a particularly sensitive area. Following the atrocities of the Second World War, where research conducted in the name of science led to terrible suffering and even the premature death of those who were involuntary research subjects, there are now extremely stringent guidelines for conducting research. Indeed, as early as 1949, the Nuremberg Code laid out 10 core requirements for conducting research on human subjects (Table 4.11).[79]

Table 4.11 The Nuremberg Code's 10 directives for human experimentation.

(1) The voluntary consent of the human subject is absolutely essential.

(2) The experiment should be such as to yield fruitful results for the good of society, unprocurable by other methods or means of study, and not random and unnecessary in nature.

(3) The experiment should be so designed . . . that the anticipated results will justify the performance of the experiment.

(4) The experiment should be so conducted as to avoid all unnecessary physical and mental suffering and injury.

(5) No experiment should be conducted where there is an *a priori* reason to believe that death or disabling injury will occur; except, perhaps, in those experiments where the experimental physicians also serve as subjects.

(6) The degree of risk to be taken should never exceed that determined by the humanitarian importance of the problem to be solved by the experiment.

(7) Proper preparations should be made and adequate facilities provided to protect the experimental subject against even remote possibilities of injury, disability or death.

(8) The experiment should be conducted only by scientifically qualified persons.

(9) During the course of the experiment the human subject should be at liberty to bring the experiment to an end if he has reached the physical or mental state where continuation of the experiment seems to him to be impossible.

(10) During the course of the experiment the scientist in charge must be prepared to terminate the experiment at any stage, if he has probable cause to believe, in the exercise of the good faith, superior skill and careful judgment required of him that a continuation of the experiment is likely to result in injury, disability or death to the experimental subject.

Adapted from *Trials of War Criminals before the Nuremberg Military Tribunals under Control Council Law No. 10*, Vol. 2. Washington, DC: US Government Printing Office, 1949, pp. 181–2.

Following the Nuremberg Code, many other guidelines for the ethical conduct of research have been produced, including the Declaration of Helsinki of the World Medical Association and the Canadian Tri-Council Policy Statement.[80, 81] Prior to carrying out a research study, the research protocol must be approved by an Institutional Review Board (IRB) or Ethics Committee. An IRB is a committee whose primary responsibility is to protect the rights and welfare of the people who participate in research studies. In many countries, institutions conducting research on human subjects are federally mandated to have an IRB. In particular, IRBs ensure that informed consent is obtained prior to recruitment into the study. According to the Declaration of Helsinki:

> in medical research involving competent human subjects, each potential subject must be adequately informed of the aims, methods, sources of funding, any possible conflicts of interest, institutional affiliations of the researcher, the anticipated benefits and potential risks of the study and the discomfort it may entail, and any other relevant aspects of the study. The potential subject must be informed of the right to refuse to participate in the study or to withdraw consent to participate at any time without reprisal.

Research ethics becomes even more complicated when conducting research in low- and middle-income countries. According to Marcia Angell:

> Our ethical standards should not depend on where the research is performed. . . the nature of investigators' responsibility for the welfare of their subjects should not be influenced by the political and economic conditions of the region. . . any other position could lead to the exploitation of people in developing countries in order to conduct research that could not be performed in the sponsoring countries.[82]

Therefore, without going into too much detail here (indeed, entire books are written on the subject of research ethics), suffice it to say that, while high-quality evidence is important, RCTs and other forms of experimentation are particularly prone to ethical concerns. Thus, it is necessary to protect those participating in research to ensure that they are not harmed in the evidence-gathering process, even if it sometimes means that the research does not take place.

Steps 4 and 5: Implementing interventions and evaluating outcomes

The final steps in the research cycle are the implementation and evaluation of the intervention in "real world" settings rather than controlled research settings. Again, many different types of research questions can be answered in relation to this, using a number of different research methodologies (Table 4.12).

Of course, one would not expect an intervention to have an impact on the health of the population if the intervention was not properly implemented to begin with. Therefore, it is often advisable to collect information on various "process outcomes" that can be used to determine the adequacy of implementation. If the intervention involves behavioural counselling, for example, then how many health workers were trained to provide such counselling, were the trainings sufficient to allow them to develop the adequate knowledge and skills needed for such counselling, how many printed leaflets were produced to be handed out to patients to reinforce the counselling messages, were these leaflets readily available in the clinic waiting rooms and so forth. To give another example, if the intervention is a policy change, then were key players aware of the change in policy, to what extent was the policy enforced in that jurisdiction and so forth. If the implementation proves to be less than adequate, we would want to know why this was so and,

Table 4.12 Research evidence on intervention implementation and evaluation of health outcomes

Question	Research	Study type	Evidence
Intervention implementation			
Was the intervention properly implemented?	Mixed methods research	Cross-sectional surveys, interviews, focus groups, etc.	Process outcomes
Was the intervention well-adapted to the local context?	Mixed methods research	Cross-sectional surveys, interviews, focus groups, etc.	Contextual adaptation
What were the barriers and facilitators to implementation?	Mixed methods research	Cross-sectional surveys, interviews, focus groups, etc.	Barriers Facilitators
Did the intervention reach the target population?	Epidemiological research	Cross-sectional surveys, etc.	Access to the intervention
Was there good uptake and ongoing use of the intervention?	Epidemiological research	Interviews, focus groups, etc.	Uptake rates Dropout rates
If uptake and/or compliance were low, why is that?	Qualitative research	Interviews, focus groups, etc.	Reasons for low uptake and/or poor compliance
Evaluation of health outcomes			
Did the intervention improve the health of the population?	Epidemiological research	Quasi-experimental study, etc.	Health outcomes (e.g. mortality, morbidity, etc.)
What impact did the intervention have on reducing health inequities?	Epidemiological research	Quasi-experimental study, etc.	Disparities in health outcomes
Were there any unintended consequences as a result of implementing the intervention?	Mixed methods research	Cross-sectional surveys, interviews, focus groups, etc.	Harm
What could be improved to make the intervention more effective and to further minimise harm?	Mixed methods research	Cross-sectional surveys, interviews, focus groups, etc.	Suggestions for improvements
What is the overall cost of implementing the intervention in a real-life setting and what is the incremental cost per incremental improvement in health?	Economic evaluations	Cost analysis, cost-benefit analysis, cost-effectiveness analysis, cost-utility analysis, etc.	Cost Cost-benefit ratio Cost-effectiveness ratio Cost-utility ratio

vice versa, what increases the chances that a programme or policy will be well implemented? This can involve research into the barriers and facilitators surrounding the implementation process, including whether and how the intervention was adapted to the local cultural and social context.

However, even if the intervention is well implemented, did it reach the people it was supposed to reach? An opportunistic screening programme that waits for patients to present to a clinic or health centre may not reach certain vulnerable groups within the target population due to various barriers such as language barriers, distance barriers, financial barriers and so on. Thus, even if the screening programme has been well implemented, only those who present to the health centre will access this service, disadvantaging a certain proportion of the target population and potentially even increasing health inequities as a result. Another example is a school programme on sexual health delivered in grade 10. If the local high-school dropout rate is over 50%, then even if the programme is well implemented in all schools across the region, less than half of the target population will have access to the programme. Yet, even if everyone in the target population is offered the intervention (i.e. through outreach or other means), not everyone will agree to try the intervention. This is probably a good thing, demonstrating that people have given their free and informed consent to participate in the programme.[83] Moreover, even if people do agree to try the intervention, they may not continue to use the intervention due to side effects or other reasons. Qualitative research can help us to understand why people choose not to try an intervention or to abandon an intervention. Such information is important since, unless there is wide-scale uptake and adherence, the intervention will not be used and therefore will have little impact on health.

Ultimately, what we really want to know is whether an intervention has improved the health of the population and has reduced health inequities. This does not entail process indicators measuring the adequacy of implementation, but rather an assessment of the actual impact of the intervention on health outcomes in a real-life setting. Commonly used ways of assessing whether there has been a positive change in population health are quasi-experimental studies such as pre–post studies and natural experiments. These studies are called "quasi"-experimental because people are not recruited and assigned to two different groups (i.e. the intervention arm and the control arm) as with RCTs. Rather, in pre–post studies, the health of the entire target population is measured as a baseline (using a cross-sectional survey, for instance), and then the intervention is implemented across the entire population, followed by measuring how health outcomes (including health inequities) have changed as a result. Thus the population acts as its own control group whereby the data collected prior to the implementation of the intervention serve as a basis for comparison with the data collected after implementation. However, there could have been other factors that also changed over time which could explain the changes in health outcomes. Another approach is therefore to use a natural experiment.

In a natural experiment, a new programme or policy is implemented in Jurisdiction A but not in Jurisdiction B. It is therefore possible to assess the health of both jurisdictions prior to implementation and following implementation. If there is an improvement of the health of the population in Jurisdiction A but not in Jurisdiction B, that provides evidence that the policy or programme has had a positive impact. If there are improvements in health in both jurisdictions but no difference between the health of Jurisdiction A and B, then some external factor may have led to the health improvements, but it is unlikely that the intervention under study has had an impact on health. Of course, reasons for equivocal results could include that the intervention in Jurisdiction A was not well implemented, that uptake rates were low, that dropout rates were high, or that another programme or policy in Jurisdiction B improved health to the same degree. As noted previously, each research study is just another piece in the puzzle and needs to be considered as part of the larger body of evidence before jumping to any conclusions.

Finally, if an intervention has been shown to produce a positive impact on health, then prior to wide-scale implementation (i.e. scaling up across multiple jurisdictions within a country or even across countries), there are still many questions that need to be answered (see Chapter 6). For instance, policy-makers would likely want to know how much the actual implementation of the intervention will cost, and what is the incremental cost per additional health benefit produced. Economic evaluations, for instance, can provide this information. Since resources are finite, and even if there is very strong evidence that an intervention is beneficial, it does not necessarily follow that the intervention is affordable or feasible in a given context. Moreover, demonstrating that an intervention is inexpensive and able to produce a health benefit in a controlled research setting is very different from ensuring that the health benefit can be realised within a given budget when the intervention is implemented on a larger scale in a "real world" setting.

The overlap between research, implementation and evaluation

The tail end of the research cycle, which deals with implementation and evaluation, is a grey zone where research blends into practice. In research, the purpose is to generate new knowledge and to develop and test hypotheses. This entails using the various research study designs described above and it also requires IRB approval to protect research participants (regardless of the study design chosen, even if certain studies such as RCTs are generally associated with greater risks than other studies such as qualitative interviews). In contrast, the purpose of implementation and evaluation is to improve the effectiveness and efficiency of programmes and policies. The methods are very context sensitive and generally there is no IRB approval required.

There are many different types of evaluation.[84] Formative evaluation is carried out during the intervention development stage to ensure that the basis for the intervention is sound and that there is adequate piloting and testing prior to large-scale implementation. Process evaluation monitors the implementation of the intervention and whether or not it reaches the intended target audience. Outcome evaluation examines whether the stated intervention objectives were met in the short or medium term (e.g. changes in knowledge, attitudes and behaviours). Impact evaluation looks at whether the intervention made a difference in improving health in the long term (i.e. disease incidence, mortality rates, etc.). In practice, however, the focus is often on two categories: process and outcomes (broadly defined) – and generally elements of both are integrated.[85]

For example, clinical preventive practices include interventions such as behaviour change counselling to reduce exposure to risk factors as a means of preventing disease and improving health. Clinical audit can therefore be regarded as a form of evaluation that uses specific criteria to compare a clinical service or clinical preventive practice to the gold standard to see where standards are met and where there is room for improvement. Clinical audit can look at both process and outcome measures. For instance, a chart review may be carried out to determine the number of patients who are smokers and who were seen by a health worker in the previous year. Of those, the audit would determine what proportion of patients received the gold standard of care as defined by national or international clinical practice guidelines. As well, the audit could also determine whether patients who received the best quality care had better health outcomes. The specific process-related criteria might be the proportion of smokers who had been: (1) asked whether they smoke, (2) advised by their health provider to quit smoking, (3) prescribed smoking cessation therapy (e.g. nicotine patch), and (4) referred for smoking cessation support (e.g. telephone helpline). The specific outcome-related criteria could be the proportion of smokers who successfully quit smoking among those receiving the best standard of care as compared to those who received substandard care. The report of the audit would then be used to provide feedback to the health care providers working in that clinic with recommendations for improving performance to be able to reach the predetermined standards and to improve the health of smokers in their practice.

Similar to the clinical setting, the evaluation of interventions can also be carried out on population-level policies and programmes. For instance, the US Centers for Disease Control and Prevention (CDC) established a six-step framework for the evaluation of programmes in public health.[86] The first step is to engage the key stakeholders involved (i.e. the people running the programme, the target population served and, in particular, those who will be using the findings of the evaluation). The second step is to describe the programme in detail (including the rationale, goals and objectives, target population, activities, resources, context and so on). The third step is to determine the scope of the evaluation depending on why the evaluation is being carried out and how the results will be used (i.e. are there concerns that the programme is not reaching certain target audiences, does the programme go over budget, etc.). The fourth step involves gathering credible evidence (which generally involves collecting data on both process and outcome indicators). The fifth step is to use the data collected to draw conclusions and make recommendations for change (i.e. was the programme well implemented? Were the goals and objectives met? What improvements can be made?). Finally, the sixth step is to share the lessons learned and ensure that the findings of the evaluation are used to change policy and practice.

Although evaluation is intended to be part of a cycle of continuous quality improvement, there are often multiple barriers to evaluation. These include: lack of management support and resources to carry out an evaluation, lack of time and skills of the workers who are too busy implementing the programme to take a step back and evaluate what works well and what could be improved, lack of data when evaluations are not planned from the outset and therefore there is no baseline data to compare to, and fear that the results of the evaluation may lead to criticism and even losing one's job. Therefore a culture of evaluation needs to be cultivated so that this becomes part of the routine. Of course, that is often easier said than done. Since there are an increasing number of tried and tested interventions in the research setting that are not being used in practice to improve health, how to improve implementation and evaluation are in themselves becoming important fields of inquiry – further blurring the lines between research, implementation and evaluation.

Implementation research

Implementation research has been defined as the study of methods to promote the uptake of research findings into routine practice.[87] According to the WHO, most research to date has focused on the development of new interventions rather than optimising the delivery of existing interventions:

> New tools and interventions are not enough to tackle disease in the developing world – there is a growing gap between the availability of tools/knowledge about disease and what is actually done to make use of these in disease settings. To be effective, they need to be usable within the available health system framework and implemented appropriately so that the end user is able to benefit from them. This is where research into health systems and implementation fits in. Lack of resources – both financial and in terms of staffing levels – means that disease endemic countries need to find ways to best use the resources they have available; health systems research can help identify best practices and prioritize areas that need strengthening. Meanwhile, implementation research focuses on studying how research outcomes can be translated into practice; an important part of this is the development of community-based interventions.[88]

An implementation research platform has therefore been developed to address these delivery issues, exploring the challenges of generalising research findings in the real world and contextualising interventions for implementation in specific settings.[89]

Evaluation research

According to the *Oxford English Dictionary*, the term "evaluation research" has been in use for many decades. In the 1960s, evaluation research was used for assessing the impact of training programmes in the field of business and management, and soon after was also adapted for evaluating the effectiveness of social programmes. While there are many different definitions and interpretations of what evaluation research is and does, it has been defined by Rutman as "the use of scientific methods to measure the implementation and outcomes of programmes for decision-making purposes"[90] (e.g. using pre-post study designs or natural experiments as described earlier). Thus the purpose of evaluation research is to assist decision-makers in making better-informed choices about whether or not to continue, modify or discontinue a certain policy or programme. Not only is this important for performance management by demonstrating accountability and the judicious use of public funds,[91] but, ultimately, evaluation research is important to ensure that the interventions implemented are indeed improving the health and well-being of individuals and populations.

Ensuring that the research cycle goes full circle

We have now reached the end of the research cycle (Fig. 4.2). Indeed, there are many different types of research studies that can be used to answer a wide variety of research questions. However, in practice, there are certain types of studies that generally prevail whereas other types of studies are few and far between. For instance, until recently, there was relatively little done in the health field in the area of implementation and evaluation research as most research was focused on earlier stages of the research cycle. Researchers would develop research protocols, apply for funding, conduct their research studies to measure disease or understand causes or test interventions, prepare manuscripts for publication in high-impact, peer-reviewed journals often concluding that "more research is needed", and then start the process all over again – essentially bypassing the implementation and evaluation stages (Fig. 4.5).

Applying research evidence to make a positive impact on health was not traditionally considered to be part of the "job" of researchers. There is still very little kudos and few incentives for researchers to become engaged in such activities. Indeed, entire books have been written on how to increase the interaction between knowledge producers (i.e. researchers) and knowledge users (i.e. practitioners and policy-makers).[92] However, this disconnect is not at all surprising if one looks at the world that researchers inhabit. Researchers, who are generally affiliated with a university or research institution, are promoted and receive merit-based salary increases if they can demonstrate that they are productive as researchers. Proof of this productivity includes how much money has been secured through successful research grants, how many research students have been supervised at the Masters and PhD levels, and how many research articles have been published, particularly in high-impact, peer-reviewed journals. Moreover, researcher-practitioners who have one foot in the "ivory tower" of academia and one foot in the "real world" can find it difficult to compete with full-time researchers who devote the majority of their time to teaching and research (i.e. applying for

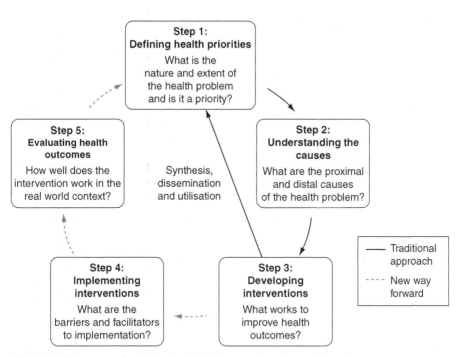

Figure 4.5 The new way forward: ensuring that the research cycle goes full circle.

grants, publishing papers, etc.). Thus, to encourage greater use of the research evidence in practice, the entire incentive system has to change. Slowly, there is some progress in this area.

For instance, it is increasingly being recognised that research evidence will have very little impact if it does not reach the key knowledge users who are in a position to apply this information to motivate change. Ideally, according to Parry and colleagues, these knowledge users should be engaged in the research process from the very outset, to help identify the key knowledge gaps that need to be addressed and to then "translate" the evidence into policy and practice.[93] This increased emphasis on "integrated knowledge translation" certainly requires more time and effort to build up the required interdisciplinary and intersectoral partnerships, but it also increases the chances that the research findings will be applied and used in practice and will be more likely to yield tangible results in the long run.

Even if researchers are progressively being encouraged to think about how the research findings can be applied in practice and can now apply for a growing number of knowledge dissemination grants, there nonetheless remain perverse incentive systems in the way that research is funded that leads to some types of research being prioritised over other types of research; not because it is more important, nor because it will lead to more significant health gains, but due to financial motives and self-interest. Pratt and Loff argue that research legislation and policies used in high-income countries have increasingly led these countries to invest in health research aimed at boosting national economic competitiveness rather than reducing health inequities:

> the regulation of research has encouraged a model that leads to products that can be commercialized; targets health needs that can be met by profitable, high-technology products; has the licensing of new products as its endpoint; and does not entail significant research capacity strengthening in other countries. Accordingly, investment in international

research is directed towards pharmaceutical trials and product development public–private partnerships for neglected diseases. This diverts funding away from research that is needed to implement existing interventions and to strengthen health systems, i.e. health policy and systems research.[94]

Whereas the goals of health research are to improve health and reduce health inequities, as mentioned previously, there are many different players involved in the health arena, each with their own vested interests. All too often, these interests (sometimes with the help of powerful lobbies) can shift the direction of research spending, which ultimately determines which research is being carried out.

To ensure that we do not lose sight of the true goals of health research, it is important to look at the big picture and not be blinded by the hype surrounding new technologies.[95] There are no "magic bullets" or easy cures for the world's health problems, which are largely a reflection of underlying economic, social and political problems. Indeed, in 1990, the Commission on Health Research for Development estimated that less than 10% of the world's resources for health research are directed at better understanding and addressing health problems in low- and middle-income countries where over 90% of the world's preventable deaths occur.[96] This was coined the *10/90 gap* by the Global Forum for Health Research, a non-governmental organisation based in Geneva which advocates for redressing the tremendous imbalance between need and investment in health research.

Governments and universities must therefore be strong leaders enacting laws and policies to ensure that the research agenda is not side-tracked by vested interests, but rather stays focused on alleviating the gross inequities of our time. Indeed, there is little point in producing all of this research evidence if it is not used to make better-informed decisions to improve health. Incentive systems are therefore required which recognise the importance of applying research in practice. Beyond the amount of research dollars awarded and publications produced, what if researchers were instead judged based on the number of lives saved or the inequities that were averted? Perhaps then we really would see the benefits of research in practice.

Returning to the example of the Minister of Health who wants to build up a case in support of tobacco control, clearly there is a wealth of research evidence to draw from, and even more research of all kinds that could be done. However, the Minister is busy with many different concerns and simply does not have the time or the expertise to wade through all that has been written on the subject. The next chapter therefore discusses how the overall body of research evidence can be synthesised and disseminated, as well as other facilitators and barriers to using this evidence to improve health and reduce health inequities.

References

1. Oxford Dictionaries Online project team. Evidence. *Oxford English Dictionary Online*, Oxford University Press, 2012. Available at: www.oxforddictionaries.com.

2. Lind J. *A Treatise of the Scurvy. In Three Parts. Containing an Inquiry into the Nature, Causes and Cure, of that Disease. Together with a Critical and Chronological View of What Has Been Published on the Subject.* Edinburgh: Printed by Sands, Murray and Cochran for A Kincaid and A Donaldson, 1753.

3. Cartier J. *Bref Récit et Succincte Narration de la Navigation Faite en 1535 et 1536 par le Capitaine Jacques Cartier aux Iles de Canada, Hochelaga, Saguenay et Autres. Réimpression Figurée de l'Edition Originale Rarissime de 1545 avec les Variantes des ms de la Bibliothèque Impériale, Précédée d'une Brève et Succincte Introduction Historique*

par M. d'Avezac. Paris: Librairie Tross, 1863.

4. Lind J. *An Essay on the Most Effectual Means of Preserving the Health of Seamen, in the Royal Navy.* London: D Wilson, 1762.

5. Dawkins R. *The God Delusion.* London: Houghton Mifflin Harcourt, 2006.

6. Desmond A. *The Politics of Evolution: Morphology, Medicine and Reform in Radical London.* Chicago: University of Chicago Press, 1989.

7. Fraenkel C. God's existence and attributes. In: Nadler S, Rudavsky T (eds.). *The Cambridge History of Medieval Jewish Philosophy.* Cambridge: Cambridge University Press, 2009, pp. 561–98.

8. Plato. *Plato in Twelve Volumes,* Vol. 12 translated by Harold N. Fowler. Cambridge, MA: Harvard University Press; London: William Heinemann Ltd., 1921. Available at: http://www.perseus.tufts.edu/hopper/text?doc=Perseus%3Atext%3A1999.01.0172%3Atext%3DTheaet.

9. Oxford Dictionaries Online project team. Epistemology. *Oxford English Dictionary Online,* Oxford University Press, 2012. Available at: www.oxforddictionaries.com.

10. Von Staden H. Experiment and experience in Hellenistic medicine. *Bull Inst Class Stud* 1975; 22: 178–99.

11. Oxford Dictionaries Online project team. Scientific method. *Oxford English Dictionary Online,* Oxford University Press, 2012. Available at: www.oxforddictionaries.com.

12. Kuhn T. *The Copernican Revolution. Planetary Astronomy in the Development of Western Thought.* Cambridge, Massachusetts: Harvard University Press, 1957.

13. Newton I. *Philosophiæ Naturalis Principia Mathematica.* London: S Pepys, 1867.

14. Huxley T. *On the Educational Value of the Natural History Sciences* (an address given in St Martin's Hall to the students in the Faculty of Medicine of University College). London, 1854.

15. Mill J. *A System of Logic: Ratiocinative and Inductive being a Connected View of the Principles of Evidence and the Methods of Scientific Investigation.* New York: Harper and Brothers Publishers, 1850.

16. Woolgar S, Latour B. *Laboratory Life: the Social Construction of Scientific Facts.* Princeton, NJ: Princeton University Press, 1986.

17. Fleck L. *The Genesis and Development of a Scientific Fact* (edited by T.J. Trenn and R. K. Merton, foreword by Thomas Kuhn). Chicago: University of Chicago Press, 1979.

18. Kuhn T. *The Structure of Scientific Revolutions,* 2nd edn. Chicago: University of Chicago Press, 1970.

19. Straus S, McAlister F. Evidence-based medicine: a commentary on common criticisms. *CMAJ* 2000; 163: 837–41.

20. Sackett D, Richardson W, Rosenberg W, Haynes R. *Evidence-Based Medicine: How to Practice and Teach EBM.* London: Churchill Livingstone, 1996.

21. Gray J. Evidence based policy making. *BMJ* 2004; 329: 988.

22. Saarni S, Gylling H. Evidence based medicine guidelines: a solution to rationing or politics disguised as science? *J Med Ethics* 2004; 30(2): 171–5.

23. Rodwin M. The politics of evidence-based medicine. *J Health Polit Policy Law* 2001; 26(2): 439–46.

24. Sackett DL, Rosenberg W, Gray J, Haynes R, Richardson W. Evidence based medicine: what it is and what it isn't. *BMJ* 1996; 312(7023): 71–2.

25. Cochrane A. *Effectiveness and Efficiency: Random Reflections on Health Services.* London: Nuffield Provincial Hospitals Trust, 1972.

26. Greenhalgh T. Book review: Effectiveness and Efficiency: Random Reflections on Health Services. *BMJ* 2004; 328: 529.

27. Bombardier C, McClaran J, Sackett D. Periodic health examinations and multiphasic screening. *CMAJ* 1973; 109(11): 1123–27.

28. The Cochrane Collaboration. *A Chronology of the Cochrane Collaboration.* Oxford: The Cochrane Collaboration, 2011. Available at: http://www.cochrane.org/about-us/history.

29. Spitzer W, Sackett D, Sibley J et al. 1965–1990: 25th anniversary of nurse practitioners. A classic manuscript reprinted in celebration of 25 years of progress. The Burlington randomized trial

of the nurse practitioner, 1971–2. *J Am Acad Nurse Pract* 1990; 2(3): 93–9.

30. Sackett D, Haynes R, Gibson E *et al.* Randomised clinical trial of strategies for improving medication compliance in primary hypertension. *Lancet* 1975; 1(7918): 1205–7.

31. Hull R, Hirsh J, Sackett D *et al.* Replacement of venography in suspected venous thrombosis by impedance plethysmography and 125I-fibrinogen leg scanning: a less invasive approach. *Ann Intern Med* 1981; 94(1): 12–15.

32. Sauvé J, Thorpe K, Sackett D *et al.* Can bruits distinguish high-grade from moderate symptomatic carotid stenosis? The North American Symptomatic Carotid Endarterectomy Trial. *Ann Intern Med* 1994; 120(8): 633–7.

33. Gent M, Barnett H, Sackett D, Taylor D. A randomized trial of aspirin and sulfinpyrazone in patients with threatened stroke. Results and methodologic issues. *Circulation* 1980; 62: V97–105.

34. Sackett D. Rational therapy in the neurosciences: the role of the randomized trial. *Stroke* 1986; 17(6): 1323–9.

35. Oxman A, Sackett D, Guyatt G. Users' guides to the medical literature. I. How to get started. The Evidence-Based Medicine Working Group. *JAMA* 1993; 270(17): 2093–5.

36. Haynes R, McKibbon K, Fitzgerald D *et al.* How to keep up with the medical literature: V. Access by personal computer to the medical literature. *Ann Intern Med* 1986; 105(5): 810–16.

37. Chalmers I. Unbiased, relevant, and reliable assessments in health care: important progress during the past century, but plenty of scope for doing better. *BMJ* 1998; 317(7167): 1167–8.

38. Greenhalgh T. How to read a paper: getting your bearings. *BMJ* 1997; 315: 243.

39. Guyatt G, Sackett D, Sinclair J *et al.* Users' guides to the medical literature. IX. A method for grading health care recommendations. Evidence-Based Medicine Working Group. *JAMA* 1995; 274(22): 1800–4.

40. Oakley A. Experimentation and social interventions: a forgotten but important history. *BMJ* 1998; 317(7167): 1239–42.

41. Concato J, Shah N, Horwitz R. Randomized, controlled trials, observational studies, and the hierarchy of research designs. *N Engl J Med* 2000; 342(25): 1887–92.

42. Killoran A, Kelly M (eds.). *Evidence-Based Public Health: Effectiveness and Efficiency.* Oxford: Oxford University Press, 2010.

43. Bell E. *Research for Health Policy.* Oxford: Oxford University Press, 2010.

44. Bogenschneider K, Corbett T, Corbett T. *Evidence-Based Policymaking: Insights from Policy-Minded Researchers and Research-Minded Policymakers.* London: Routledge, 2010.

45. Wyckoff P. *Policy and Evidence in a Partisan Age: The Great Disconnect.* Washington, DC: The Urban Institute Press, 2009.

46. Testa M, Poertner J (eds.). *Fostering Accountability: Using Evidence to Guide and Improve Child Welfare Policy.* Oxford: Oxford University Press, 2010.

47. Beaglehole R, Bonita R, Horton R *et al.* on behalf of the NCD Action Group and the NCD Alliance. Priority actions for the non-communicable disease crisis. *Lancet* 2011; 377(9775): 1438–47.

48. Fausto N. Atherosclerosis in young people: the value of the autopsy for studies of the epidemiology and pathobiology of disease. *Am J Pathol* 1998; 153(4): 1021–2.

49. Knudson A. Two genetic hits (more or less) to cancer. *Nature Reviews Cancer* 2001; 1(2): 157–62.

50. Liu S, Wang W, Zhang J *et al.* Prevalence of diabetes and impaired fasting glucose in Chinese adults, China National Nutrition and Health Survey, 2002. *Prev Chronic Dis* 2011; 8(1): A13.

51. Abbas S, Alam A, Majid A. To determine the probable causes of death in an urban slum community of Pakistan among adults 18 years and above by verbal autopsy. *J Pak Med Assoc* 2011; 61(3): 235–8.

52. Cecil R, Mc Caughan E, Parahoo K. 'It's hard to take because I am a man's man': an ethnographic exploration of cancer and masculinity. *Eur J Cancer Care* 2010; 19(4): 501–9.

53. Green L, Kreuter M. *Health Program Planning: An Educational and Ecological Approach*, 4th edn. New York: McGraw-Hill, 2005.

54. Theodorou M, Samara K, Pavlakis A *et al.* The public's and doctors' perceived role in participation in setting health care priorities in Greece. *Hellenic J Cardiol* 2010; 51(3): 200–8.

55. Gruskin S, Daniels N. Process is the point: justice and human rights: priority setting and fair deliberative process. *Am J Public Health* 2008; 98(9): 1573–7.

56. Smith A, Adams R, Bushell F. Qualitative health needs assessment of a former mining community. *Community Pract* 2010; 83(2): 27–30.

57. IARC Working Group on the Evaluation of Carcinogenic Risks to Humans. *Tobacco Smoke and Involuntary Smoking. IARC Monographs on the Evaluation of Carcinogenic Risks to Humans*, Vol. 83. Lyon: International Agency for Research on Cancer, 2002. Available at http://monographs.iarc.fr/ENG/Monographs/vol83/volume83.pdf.

58. Catassi A, Servent D, Paleari L, Cesario A, Russo P. Multiple roles of nicotine on cell proliferation and inhibition of apoptosis: implications on lung carcinogenesis. *Mutat Res* 2008; 659(3): 221–31.

59. King James I. *A Counterblaste to Tobacco.* London: R.B., 1604.

60. Doll R, Hill A. Smoking and carcinoma of the lung. Preliminary report. *BMJ* 1950; ii: 739–48. Available at http://www.who.int/bulletin/archives/77(1)84.pdf.

61. Doll R, Peto R, Boreham J, Sutherland I. Mortality in relation to smoking: 50 years' observations on male British doctors. *BMJ* 2004; 328: 1519–28. Available at http://www.bmj.com/cgi/reprint/328/7455/1519.

62. Hill A. The environment and disease: association or causation? *Proc R Soc Med* 1965, 58: 295–300.

63. Sterne J, Davey Smith G. Sifting the evidence – what's wrong with significance tests. *BMJ* 2001; 322: 226–31.

64. Last J (ed.). *A Dictionary of Epidemiology*, 4th edn. Oxford: OUP, 2001.

65. Stampfer M, Colditz G. Estrogen replacement therapy and coronary heart disease: a quantitative assessment of the epidemiologic evidence. *Int J Epidemiol* 2004; 33: 445–53 (reprint 1990).

66. Rossouw J, Anderson G, Prentice R *et al.;* Writing Group for the Women's Health Initiative Investigators: Risks and benefits of estrogen plus progestin in healthy postmenopausal women: principal results from the Women's Health Initiative randomized controlled trial. *JAMA* 2002; 288(3): 321–33.

67. Taubes G. Do We Really Know What Makes Us Healthy? *The New York Times Magazine* September 16, 2007. Available at: http://www.nytimes.com/2007/09/16/magazine/16epidemiology-t.html.

68. Lawlor D, Davey Smith G, Ebrahim S. Commentary: The hormone replacement–coronary heart disease conundrum: is this the death of observational epidemiology? *Int J Epidemiol* 2004; 33: 464–7.

69. Sackett D. Uncertainty about clinical equipoise. There is another exchange on equipoise and uncertainty. *BMJ* 2001; 322(7289): 795–6.

70. Rose G, Colwell L. Randomised controlled trial of anti-smoking advice: final (20 year) results. *J Epidemiol Community Health* 1992; 46(1): 75–7.

71. Sasco A, Secretan M, Straif K. Tobacco smoking and cancer: a brief review of recent epidemiological evidence. *Lung Cancer* 2004; 45(Suppl 2): S3–9.

72. Smith L, Paszkiewicz G, Hutson A, Pauly J. Inflammatory response of lung macrophages and epithelial cells to tobacco smoke: a literature review of ex vivo investigations. *Immunol Res* 2010; 46(1–3): 94–126.

73. Solberg L, Strong J. Risk factors and atherosclerotic lesions. A review of autopsy studies. *Arteriosclerosis* 1983; 3(3): 187–98.

74. Petitti D. Commentary: Hormone replacement therapy and coronary heart disease: four lessons. *Int J Epidemiol* 2004; 33: 461–3.

75. Hopkins D, Briss P, Ricard C *et al.;* Task Force on Community Preventive Services. Reviews of evidence regarding interventions to reduce tobacco use and exposure to environmental tobacco smoke. *Am J Prev Med* 2001; 20(2 Suppl): 16–66.

76. Hawe P, Samis S, Di Ruggiero E, Shoveller J. Population Health Intervention Research Initiative for Canada: progress and

prospects. *N S W Public Health Bull* 2011; 22(1–2): 27–32.

77. Hawe P, Potvin L. What is population health intervention research? *Can J Public Health* 2009; 100(1 Suppl): I8–14.

78. Moher D, Hopewell S, Schulz K *et al.*, for the CONSORT Group. CONSORT 2010 Explanation and Elaboration: updated guidelines for reporting parallel group randomised trials. *BMJ* 2010; 340: c869. Available at: http://www.bmj.com/content/340/bmj.c869.full.

79. *Trials of War Criminals before the Nuremberg Military Tribunals under Control Council Law No. 10*, Vol. 2. Washington, DC: US Government Printing Office, 1949, pp. 181–2. Available at: http://history.nih.gov/research/downloads/nuremberg.pdf.

80. World Medical Association. *Declaration of Helsinki: Ethical Principles for Medical Research Involving Human Subjects*. Geneva: World Medical Association, 2008. Available at: http://www.wma.net/en/30publications/10policies/b3/index.html.

81. Interagency Advisory Panel on Research Ethics. *Tri-Council Policy Statement: Ethical Conduct for Research Involving Humans*. Ottawa: Canadian Institutes of Health Research, Natural Sciences and Engineering Research Council of Canada, Social Sciences and Humanities Research Council of Canada, 2010. Available at: http://www.pre.ethics.gc.ca/pdf/eng/tcps2/TCPS_2_FINAL_Web.pdf.

82. Angell M. Investigators' responsibilities for human subjects in developing countries. *N Engl J Med* 2000; 342: 967–9.

83. Austoker J. Gaining informed consent for screening: is difficult; but many misconceptions need to be undone. *BMJ* 1999; 319: 722–5.

84. Issel M. *Health Program Planning and Evaluation: A Practical, Systematic Approach for Community Health*, 2nd edn. Sudbury, MA: Jones & Bartlett Publishing, 2008.

85. Chen H. *Practical Program Evaluation: Assessing and Improving Planning, Implementation and Effectiveness*. Thousand Oaks, CA: SAGE Publications, 2005.

86. Centers for Disease Control and Prevention. Framework for program evaluation in public health. *MMWR* 1999; 48(No. RR-11): 1–40. Available at: ftp://ftp.cdc.gov/pub/Publications/mmwr/rr/rr4811.pdf.

87. Bhattacharyya O, Reeves S, Zwarenstein M. What is implementation research? Rationale, concepts, and practices. *Res Social Work Prac* 2009; 19: 491–502.

88. Special Programme for Research and Training in Tropical Diseases (TDR). *Health Systems Research and Implementation Research*. Geneva: World Health Organization, 2011. Available at: http://apps.who.int/tdr/svc/topics/health-systems-implementation-research.

89. Alliance for Health Policy and Systems Research. *Implementation Research Platform*. Geneva: World Health Organization, 2011. Available at: http://www.who.int/alliance-hpsr/projects/implementationresearch/en/index.html.

90. Rutman L. *Evaluation Research Methods: A Basic Guide*. Newbury Park, CA: SAGE, 1984.

91. Blalock A. Evaluation research and the performance management movement: from estrangement to useful integration? *Evaluation* 1999; 5(2): 117–49.

92. Bogenschneider K, Corbett T, Corbett T. *Evidence-Based Policymaking: Insights from Policy-Minded Researchers and Research-Minded Policymakers*. London: Routledge, 2010.

93. Parry D, Salsberg J, Macaulay A. *A Guide to Researcher and Knowledge-User Collaboration in Health Research* [online course]. Ottawa: Canadian Institutes of Health Research, 2009.

94. Pratt B, Loff B. Health research systems: promoting health equity or economic competitiveness? *Bull World Health Organ* 2012; 90: 55–62.

95. Evans P, Meslin E, Marteau T, Caufield T. Deflating the genomic bubble. *Science* 2011; 331(6019): 861–2.

96. Commission on Health Research for Development. *Health Research: Essential Link to Equity in Development*. Oxford: Oxford University Press, 1990.

Facilitators and barriers to using evidence

Producing evidence is not the same as using evidence. Notwithstanding the value of creating knowledge for its own sake, it is difficult to justify spending valuable resources on countless research studies, especially research studies where there is potential for causing harm to research subjects (whether human or animal), if it does not contribute to a deeper under-standing of the world we live in and how to make that world a better place. Yet, even the highest quality evidence is useless if it is not incorporated into decision-making for health. Indeed, the study of why health practitioners do not use evidence-based clinical practice guidelines has become a field of research in its own right.[1] A systematic review of systematic reviews found that interactive techniques such as audit, feedback, outreach and reminder systems work best to promote the uptake of evidence. Despite this, clinical practice guidelines are often used in an attempt to change physician behaviours, but with much less success.[2] There exists an entire online clearinghouse with thousands of such guidelines,[3] but what good are they if nobody uses them? Therefore, at the core of the research cycle presented in the previous chapter, there is "synthesis, dissemination and utilisation", which are the driving forces for ensuring that research evidence is used to influence decisions that can improve health. In an ideal world, this is not just an afterthought at the end of the cycle, but something that occurs every step of the way to continually move evidence into policy and practice (Fig. 5.1). However, if our goal is to make more evidence-informed decisions that improve health, it is also important to be aware of the many barriers to using research evidence, such as missing the window of opportunity, controversy over the research findings and vested interests. This chapter therefore describes in greater detail some of the facilitators and barriers to translating research evidence into improved health outcomes.

Facilitators to using evidence

Increasingly, there has been a push towards closing the "know–do" gap – i.e. the gap between what we know works based on research evidence and what we actually do in practice. An important approach to closing this gap is often referred to as knowledge translation.

Knowledge translation

Although there are many different terms to describe how research findings are used to improve health,[4] and despite a lack of consensus on which term should be used,[5] for the purpose of this book I will continue to use the term "knowledge translation". Knowledge translation (KT) has been defined as a dynamic and iterative process that includes the synthesis, dissemination, exchange and ethically sound application of knowledge to improve

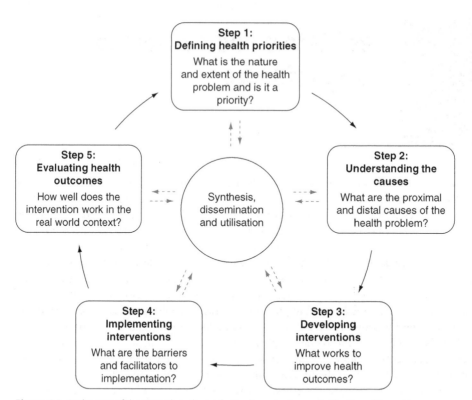

Figure 5.1 At the core of the research cycle: synthesis, dissemination and utilisation of the evidence.

health, provide more effective health services and products, and strengthen the health care system.[6]

As part of the growing effort to encourage knowledge translation, there has been an increasing number of "knowledge brokering" initiatives in recent years that promote the use of evidence by bridging the gap between knowledge producers and knowledge users.[7] According to Lomas:

> Researchers tend to see decision making as an event – they deliver their edicts to the impenetrable cardinals' retreat and await the puff of smoke that signals "decision," while grumbling about irrationality within the conclave. Decision makers – the patients, the care providers, the managers, and the policy makers – tend to see research as a product they can purchase from the local knowledge store, but too often it is the wrong size, needs some assembly, is on back order, and comes from last year's fashion line. Neither side seems to recognize that the other is managing a complex process rather than presiding over an event or manufacturing a product... one path to more research informed decision making is to focus on better linkage and exchange between the processes that create the facts (research) and the ones that incorporate the values (decision making).[8]

However, while research findings can only improve health if they are applied in practice, it does not follow that every researcher from basic scientists to policy analysts should be involved in knowledge translation.

According to Ian Graham, Vice President of the Knowledge Translation Portfolio at the Canadian Institutes of Health Research (CIHR), the "KT imperative" is "the perceived need to do everything to encourage everyone to apply their research findings".[9] However, this can be a dangerous business since, as we have seen in the previous chapter, there are many factors that can affect the internal validity of a research study (i.e. bias, chance, confounding). The results from any single study would therefore need to be considered in relation to the larger body of evidence before large-scale dissemination or implementation of a proposed intervention is carried out. According to Graham, "we need to bring common sense as well as academic rigour to bear on our decisions about the degree and intensity of KT activities warranted by a single research study". Thus it is necessary to first conduct a synthesis of the existing body of evidence.

Knowledge synthesis

Before embarking upon any research study, a synthesis of the existing literature (also referred to as a literature review) is often used to explore the current state of knowledge in the area, including which questions have been answered and where knowledge gaps remain. Thus the rationale for conducting new research is often based upon this initial review of the literature. The synthesis is generally updated at the end of the research study to ensure that any new information is included, and to be able to examine what the study adds to the existing body of knowledge and whether the research findings are coherent with or contradict what is already known.

However, knowledge synthesis is not simply a tool that is used when conducting research. Over the past few decades, there has been a growing interest in knowledge synthesis as a form of research in and of itself. Whereas primary research sets out to collect new data to answer various research questions across the research cycle, secondary research synthesises what is known from existing research studies. The main type of secondary research is called a systematic review, which can be conducted with or without meta-analysis depending on the nature and quality of the primary data available. In contrast with a simple literature review, a systematic review is "a review of a clearly formulated question that uses systematic and explicit methods to identify, select, and critically appraise relevant research, and to collect and analyse data from the studies that are included in the review".[10] Meta-analysis is "the use of statistical techniques in a systematic review to integrate the results of included studies", which are then graphically displayed using a "forest plot" or "blobbogram" to provide a visual summary of the existing body of knowledge.

The methodology for conducting systematic reviews has been developed and refined over the years by the Cochrane Collaboration and involves the following eight steps: (1) Defining the review question and developing criteria for including studies, (2) Searching for studies, (3) Selecting studies and collecting data, (4) Assessing risk of bias in included studies, (5) Analysing data and undertaking meta-analyses, (6) Addressing reporting biases, (7) Presenting results and 'Summary of findings' tables, and (8) Interpreting results and drawing conclusions. These methods are described in greater detail in the *Cochrane Handbook for Systematic Reviews of Interventions*.[11]

To take an example, in a recent Cochrane review of interventions for preventing obesity in children, while many studies show no significant difference associated with the use of physical activity and/or dietary interventions, overall, when all of the data are pooled, there is a significant reduction in obesity from physical activity interventions alone, and an even greater reduction in obesity when physical activity and dietary interventions are combined (Fig. 5.2).[12] This is an important finding, since many of the studies taken on their own would lead us to believe that there is no point investing in such interventions, which would be a

Study or subgroup	Experimental			Control			Weight	Std. mean difference IV, Random, 95% CI	Std. mean difference IV, Random, 95% CI
	Mean	SD	Total	Mean	SD	Total			
1.1.1 Physical activity									
Dennison 2004	−0.24	1.64	43	0.12	1.75	34	2.8%	−0.21 [−0.66, 0.24]	
Donnelly 2009	2	1.9	792	2	1.9	698	10.4%	0.00 [−0.10, 0.10]	
Gutin 2008	0.1	2.1	182	0.3	1.99	265	7.7%	−0.10 [−0.29, 0.09]	
Harrison 2006	−0.2	1.3	175	0.1	2	118	6.4%	−0.18 [−0.42, 0.05]	
Lazaar 2007 (1)	−0.1	0.54	69	0.2	0.49	94	4.6%	−0.58 [−0.90, −0.27]	
Lazaar 2007 (2)	−0.2	1.4	30	0.4	0.97	21	2.0%	−0.48 [−1.04, 0.09]	
Lazaar 2007 (3)	−0.1	1.13	30	0.3	0.92	21	2.0%	−0.38 [−0.94, 0.19]	
Lazaar 2007 (4)	−0.1	0.54	69	0.3	0.52	94	4.5%	−0.75 [1.07, −0.43]	
Mo-Suwan 1998 (5)	−0.67	0.85	65	−0.39	0.99	57	3.9%	−0.30 [−0.66, 0.05]	
Mo-Suwan 1998 (6)	−0.33	1.23	82	−0.44	1.06	88	4.9%	0.10 [0.21, 0.40]	
Read 2008	0.4	2.42	156	0.3	2.92	81	5.6%	0.04 [−0.23, 0.31]	
Reilly 2006	0.07	0.45	231	0.02	0.46	250	8.0%	0.11 [−0.07, 0.29]	
Simon 2008	2.38	2.2	479	2.42	2.14	475	9.6%	−0.02 [0.15, 0.11]	
Vizcaino 2008 (6)	0.4	1.64	234	0.4	1.52	280	8.1%	0.00 [−0.17, 0.17]	
Vizcaino 2008 (5)	0.2	1.61	231	0.3	1.61	299	8.2%	−0.06 [0.23, 0.11]	
Webber 2008	2	2.05	1751	2	2.05	1751	11.3%	0.00 [−0.07, 0.07]	
Subtotal (95% CI)			**4619**			**4626**	**100.0%**	**−0.11 [−0.19, −0.02]**	
Heterogeneity: Tau^2 = 0.02; Chi^2 = 44.45, df = 15 (P < 0.0001); I^2 = 66%									
Test for overall effect: Z = 2.41 (P = 0.02)									
1.1.2 Dietary									
Amaro 2006	0.13	0.68	153	0.26	0.64	88	14.6%	−0.19 [−0.46, 0.07]	
Ebbeling 2006	0.07	1.02	53	0.21	1.06	50	10.1%	−0.13 [−0.52, 0.25]	
James 2004	0.7	0.2	297	0.8	0.3	277	18.8%	−0.39 [−0.56, −0.23]	
Paineau 2008 (7)	0.05	0.94	280	0.12	0.91	197	18.1%	−0.08 [−0.26, 0.11]	
Paineau 2008 (8)	0.1	1.1	274	0.12	0.91	197	18.0%	−0.02 [−0.20, 0.16]	
Sichieri 2009	0.32	1.43	434	0.22	1.08	493	20.4%	0.08 [−0.05, 0.21]	
Subtotal (95% CI)			**1491**			**1302**	**100.0%**	**−0.12 [−0.28, 0.05]**	
Heterogeneity: Tau^2 = 0.03; Chi^2 = 20.91, df = 5 (P = 0.0008); I^2 = 76%									
Test for overall effect: Z = 1.40 (P = 0.16)									
1.1.3 Physical activity & Dietary combined									
Baranowski 2003 (5)	3.2	3.53	17	−2.2	6.93	14	1.1%	0.99 [0.23, 1.74]	
Beech 2003 (9)	−1.2	6.58	21	2.1	4.85	9	1.0%	−0.52 [−1.32, 0.27]	
Beech 2003 (10)	−1.2	6.58	21	2.1	4.85	9	1.0%	−0.52 [−1.32, 0.27]	
Caballero 2003	3	2.05	727	3.1	2.05	682	5.2%	−0.05 [−0.15, 0.06]	
Fitzgibbon 2005	0.05	0.67	179	0.14	0.68	183	4.3%	−0.13 [−0.34, 0.07]	
Fitzgibbon 2006	0.11	1.54	196	0.13	1.5	187	4.3%	−0.01 [−0.21, 0.19]	
Foster 2008	1.99	1.9	479	2.1	1.9	364	4.9%	−0.06 [−0.19, 0.08]	
Gentile 2009	0.6	2.9	582	0.5	2.8	619	5.1%	0.04 [−0.08, 0.15]	
Haerens 2006 (6)	1.48	1.55	611	1.22	1.29	120	4.4%	0.17 [−0.02, 0.37]	
Haerens 2006 (11)	1.11	1.74	381	1.66	1.61	176	4.5%	−0.32 [−0.50, −0.14]	
Haerens 2006 (5)	1.42	1.62	118	1.66	1.61	176	4.0%	−0.15 [−0.38, 0.09]	
Haerens 2006 (12)	1.31	1.63	590	1.22	1.29	119	4.4%	0.06 [−0.14, 0.25]	
Hamelink–Basteen 2008	0.83	1.03	349	0.95	0.73	77	3.9%	−0.12 [−0.37, 0.13]	
Harvey-Berino 2003 (13)	−0.27	0.52	17	0.31	0.7	20	1.3%	−0.91 [−1.59, −0.23]	
Kain 2004 (5)	0.3	1.72	996	0.2	1.7	454	5.1%	0.06 [−0.05, 0.17]	
Kain 2004 (6)	0	1.62	1145	0.3	1.44	491	5.2%	−0.19 [−0.30, −0.09]	
Keller 2009	−0.15	0.23	49	0.11	0.23	134	3.0%	−1.13 [−1.47, −0.78]	
Marcus 2009	−0.01	0.73	591	0.3	0.73	430	5.0%	−0.42 [−0.55, −0.30]	
NeumarkSztainer 2003 (5)	−0.96	3.22	84	0.75	2.59	106	3.5%	−0.59 [−0.88, −0.30]	
Peralta 2009 (6)	0.3	1.86	16	0.6	1.83	16	1.3%	−0.16 [−0.85, 0.54]	
Robinson 2003 (5)	0.5	2.43	28	0.71	2.47	33	2.0%	−0.08 [−0.59, 0.42]	
Sanigorski 2008	−0.09	0.42	833	−0.02	0.39	974	5.3%	−0.17 [−0.27, −0.08]	
Singh 2009 (5)	0.5	1.37	312	0.5	1.55	208	4.6%	0.00 [−0.18, 0.18]	
Singh 2009 (6)	0.4	1.22	276	0.4	1.3	234	4.6%	0.00 [−0.17, 0.17]	
Spiegel 2006	0.16	0.89	534	0.52	1.02	479	5.0%	−0.38 [−0.50, −0.25]	
Story 2003a (5)	−0.2	5	26	2	2.41	27	1.8%	−0.56 [−1.11, −0.01]	
Taylor 2006	0.8	1.32	201	1.4	1.77	188	4.3%	−0.39 [−0.59, −0.18]	
Subtotal (95% CI)			**9379**			**6529**	**100.0%**	**−0.18 [−0.27, −0.09]**	
Heterogeneity: Tau^2 = 0.04; Chi^2 = 148.15, df = 26 (P < 0.00001); I^2 = 82%									
Test for overall effect: Z = 3.92 (P < 0.0001)									

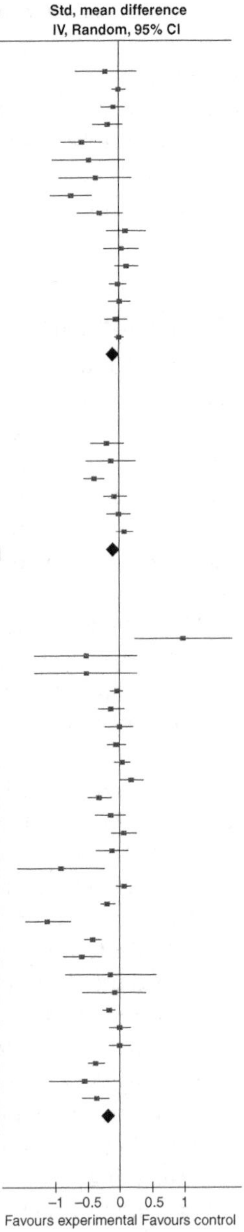

−1 −0.5 0 0.5 1
Favours experimental Favours control

Test for subgroup differences : Chi^2 =1.34, df = 2 (P = 0.51), I^2 = 0%

Legend

(1) Non-obese (males); (2) Obese (females); (3) Obese (males); (4) Non-obese (females); (5) Females; (6) Males; (7) Intervention A vs. Control;
(8) Intervention B vs. Control; (9) Child-targeted intervention (females); (10) Parent-targeted intervention (females);
(11) Intervention + Parents (females); (12) Intervention + Parents (males); (13) Weight-for-height z score

Figure 5.2 Example of a forest plot from a systematic review with meta-analysis.
Reproduced with permission from Waters E, de Silva-Sanigorski A, Hall B et al. Interventions for preventing obesity in children. *Cochrane Database Syst Rev* 2011; (12): CD001871.

missed opportunity for improving health. This illustrates why we need to consider the overall evidence base during decision-making, rather than relying on a single study to change policy and practice.

For this reason, systematic reviews, with or without meta-analysis, are at the pinnacle of the hierarchy of evidence. When well conducted, systematic reviews provide the best possible estimate of the true effect of an intervention. However, as with any study, systematic reviews can also vary in quality.[13] According to Sir Richard Peto, "epidemiology is so beautiful and provides such an important perspective on human life and death, but an incredible amount of rubbish is published".[14] Indeed, a poorly conducted study – whether a simple cross-sectional survey or an elaborate systematic review – can produce misleading results that should be used with caution when making health decisions, whether in clinical practice or in public policy. Therefore, even systematic reviews should be subject to critical appraisal to determine whether the findings are valid and reliable.

Critical appraisal

As described in Chapter 4, critical appraisal is a key component of evidence-based medicine (EBM). It provides a systematic way of assessing the validity and applicability of research studies in answering a specific clinical or policy question. During the 1990s, Oxman, Sackett and Guyatt published a series of articles in the *Journal of the American Medical Association* (*JAMA*) to guide evidence users in becoming critical readers of the scientific literature.[15] The content of this series has been adapted and integrated into various critical appraisal tools. For instance, the Critical Appraisal Skills Programme (CASP) helps people to find and interpret the best available evidence from health research by providing a series of checklists that are tailored to different types of study design.[16] Currently there are seven checklists which span the hierarchy of evidence, including: (1) systematic reviews, (2) randomised controlled trials, (3) cohort studies, (4) case-control studies, (5) diagnostic studies, (6) qualitative studies, and (7) economic evaluations. Each checklist guides the reader in answering three main questions about the research study: (A) Is the study valid? (B) What are the results? (C) Are the results applicable in this context?

For instance, in appraising a systematic review, one begins by asking whether the review addressed a clearly focused question and whether the authors looked for the appropriate types of studies. If not, then there is little point even continuing with the appraisal since it is unlikely that the results of the study will be of sufficient quality to be interpretable or usable. However, if the answers to the initial screening questions are "yes", then more detailed questions follow to further establish the rigour and reliability of the study (also known as the internal validity). For example, the checklist questions ask: Were the important and relevant studies included in the review? Did the authors sufficiently assess the quality of the studies included? If the results of the study were combined (i.e. using meta-analysis) was it appropriate to do so? And so forth.

If it is determined that the study methodology was valid, then the next step is to look at the study results, including the precision of the results. For instance, a systematic review entitled "Can nicotine replacement therapy (NRT) help people quit smoking" compared the rates of quitting smoking among smokers who used nicotine replacement versus controls (i.e. those who did not use nicotine replacement).[17] The results show that the relative risk (RR) of quitting smoking for those smokers receiving nicotine replacement versus controls was 1.58 (95% CI: 1.50 to 1.66). In terms of the precision of the results, there are very narrow confidence limits (i.e. a high level of certainty), reflecting the fact that there were over 40,000 persons enrolled across more than 100 smoking cessation trials, the data of which were pooled in this systematic review using meta-analysis to obtain this overall estimate of the effect of nicotine replacement on the likelihood of quitting smoking. In plain English, the results mean that nicotine replacement increased the chances of quitting smoking by 50 to 70%. The effects were largely independent of the duration of therapy, the intensity of additional support provided, the setting in which nicotine replacement was offered or whether it was obtained with or without a prescription.

Before running off and changing practice or policy, it is important to assess the external validity or applicability of the results to various contexts. Whereas internal validity described above is concerned with the rigour and reliability of the study findings, external validity depends upon the study population that was used and the extent to which the results can be extrapolated to other groups who were not part of the study population. For instance, it used to be common practice to conduct research on men only (e.g. Sir Richard Doll's classic study on the effects of smoking that followed a cohort of over 34,000 male British doctors), therefore it is unclear whether the results of these studies would also be applicable to women (e.g. are the effects of tobacco smoke on the development of heart disease the same for women, or do oestrogen levels counteract these effects to a certain degree prior to meno-pause?). Similarly, to protect children from potential harm associated with participating in research, there were historically far fewer studies involving children. However, increasingly, it has been argued that it is important to conduct research with children since they are not simply "small adults", and it is often difficult to extrapolate from studies conducted on adults to determine the best course of action for children.[18] Yet another example, alluded to previously, is that there are also far fewer studies conducted in low-resource settings. To what extent are research findings from high-income countries transferable to low- and middle-income countries? Even if the results of a given study have strong internal validity, whether or not the results can be applied to a specific population group or setting depends on how and where the study was conducted. It is therefore important that any extrapolation from a given study to a different population group or setting is done in an explicit and transparent way.

Using the CASP or other appraisal checklists can assist in carrying out a "critical reading" of the literature and identifying valid, unbiased research studies to ensure that decisions are made using the best-quality evidence. However, as the number of research publications continues to grow exponentially – from about 1,000 articles indexed in PubMed each year in 1891, to about 100,000 per year in 1951 and almost 1 million per year in 2011 – it is becoming virtually impossible to keep abreast of the scientific literature in any given field, let alone conduct a critical appraisal of each study. Certainly, the production of secondary research (i.e. systematic reviews) is helpful in providing "pre-appraised" information on a given question. Although, even systematic reviews now have "Cochrane Summaries", and there are many different kinds of initiatives to "digest" the evidence into more manageable and accessible "bite-size" pieces for busy decision-makers.

Knowledge dissemination

Knowledge dissemination is a key step in being able to move the research evidence into the hands of knowledge users who can then translate new knowledge into health gains. There now exists a growing number of resources that assist in synthesising, appraising and disseminating the vast amount of research evidence created each year to encourage uptake and use by practitioners and policy-makers. For clinical settings in particular, there is increasing reliance on evidence-based clinical practice guidelines and clinical preventive practices.

Task forces

Established in 1976 and initially called the Canadian Task Force on the Periodic Health Examination, the Canadian Task Force on Preventive Health Care (CTFPHC) was responsible for reviewing the vast body of research evidence and making recommendations on which preventive actions should be included in routine clinical practice. In 1994, the task force published the widely acclaimed *Canadian Guide to Clinical Preventive Health Care.*[19] Although the task force subsequently became defunct in 2005 due to lack of funding and a permanent "home", it was recently revitalised through the assistance of the Public Health Agency of Canada (PHAC).

Similarly, in the United States, the US Preventive Services Task Force (USPSTF) of the Agency for Healthcare Research and Quality (AHRQ) is "a Congressionally mandated, independent panel of experts in primary care and prevention that systematically reviews the evidence of effectiveness and develops recommendations for clinical preventive services".[20] First convened in 1984, the USPSTF conducts reviews of the scientific evidence to assess the effectiveness of a broad range of clinical preventive services, including screening, counselling and preventive medications. The USPSTF also produced a guide for clinicians, the *Guide to Clinical Preventive Services*, which was published in 1989 and is regularly updated online.[21]

However, in addition to informing practice at a clinical level, there is also a task force that synthesises the evidence to make recommendations on what works to improve health at a population level. The Task Force on Community Preventive Services is an independent, non-federal, volunteer body of public health and prevention experts whose members are appointed by the Director of the US Centers for Disease Control and Prevention (CDC). In 2005, the task force published *The Community Guide*, a free and highly recommended resource to inform the choice of programmes and policies to improve health and prevent disease in communities and populations.[22]

Whereas the CTFPHC and the USPSTF make recommendations aimed at health practitioners and notably frontline primary health care workers (e.g. The USPSTF recommends that clinicians ask all adults about tobacco use and provide tobacco cessation interventions for those who use tobacco products, as well as augmented pregnancy-tailored counselling for pregnant women who smoke), *The Community Guide* recommendations are aimed more towards health managers and policy-makers (e.g. The Community Preventive Services Task Force recommends: increasing the unit price for tobacco products, reducing client out-of-pocket costs for effective cessation therapies, provider reminder systems with a provider education programme, mass media campaigns when combined with other interventions, and cessation interventions that include telephone support).

Nonetheless, all of these task forces base their recommendations upon reviews of the evidence base and specify the grade of recommendation depending on the nature and quality of the evidence available (Table 5.1).[23] Each task force has slight variations on how recommendations are graded. For instance, *The Community Guide* recommendations fall into one of three categories: (1) "recommend" based on strong or sufficient evidence that an

Table 5.1 Grade of recommendation based on the evidence available.

Grade	Definition	Suggestions for practice
A	The USPSTF recommends the service. There is high certainty that the net benefit is substantial.	Offer or provide this service.
B	The USPSTF recommends the service. There is high certainty that the net benefit is moderate or there is moderate certainty that the net benefit is moderate to substantial.	Offer or provide this service.
C	Clinicians may provide this service to selected patients depending on individual circumstances. However, for most individuals without signs or symptoms there is likely to be only a small benefit from this service.	Offer or provide this service only if other considerations support the offering or providing the service in an individual patient.
D	The USPSTF recommends against the service. There is moderate or high certainty that the service has no net benefit or that the harms outweigh the benefits.	Discourage the use of this service.
I	The USPSTF concludes that the current evidence is insufficient to assess the balance of benefits and harms of the service. Evidence is lacking, of poor quality, or conflicting, and the balance of benefits and harms cannot be determined.	Read the clinical considerations section of USPSTF Recommendation Statement. If the service is offered, patients should understand the uncertainty about the balance of benefits and harms.

Adapted from the US Preventive Services Task Force (USPSTF) definitions.

intervention has beneficial effects, (2) "recommend against" based on strong or sufficient evidence that the intervention is harmful or not effective, and (3) "insufficient evidence" when available studies do not provide sufficient evidence to determine whether the intervention is, or is not, effective. As noted by Altman and Bland, "absence of evidence is not evidence of absence".[24] Just because there is insufficient evidence does not imply that an intervention is ineffective. Indeed many important interventions (e.g. interventions for the prevention of gender-based violence) simply haven't been sufficiently researched to be able to draw meaningful conclusions. Additional research is therefore needed before it will be possible to make evidence-based recommendations for action in these areas. Yet, in the meantime, it will still be necessary to make decisions and to take action using the best available evidence and expert advice.

Health technology assessment

In addition to task forces, Health Technology Assessment (HTA) is also a burgeoning field that relies heavily on the use of evidence for making policy recommendations. According to Banta and Luce, "technology assessment is a form of policy research that examines short- and long-term social consequences of the application of technology with the goal of providing policy-makers with information on policy alternatives".[25] Having emerged in the 1960s and 1970s, and responding to the growing need to ensure the sustainability of publicly funded health care systems, the number of HTA agencies has increased dramatically in recent years. The International Network of Agencies for Health Technology Assessment (INAHTA), established in 1993, now has 53 member agencies from 29 countries across 6 continents, including North and South America, Europe, Africa, Asia, Australia and New Zealand.[26] All member agencies are non-profit organisations linked to regional or national government, although HTA also occurs in academia as well as in the private sector.

Best practices for conducting and reporting HTA reviews include defining the policy question, developing an HTA protocol to answer the question and making policy recommendations by addressing five main areas: (1) safety, (2) efficacy/effectiveness, (3) social, psychological and ethical considerations, (4) organisational and professional implications, and (5) economic issues (Fig. 5.3).[27] The Centre for Reviews and Dissemination at the University of York in the United Kingdom now has a database of over 10,000 completed and ongoing HTA reviews from around the world.[28] Indeed, the HTA database is a valuable resource for identifying the grey literature (i.e. unpublished studies), as most of the documents contained in the database are generally only available directly from individual HTA agencies or their funding bodies.

Increasingly, HTA is being used not only to answer questions relating to new technologies, but also to address issues surrounding health planning and reducing health inequities in resource-poor settings. The WHO Collaborating Center for Knowledge Translation and Health Technology Assessment in Health Equity was founded in 1997 and is based in the Centre for Global Health at the University of Ottawa. The centre has developed an Equity-Oriented Toolkit for HTA which provides an evidence-based framework for matching the identified health needs of a population to the most appropriate interventions, as well as assessing the impact of health policies and interventions on the rich–poor gap.[29]

International networks

Beyond task forces and HTA agencies, there are also international networks for the synthesis and dissemination of evidence. As mentioned in the previous chapter, the Cochrane Collaboration is an international network of over 28,000 people across 100 countries, which aims to help health care providers, policy-makers and patients make well-informed decisions about health care based on the best available research evidence. They do so by preparing, updating and promoting the accessibility of Cochrane reviews – which are essentially well-conducted systematic reviews of the literature as described in the section on knowledge synthesis above. Their sister organisation is called the Campbell Collaboration, which similarly prepares, maintains and disseminates systematic reviews in areas such as education, criminal justice, social policy and social care. As of January 2011, the Cochrane Collaboration even holds a seat at the World Health Assembly, the decision-making body of the World Health Organization (WHO), to provide input on WHO resolutions and to influence the way that evidence is produced and used to improve health and promote health equity.[30]

Another WHO initiative launched in 2005 is the Evidence-Informed Policy Network (EVIPNet), which promotes the systematic use of research evidence in policy-making, especially in low- and middle-income countries. Indeed, access to high-quality evidence should not be considered a luxury good that is only used by wealthy decision-makers in the North. Rather, "if you are poor . . . you need more evidence" before you invest in health because poor countries cannot afford to waste money on interventions that do not address the root causes of health problems or that simply do not work.[31] The EVIPNet partners therefore envision a world in which policy-makers in low- and middle-income countries use the best scientific

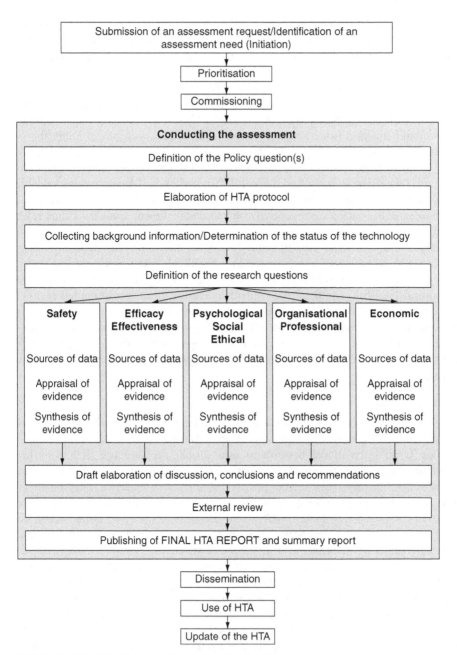

Figure 5.3 Best practice in conducting and reporting an HTA review.
Reproduced with permission from: Busse R, Orvain J, Velasco M *et al*. Best practice in undertaking and reporting health technology assessments. *Int J Technol Assess Health Care* 2002; 18: 361–422.

evidence, contextualised to the reality of their nation, to inform policy-making and policy implementation.

There are therefore a growing number of organisations, agencies and even global networks devoted to disseminating research evidence with the goal of improving health and reducing inequities. However, while finding, appraising and synthesising the evidence and "putting it out there" on a website or in a database is important, it is often not sufficient to ensure that the evidence will be used to influence policy and practice.

Promoting evidence uptake

Increasingly it is being recognised that evidence needs to be packaged in such a way so as to actively promote uptake, since passive diffusion measures are much less likely to have an impact.[32] Many different models are being developed to increase the uptake and use of evidence in practice.[33] These often involve some form of evidence summaries or decision-support tools.

Policy briefs and evidence summaries

While still a work in progress, the EVIPNet Portal (http://global.evipnet.org/) is building up a repertory of EVIPNet Policy Briefs which synthesise the research evidence and offer evidence-informed and contextualised policy options in a user-friendly format to support well-informed policy decisions. Indeed, such policy briefs, which are free from technical jargon and highlight key messages in a brief executive summary, dramatically increase the likelihood that policy-makers will read, consider and apply the evidence where appropriate. The EVIPNet partners with multiple organisations to produce these policy-relevant evidence syntheses, including the Alliance for Health Policy and Systems Research (AHSPR), the Health Evidence Network (HEN), and the international collaboration Supporting Policy Relevant Reviews and Trials (SUPPORT). Similarly, the Cochrane Collaboration produces "Cochrane Summaries" to make their systematic reviews more readily accessible to a wider audience of knowledge users.[34] These "free-form" half-page summaries provide the main conclusions of the Cochrane Review in lay terms, and also have a link to the more structured abstract.

Checklists and decision aids

Changing practice and policy, however, may require more than just browsing for evidence-based summaries online. Indeed, there are a growing number of evidence-based computerised decision support tools for busy health practitioners to ensure that they can find the answer to their questions in an easily accessible format where and when they need it – a kind of "one stop shop" for evidence. For instance, Up to Date (http://www.utdol.com) is a clinical decision support system that uses current evidence to answer clinical questions quickly and easily at the point of care. However, providing this service comes at a cost of almost $500 per year for an individual subscription. Another such service is MD Consult (http://www.mdconsult.com), which brings the leading medical resources together into one integrated online service to help health workers efficiently find answers to pressing clinical questions. Once again, this too comes at a cost of about $400 per year.

Yet, all of the above decision support resources require the decision-maker to ask a clinical question and actively search for the evidence (even if the evidence is made available in a pre-digested format). However, there are also tools such as evidence-based checklists that actually prompt health care workers to think about clinical preventive practices when they are overwhelmed by many other acute care issues and might not otherwise make time for prevention. For instance, the recommendations of the Canadian Task Force on Preventive Health Care (CTFPHC) have been integrated into numerous clinical practice tools that act as memory aids for busy practitioners (Table 5.2). For example, the Rourke Baby Record

Table 5.2 Links to evidence-based checklists for use by frontline health care providers.

Infants and young children 0–5 years

Rourke Baby Record (children 0–5 years)
http://www.cps.ca/english/statements/CP/Rourke/RBRNational.pdf

WHO growth charts for Canada
http://www.dietitians.ca/Secondary-Pages/Public/Who-Growth-Charts.aspx

Older children and youth 6–17 years

Greig Health Record (children 6–9 years)
http://www.cps.ca/english/statements/CP/PreventiveCare/GreigHealth-Age6to9.pdf

Greig Health Record (children 10–13 years)
http://www.cps.ca/english/statements/CP/PreventiveCare/GreigHealth-Age10to13.pdf

Greig Health Record (children 14–17 years)
http://www.cps.ca/english/statements/CP/PreventiveCare/GreigHealth-Age14to17.pdf

Explanation of checklists
http://www.cps.ca/english/statements/CP/PreventiveCare/GHRPage1.pdf
http://www.cps.ca/english/statements/CP/PreventiveCare/GHRPage2.pdf
http://www.cps.ca/english/statements/CP/PreventiveCare/GHRPage3.pdf

Adults 18+ years

Preventive Care Checklist (Adult male, 18+ years)
http://www.cfpc.ca/uploadedFiles/Resources/Resource_Items/Male_Preventive_Care_Checklist_Form.pdf

Preventive Care Checklist (Adult female, 18+ years)
http://www.cfpc.ca/uploadedFiles/Resources/Resource_Items/Female_Preventive_Care_ChecklistForm.pdf

Explanation of checklists
http://www.cfpc.ca/uploadedFiles/Resources/Resource_Items/Preventive_Care_Checklist_Form_Explanations.pdf

incorporates dozens of evidence-based recommendations for the care of newborns, infants and children aged 0 to 5 years. This helps to ensure that busy practitioners remember to provide anticipatory guidance to prevent injuries – one of the leading causes of death in this age group, screen for developmental delay, provide age-appropriate vaccines and so forth. The more recent Greig Health Record is a similar checklist for older children and adolescents aged 6 to 17 years. Finally, there are also Preventive Care Checklists for men and women aged 18 and over, including specific guidance for those over the age of 65 years. These checklists have been approved by the College of Family Physicians of Canada (CFPC) and the Canadian Paediatric Society (CPS) and are used by health professionals across Canada to improve the quality of care provided to patients with the aim of improving health outcomes. Moreover, these checklists can be downloaded from the internet, are available free of charge and are also potentially adaptable to other contexts and settings.

In addition to using evidence to help practitioners and policy-makers make better-informed decisions, there are also evidence-based resources available for patients and the public. More recently, the CTFPHC has started to produce decision aids and fact sheets for patients which accompany the clinical practice guidelines produced for health profession-als. For instance, alongside a recent review on breast cancer screening, the task force prepared a one-page algorithm that guides patients through the decision process of whether or not to undergo mammography screening.[35] The algorithm begins by asking whether the woman is at increased risk of developing breast cancer due to family history, *BRCA* mutation or history of chest wall radiation. If "yes", then the advice is to talk to a doctor to find out what screening options are most appropriate under these specific circumstances. However, if "no", for women at general risk of developing breast cancer, the advice of what to do and why depends on the woman's age (i.e. screening is recommended for all women aged 50 to 74 years). An accompanying fact sheet for patients describes in greater detail the potential benefits and harms of breast cancer screening to further assist them in making informed choices.

Thus, while there are certainly a growing number of initiatives as described above to promote the use of evidence in making better-informed decisions, a great many obstacles must still be overcome.

Barriers to using evidence

Barriers to using evidence in decision-making range from missing the window of opportunity and knowledge gaps to conflicting evidence and conflicts of interest. At times these barriers stem from the complexity inherent to producing knowledge and creating facts (as described in the previous chapter), at times they are due to the disconnect between the worlds of researchers and policy-makers, at times there is intentional subverting of the evidence for political or economic gain, and at times it is a combination of the above.

Missing the window of opportunity

The window of opportunity for incorporating evidence into clinical decision-making is often very narrow. For instance, a pregnant woman goes to see her doctor for the first time at 12 weeks' gestation. The doctor offers her the option of prenatal screening for Down syndrome. The blood tests and ultrasound examination involved are time sensitive and must be done during the next couple of weeks to be valid. If the screening tests are positive, then the confirmatory test to diagnose Down syndrome in the fetus should be conducted between 16 and 18 weeks' gestation. Since the results of this test can take a few weeks to process (although there are some newer tests on the market using fluorescent in-situ hybridisation which provide a rapid answer in 24–48 hours), if the test result comes back positive, there is a limited window to decide whether or not to terminate the pregnancy. Thus there is a time pressure to make these very difficult, morally charged and potentially life-changing decisions, and not much leeway for examining the large body of evidence in this area unless the "work" of having synthesised and packaged the evidence into a usable format has already been done beforehand. This explains why busy clinicians often turn to "pre-digested" evidence-based resources such as Up to Date, JAMA evidence and MD Consult, since these are quick and easy to use, as well as being clinically relevant, even if they come at a price. However, patients rarely have access to such tools, or even to information leaflets intended for patients, which are not always distributed in practice, and therefore they must rely on what they can recall from the medical visit or else risk the information minefield which is the Internet. While "Googling" for answers is certainly an option, there is a great deal of misleading information on the Internet. At the very least, it is important to use reputable websites, and ideally sites that adhere to the HONcode principles, which is a code of ethics for high-quality health and medical information on the Internet.[36]

In the policy world, the window of opportunity for decision-making can also be very narrow. Whether a controversy erupts in the media or an outbreak occurs, decisions must often be made under pressure. Therefore, while there are occasions when governments have the luxury of commissioning research from health technology assessment agencies to aid decision-making, there are also occasions when the evidence is needed before the 5 p.m. press conference and there is simply no time to embark upon a systematic synthesis of the literature, even if one could call upon the experts to do so.

Thus, being able to influence health decisions requires forethought and planning. Once the decision arises, it is often too late to start collecting and collating the information. Nonetheless, it is possible to foresee common and/or important decisions that must be made – whether in a clinical setting or in a political context – and collect the best available evidence in advance to lay out the options and guide decision-makers through the pros and cons of these various options.

Using the Down syndrome screening example above, this is a daily occurrence in high-income contexts. In an ideal world, population-based screening programmes would have evidence-based patient information materials available to guide choices. These materials can even be provided to women who present for pre-conception counselling, as it would allow them even more time to digest the information and consider their options. In terms of policy decisions, these may not be regularly occurring events, yet it is also possible to forecast important opportunities for ensuring that evidence is used in making decisions that can influence the health of the population, and to prepare the necessary materials in advance (just as many major newspapers keep on file obituaries of famous people so that they are ready to go to print within hours when the time comes).

Health impact assessments (HIAs) are increasingly being used as tools for informing complex policy decisions. For instance, an HIA can be carried out to assess the potential benefits and harms associated with a proposed policy before it is put in place. In this way, the HIA can recommend various policy alternatives that can maximise the benefits while minimising harms. While it is certainly helpful to rely upon the best-available evidence to determine the optimal course of action in a rational and systematic way, as we saw in Chapter 3, decision-making, especially in politics, is not straightforward, but rather a dynamic and non-linear process.[37] Certainly, evidence can be misused as a tactic to stall decision-making (i.e. more research is needed before we can conclude...) or to justify decisions that have already been made (i.e. selectively citing studies that support the decision and ignoring research findings that are in conflict with the decision). However, even when evidence is not misused in this way, it is rare for the evidence to provide the entire basis for making a decision. Quite often the decision also relies upon value judgements and knowledge of the specific context. Therefore, evidence is generally only one type of input into the decision-making process, which also integrates many other considerations such as preferences, feasibility and so forth. Nonetheless, evidence is more likely to be used when it is available during the window of opportunity, if it points to options which are actionable and if the resources and infrastructure exist to make it happen.

Knowledge gaps and uncertainty

Another major barrier to using evidence for informing policy and practice is the lack of available evidence in specific areas. This can be extremely problematic. Particularly as we move away from strictly clinical questions such as the best pharmaceutical treatment for hypertension or the best diagnostic test for colon cancer, and attempt to address broader social questions such as how to tackle gender-based violence and how to create supportive environments for health, we enter a realm where it is often difficult to be entirely evidence based because the evidence has not been produced to the same extent. Since research requires funding, and a great deal of research is privately funded in part or in whole, it is not surprising that there is relatively little research on issues such as gender-based violence, since there is no pill or product associated with this health problem. Similarly, when dealing with health problems in specific under-serviced populations, such as immigrants or Aboriginal groups, one may also run into the same problem that there is often relatively little research evidence on "what works" to guide action in these specific populations.

As mentioned previously, lack of evidence does not mean that the interventions or strategies in question are not effective. It simply means that they have not been sufficiently investigated. The bottom line is that in the absence of evidence one is left with a great deal of uncertainty, despite which decisions must nonetheless be made. Therefore, at the very least, it is necessary to gather together the best possible evidence and to at least make explicit the knowledge gaps. Indeed, there is no such thing as zero uncertainty, and so it is simply a matter of degree. Often pleas for more research, while helpful, will generally not provide the additional evidence required within the timeline necessary to make decisions. In the mean-time, decision-makers must resort to examining best practices or examples of what has worked in different contexts to make the best possible decisions in spite of a lack of guidance from the existing body of research evidence.

Controversy and conflicting evidence

Sometimes there is not a lack of evidence altogether but rather a disagreement on the interpretation and use of the evidence. While, generally, evidence-based recommendations are quite similar across jurisdictions and contexts,[38] there are occasions when certain groups put out recommendations based on the same international body of evidence which are clearly at odds with the recommendations made elsewhere. This can lead to significant confusion and contentious debate in determining where the truth lies, and is a major barrier to the uptake and use of evidence.

The mammography controversy is a case in point.[39] When the Nordic Cochrane Centre published a systematic review in 2001 stating that "currently available reliable evidence does not show a survival benefit of mass screening for breast cancer", it caused a great outcry.[40] There were many articles written condemning anyone who dared to question the clinical utility of breast screening as being part of an "active anti-screening campaign... based on erroneous interpretation of data from cancer registries and peer-reviewed articles".[41] Indeed, unlike the other reviews of breast cancer screening, the Nordic review excluded certain studies for methodological reasons and included others, thereby arriving at a different conclusion. A few years later, the Nordic Cochrane Centre updated their analysis and revised their conclusions to be more nuanced. The most recent update of the review in 2011 states that "screening is likely to reduce breast cancer mortality" – but, they qualify this statement with an explanation.[42] The authors conclude that the mortality reduction attributable to screening is much lower than previously suggested by reviews of the mammography literature (i.e. 15% versus 30%). As well, overdiagnosis and overtreatment are much more common than is generally acknowledged. Thus, without rejecting breast screening alto-gether, the Nordic Cochrane Centre provides the data for patients and policy-makers to better weight the benefits and harms. If people invited for screening only knew that, out of

2,000 women screened for 10 years, only one will avoid dying from breast cancer, whereas 10 will receive unnecessary treatment, and over 200 will experience a false alarm requiring repeat testing and invasive diagnostic procedures, they would be better equipped to judge for themselves the merits of participating in the screening programme.[43] Indeed, if they choose to participate, they may even find this information reassuring by knowing in advance that false alarms are common and that only a small proportion of women who are recalled for additional testing actually have cancer.

However, the mammography controversy does not end here. There is also the issue of the age at which to begin mass screening. In many countries, the evidence-based recommendations are to begin mammography screening at 50 years of age. However, in 2002, the United States lowered the recommended starting age to 40 years.[44] Then, in 2009, the US Preventive Services Task Force (USPSTF) revised their recommendations based on new evidence from a British RCT which found no mortality benefit when screening women before the age of 50 years.[45] Once again, there was a huge outcry. Many proponents of breast cancer screening believe that more and earlier is better, and were outraged by the change in the recommendations. As a result, the USPSTF unanimously voted to update the language of their recommendation regarding women under 50 years of age. While they still do not recommend mass screening before the age of 50, they leave the door open for women to choose: "the decision to start regular, biennial screening mammography before the age of 50 years should be an individual one and take patient context into account, including the patient's values regarding specific benefits and harms".[46]

Therefore, even though we all share the same international body of research evidence, there are nonetheless times when the interpretation of that evidence leads to various controversies and disagreements which act as barriers to the uptake of evidence. Certainly, the body of evidence is not static, and as new information becomes available it can make knowledge users quite uncomfortable when there are changes to evidence-based recommendations over time. Yet this is a product of the knowledge base, which is constantly being revised and refined. Of course, another reason for disagreements between different clinical practice guidelines is also the quality and rigour of the process used in developing these guidelines. This is of much greater concern. Indeed, Dinnes and colleagues used the Appraisal of Guidelines for Research and Evaluation (AGREE) framework[47] to assess the validity of nine published guidelines on prostate cancer screening.[48] They conclude that the guidelines are inconsistent, and that the recommendations for "when to take action" are primarily based on consensus rather than scientific evidence. However, of even greater concern is when the evidence base is deliberately manipulated and misused with the intention of promoting certain vested interests. This is discussed separately in the following section.

Vested interests and conflicts of interest

The degree to which vested interests have infiltrated the international body of evidence is not to be underestimated. In areas such as cigarette smoking, prescribing pharmaceuticals and asbestos use, the research evidence can make or break an industry, with millions of dollars as well as thousands of jobs at stake. Therefore, there is a great deal to lose and tremendous incentive for these mega-industries to at the very least prevent the diffusion of studies which go against their commercial interests or even to actively infuse the larger body of evidence with conflicting studies to raise some doubt as to whether their product is indeed harmful – sufficient doubt to allow the money-making enterprise to continue reaping profits, even if only for a few more years. This sounds very sinister and hard to believe, yet, there are regular accounts of just this.

Indeed, a great deal has been written over the years about how the tobacco industry has attempted in various ways to call into question the link between smoking and cancer by producing their own evidence – often flawed or misinterpreted to their own ends.[49] For example, in 1988, three tobacco companies in the United States established the Center for Indoor Air Research (CIAR), which claims to be conducting objective and unbiased research. While in part this may be true, it has been suggested that at least some of the research funding is going towards producing research evidence that diverts attention away from environmental tobacco smoke (ETS) as an indoor air pollutant and supports the stance of tobacco companies that smoking should not be regulated in public places.[50] Even accepting "tobacco money" (i.e. in the form of research grants, endowed chairs, etc.) is in itself a highly contentious issue since it places researchers in a situation of compromise, reluctant to "bite the hand that feeds you". According to Chapman and Shatenstein:

> For decades, the tobacco industry's seductive international programme of research benefaction masqueraded behind the legitimising language of independence, dispassionate enquiry, and respect for scholarship. But, as revealed in the avalanche of internal industry documents now available on the World Wide Web, the industry was peerless in its proclivity for cultivating venal or naive scientists into a massively funded public relations campaign. The sole purpose of the exercise was to sow doubt among the public. Tobacco industry grant recipients often unwittingly reinforced the industry argument that it was genuinely seeking to define more precisely the relation between smoking and illness. 'If only we could do this, we might then be prepared to agree that our tobacco kills and is addictive' . . . that the issue of smoking and disease needed to be seen as wide open, therefore allowing the industry to remain blameless and unfettered in promoting its products.[51]

The tobacco industry has even gone so far as to commission consultants to write review articles for publication in the medical literature to call into question the link between secondhand smoke (SHS) and sudden infant death syndrome (SIDS). According to internal memos made public during legal action against the tobacco industry, there is proof that tobacco company executives "successfully encouraged one author to change his original conclusion that SHS is an independent risk factor for SIDS to state that the role of SHS is 'less well established'".[52] The author's disclosure of industry funding did not reveal the full extent of the company's involvement in shaping the content of the article. Yet another example of how accepting industry funds can disrupt the integrity of the scientific process with little or no regard for the lives that are at stake.

However, the tobacco industry is not the only culprit. A great deal has also been written in the medical literature about the pharmaceutical industry, which funds the bulk of clinical research that is carried out on medications. The success of these research studies can make all the difference between a "top-selling drug" and "going back to the drawing board". It is therefore unsurprising that there are incentives for introducing bias which could have a favourable impact on medication sales and ultimately increase profits for shareholders. According to Lexchin:

> Biases are introduced through a variety of measures including the choice of comparator agents, multiple publication of positive trials and non-publication of negative trials, reinterpreting data submitted to regulatory agencies, discordance between results and conclusions, conflict-of-interest leading to more positive conclusions, ghostwriting and the use of

"seeding" trials. Thus far, efforts to contain bias have largely focused on more stringent rules regarding conflict-of-interest (COI) and clinical trial registries. There is no evidence that any measures that have been taken so far have stopped the biasing of clinical research and it's not clear that they have even slowed down the process.[53]

How is it that this deliberate contamination of the body of evidence is allowed to continue? Well, as the saying goes, "money talks" and industries are not the only ones who are hungry for more.

Increasingly, cash-strapped universities are looking for alternative routes to fund-raising, and attempt to capitalise on the production of intellectual property. Indeed, some universities have even developed special venture capital teams to support the rollout and marketing of scientific discoveries and technological innovations developed on their campuses. Yet, a commitment to open scientific inquiry and the pursuit of financial gains are two goals that are very difficult to reconcile. Nonetheless, the growth of public–private partnerships (PPPs) is on the rise. These partnerships, while gaining in popularity, are inherently faced with multiple tensions and should therefore be entered into with great caution – if at all.

At times, amidst all of these vested interests, researchers can end up being caught in the middle. Even though industry goes to great lengths to create "an impression of legitimate, unbiased scientific research",[54] their primary accountability is to their shareholders in terms of increased profits, not the public good. It is therefore our responsibility to be vigilant in monitoring both the affiliations of the researchers and where they obtain their research funding. These links can seriously compromise a researcher's scientific integrity as well as their academic freedom to release research results which go against private interests. Indeed, there have been several scandals related to this. In one highly publicised case, Dr. Nancy Olivieri discovered that a treatment which was being tested on children at the Toronto Sick Kids Hospital was harmful to patients, and, despite having signed a non-disclosure agreement, she wanted to warn physicians and stop the study. However, the drug company which was funding the research and supplying the drugs threatened her with legal action if she spoke out. Sensing the ethical imperative to go against these legal threats out of the primacy of the well-being of patients, Olivieri soon found herself caught up in a maelstrom. Rather than being supported by her academic institution for protecting the public good, Olivieri was made out to be a scapegoat and fired. The Ontario College of Physicians eventually vindicated Olivieri of any wrongdoing, but she had to suffer through a very unpleasant experience. According to Arthur Shafer, a biomedical ethicist:

> With seeming indifference to the campaign of vilification against Olivieri – a campaign which questioned her scientific competence, her ethics, her personality, and even her sanity – both the scientific community and the general public appeared intuitively to understand that when Olivieri spoke out publicly about perceived dangers to her patients, she was acting in a manner consistent with the highest traditions of her profession.[55]

Indeed, Shafer and others call for an end to corporate sponsorship of research. However, until that day comes, the importance of critical appraisal is particularly important. As well, there is also increasing emphasis on rules of conduct to manage these thorny partnerships, including the routine disclosure and management of conflicts of interest.[56] Unfortunately these safeguards are essential when "dancing with the porcupine", as we have seen how easily ulterior motives and private interests can jeopardise the reliability and validity of research evidence.

However, even beyond academia – the bastion of knowledge production – governments are also implicated. In the interest of keeping the economy running and creating more jobs, governments are often eager supporters of new industrial sectors. For instance, the Canadian government is pouring money into genome research,[57] even though personalised medicine on the whole shows little promise for improving population health outcomes, as discussed previously in Chapter 3.[58] At times, these business ventures are even shown to have serious negative consequences for human health and well-being. Yet, any evidence of such links must be quashed as it risks interfering with economic gains and even with re-election. Therefore, in certain situations, governments have been accused of obfuscating the truth. The ongoing export of asbestos to low- and middle-income countries is a good example of this. According to Kazan-Allen:

> That asbestos is still being sold despite overwhelming evidence linking it to debilitating and fatal diseases is testament to the effectiveness of a campaign, spear-headed by Canadian interests, to promote a product already banned in many developed countries. Blessed by government and commercial support, asbestos apologists have implemented a long-term coordinated strategy targeting new consumers in Asia, the Far East and Latin America. At industry-backed 'conferences' and on government-funded junkets, they spin a web of deceit, telling all who will listen that 'chrysotile (white asbestos) can be used safely.' The fact that Canada exports over 95% of all the chrysotile it mines suggests that while chrysotile is supposedly safe enough for foreigners, it is not safe enough for Canadians. Asbestos victims in many countries have struggled to gain public recognition of the human cost of asbestos use. In recent years, nongovernmental organisations working with these groups have created a global anti-asbestos virtual network; with the commitment and support of thousands of 'virtual members,' this network challenges industry's propaganda and exposes the forces that support its cynical attempt to offload this dangerous substance on developing countries.[59]

Although the use of asbestos (including chrysotile asbestos) is banned in over 50 countries, the Canadian government has been actively blocking the addition of asbestos to the Rotterdam Convention, which lists pesticides and industrial chemicals that are banned or severely restricted for health or environmental reasons. Indeed, the government has refused to heed the recommendations of the public health community and even their own senior advisors within the Ministry of Health, who recommend that asbestos – a known carcinogen – should at the very least be added to Annexe III of the convention, which requires exporters to inform importers of the risks and precautionary measures for safer handling of the hazardous product.[60] According to an editorial in the *Canadian Medical Association Journal*, "Canada is the only Western democracy to have consistently opposed international efforts to regulate the global trade in asbestos. And the government of Canada has done so with shameful political manipulation of science".[61]

For years, the government liberally funded the Chrysotile Institute – the main lobby group for the asbestos industry – and sees no irony in spending millions of dollars scraping asbestos out of Canadian public buildings (including the parliament buildings and the Prime Minister's house at 24 Sussex Drive) while continuing to export asbestos to resource-poor countries.[62] To add insult to injury, a sizeable proportion of the exported asbestos is being used to make low-cost roofing for slum dwellers in places such as India. According to one asbestos exporter:

> Chrysotile usage in India alone has gone up nine per cent in the past year. That country's government and institutions have the same information we have. They are obviously of the

opinion that chrysotile answers important basic needs of their population, providing affordable roofing for the poor, for whom the choice is having a chrysotile cement roof or having no roof.[63]

As if choosing between having a roof over one's head and dying of lung cancer is a truly free and informed choice. However, there are members of parliament who are vocal opponents to the continued export of asbestos. Pat Martin, a former miner who has led a longstanding crusade to ban asbestos, says:

Claims that chrysotile asbestos is harmless are entirely bogus. Industry-funded junk science doesn't stand up to the facts. Canada has dumped 750,000 tonnes of asbestos on world markets since ignoring Health Canada's advice and it's still the world's leading industrial killer, claiming over 100,000 lives every year.[64]

Indeed, an internal memo to the environment minister that was recently obtained under access to information reveals that the government has known all along that the criteria have been met for the inclusion of chrysotile asbestos on the Rotterdam Convention list, and yet the addition has nonetheless been repeatedly blocked. According to Martin: "They didn't just deny the science. They acknowledged it but yet ignored it. . . They've put commercial and political interests ahead of scientific interests, and in doing, compromised and undermined the whole purpose and intent of the convention".[65] Although there is mounting pressure locally and internationally to end the production and export of asbestos, a $58 million provincial government loan was recently approved to reopen an asbestos mine in Quebec. Then, following the Quebec elections where the newly elected leader had promised to revoke the loan, the federal government reacted by grudgingly reversing their longstanding position on asbestos and finally announced that they would no longer veto the ban. Concurrently, the asbestos question is also being hotly debated in Brazil's Supreme Court. Thus, there is renewed optimism, but the battle is not yet over.

Even beyond the corporate interests of powerful manufacturers (i.e. tobacco, pharmaceuticals, asbestos, etc.) who compromise the integrity and reliability of the body of evidence, there are also many vested interests in the service sector who attempt to spin the evidence for their financial advantage. The health care sector in particular is a multi-billion-dollar industry, and everyone wants a piece of the pie. Although there is a great deal of evidence that demonstrates the power of universal access to publicly funded health care as an important determinant of health, and the need to have primary health care as the bedrock of all health systems,[66] there is a great deal of resistance to this model. What about free enterprise? Is health care a public good or a profitable way of doing business? Indeed, privatisation finds a way of creeping in wherever there is the smallest loophole because it is quite simply an extremely lucrative business. There is a burgeoning of "boutique" health services and medical tourism for the wealthy that include private jet travel, beachside villas and personal chefs, while poor people in many countries around the world cannot even access the most basic health services and often rely upon a network of informal health providers. Moreover, it is debatable whether luxury health care will even improve one's health, since any epidemiologist will tell you that the more tests that you do, especially among those who are not at high risk for developing a given disease (i.e. where prevalence is low), the greater the likelihood that you will have false-positive results that can lead you down the path to even more invasive diagnostic testing and all the needless anxiety and discomfort that goes along with it. For instance, one high-end health service provider offers dozens of tests in a single day, a kind of medical "fishing expedition" with a large price tag attached:

You might call it the Mercedes-Benz of checkups and it doesn't come cheap. The one-day 'premium check-up' booked through [company A] starts from €2,405 and consists of the following: a clinical examination (physical, orthopaedic and basic neurological examinations); laboratory tests; examination of the stomach and pelvic organs as well as the thyroid; colour ultrasound of the liver, gall bladder, spleen, kidneys, stomach, intestines, pancreas, bladder, abdominal artery, vena cava, thyroid, prostate for men, uterus and ovaries for women; cardio-respiratory diagnostics for stroke prevention; screening for skin cancer; lung diagnostics; and, a final consultation with the doctor who gives the patient a detailed written report. Depending on the test results, additional modules in urology, gynaecology, gastroenterology and neurology may be recommended. Eyes, ears, nose and throat checks also cost extra.[67]

Indeed, there is a large and growing literature on the impact of privatised health care. At the individual doctor–patient level, there is a great deal that has been written on personal interests and financial motivations leading private providers to over-prescribe[68] and over-treat,[69] unless there are regulations in place and competing incentive structures to prevent this from happening.[70] The fact that poor people desperate to preserve themselves and their loved ones pay for health services out of pocket is not the same as "ability to pay" since there are many sacrifices that result from these payments, including removing children from schools, entering into bonded labour and other forms of debt, selling off homes and farms – anything to cover the immediate costs of accessing care – but ultimately placing themselves and their families in an even more precarious situation. Indeed, catastrophic illness can throw an entire family deeper and deeper into poverty.

Proponents of privatisation, such as the World Bank, attempt to take a "harm reduction" approach and suggest that private sector involvement can be a lever for attaining population health goals if only there is greater public stewardship on the part of national governments.[71] Yet there is widespread consensus that "a privatised, 'American-style' health financing and provision system is neither a feasible nor desirable model for developing countries".[72] Given the many challenges that governments face regulating the private sector even in high-income settings, it is questionable the extent to which adequate national-level stewardship is possible around the world, especially with the growing globalisation of private-sector health care services. Margaret Whitehead and colleagues warn that private interests threaten to worsen health inequities for the world's most poor and vulnerable:

In the past two decades, powerful international trends in market-oriented health-sector reforms have been sweeping around the world, generally spreading from the northern to the southern, and from the western to the eastern hemispheres. Global blueprints have been advocated by agencies such as the World Bank to promote privatisation of health-service providers, and to increase private financing – via user fees – of public providers. Furthermore, commercial interests are increasingly promoted by the World Trade Organisation, which has striven to open up public services to foreign investors and markets. This policy could pave the way for public funding of private operators in health and education sectors, especially in wealthy, industrial countries in the northern hemisphere. Although such attempts to undermine public services pose an obvious threat to equity in the well-established social-welfare systems of Europe and Canada, other developments pose more immediate threats to the fragile systems in middle-income and low-income countries. Two of these trends – the introduction of user fees for public services, and the growth of out-of-pocket expenses for private services – can, if combined, constitute a major poverty trap.[73]

The authors therefore call for an evidence-based approach to health-sector reform. Rather than promoting mass privatisation of health care services and charging poor people user fees, which have been shown time and again to have negative impacts on health,[74,75] alternative approaches are needed. For instance, it has been suggested that taxing the funds that are currently hidden in tax-free offshore accounts could generate an estimated $160 billion per year.[76] While this would almost certainly provoke an outcry from the wealthy who take advantage of these tax loopholes, this amount would go a long way in providing health and social care to people in low- and middle-income countries who are most in need.

Thus, readers of the scientific literature should be aware of the various ways in which the research evidence can be influenced and misused for various aims and agendas. That is not to say that we should throw out the whole "evidence-based" enterprise, but a healthy dose of scepticism and critical thinking is advisable. It is not enough to simply produce evidence, nor even to synthesise and package evidence into a more user-friendly format. Particularly at the policy level, political savvy is also needed to ensure that vested interests do not undermine decisions that can impact the health of individuals and populations. Whether it is tobacco companies trying to flood the literature with contradicting evidence, or pharmaceutical companies hiding research demonstrating that their products have no effect or lead to harm, these conflicts of interest can lead us to make erroneous conclusions and misinformed decisions. Ultimately, the public pays the price, whether through poor health or misspent money. In the next chapter, a model for ensuring more participatory, transparent and evidence-informed decisions will be presented and discussed.

References

1. Cabana M, Rand C, Powe N et al. Why don't physicians follow clinical practice guidelines? A framework for improvement. JAMA 1999; 282: 1458–65.

2. Bloom B. Effects of continuing medical education on improving physician clinical care and patient health: A review of systematic reviews. Int J Technol Assess Health Care 2005; 21(3): 380–5.

3. Agency for Healthcare Research and Quality. National Guideline Clearinghouse. Rockville, MD: Agency for Healthcare Research and Quality, 2012. Available at: http://www.guideline.gov/.

4. Graham I, Logan J, Harrison M et al. Lost in knowledge translation: time for a map? Contin Educ Health Prof 2006; 26: 13–24.

5. Greenhalgh T, Wieringa S. Is it time to drop the 'knowledge translation' metaphor? A critical literature review. J R Soc Med 2011; 104(12): 501–9.

6. Straus S, Tetroe J, Graham I. Defining knowledge translation. CMAJ 2009; 181: 165–8.

7. Denis J, Lomas J, Stipich N. Creating receptor capacity for research in the health system: the Executive Training for Research Application (EXTRA) program in Canada. J Health Serv Res Policy 2008; 13 (Suppl 1): 1–7.

8. Lomas J. The in-between world of knowledge brokering. BMJ 2007; 334 (7585): 129–32.

9. Graham I. Knowledge translation at CIHR [PowerPoint presentation]. Ottawa: Canadian Institutes for Health Research, 2009. Available at: http://www.cihr-irsc.gc.ca/e/documents/knowledge_translation_at_cihr_general_slide_deck_internet_english_2009_04_20.pdf.

10. The Cochrane Collaboration. Glossary. Oxford: The Cochrane Collaboration, 2012. Available at: http://www.cochrane.org/glossary/.

11. Higgins J, Green S (eds.). Cochrane Handbook for Systematic Reviews of Interventions. Version 5.1.0, Oxford: The Cochrane Collaboration, 2011. Available at: http://www.cochrane-handbook.org/.

12. Waters E, de Silva-Sanigorski A, Hall B, et al. Interventions for preventing obesity in children. Cochrane Database Syst Rev 2011; (12): CD001871.

13. Rosen L, Ben Noach M, Rosenberg E. Missing the forest (plot) for the trees? A critique of the systematic review in tobacco control. BMC Med Res Methodol 2010; 10: 34.

14. Taubes G. Do we really know what makes us healthy? *The New York Times Magazine.* September 16, 2007. Available at: http://www.nytimes.com/2007/09/16/magazine/16epidemiology-t.html.

15. Oxman A, Sackett D, Guyatt G. Users' guides to the medical literature. I. How to get started. *JAMA* 1993; 270(17): 2093–5.

16. Critical Appraisal Skills Programme (CASP). *Appraising the Evidence.* Oxford: CASP UK, 2012. Available at: http://www.casp-uk.net/find-appraise-act/appraising-the-evidence/.

17. Stead L, Perera R, Bullen C, Mant D, Lancaster T. Nicotine replacement therapy for smoking cessation. *Cochrane Database of Syst Rev* 2008; (1): CD000146. DOI: 10.1002/14651858.CD000146.pub3. Available at: http://summaries.cochrane.org/CD000146/can-nicotine-replacement-therapy-nrt-help-people-quit-smoking.

18. Budetti P. Ensuring safe and effective medications for children. *JAMA* 2003; 290: 950.

19. Canadian Task Force on the Periodic Health Examination. *Canadian Guide to Clinical Preventive Health Care.* Ottawa: Health Canada, 1994. Available at: http://www.canadiantaskforce.ca/recommendations__current_eng.html.

20. US Preventive Services Task Force (USPSTF). Rockville, MD: Agency for Healthcare Research and Quality, 2012. Available at: http://www.uspreventiveservicestaskforce.org/.

21. US Preventive Services Task Force (USPSTF). *Guide to Clinical Preventive Services, 2010–2011.* Rockville, MD: Agency for Healthcare Research and Quality, 2010. Available at: http://www.ahrq.gov/clinic/pocketgd.htm.

22. Task Force on Community Preventive Services; Zaza S, Briss P, Harris K (ed.). *The Guide to Community Preventive Services: What Works to Promote Health?* Oxford: Oxford University Press, 2005. Available at: http://www.thecommunityguide.org/library/book/index.html.

23. US Preventive Services Task Force (USPSTF). *Grade Definitions After May 2007.* Rockville, MD: USPSTF Program Office, 2008. Available at: http://www.uspreventiveservicestaskforce.org/uspstf/gradespost.htm#arec.

24. Altman D and Bland J. Absence of evidence is not evidence of absence. *BMJ* 1995; 311: 485.

25. Banta H, Luce B. *Health Care Technology and Its Assessment: An International Perspective.* New York, NY: Oxford University Press, 1993.

26. International Network of Agencies for Health Technology Assessment (INAHTA). Secretariat. *Members.* Cologne, Germany: International Network of Agencies for Health Technology Assessment, 2012. Available at: http://www.inahta.net/.

27. Busse R, Orvain J, Velasco M *et al.* Best practice in undertaking and reporting health technology assessments. *Int J Technol Assess Health Care* 2002; 18: 361–422.

28. Centre for Reviews and Dissemination (CRD). *HTA Database.* York: University of York, 2012. Available at: http://www.crd.york.ac.uk/crdweb/AboutPage.asp.

29. Ueffing E, Tugwell P, Roberts J *et al.* Equity-oriented toolkit for health technology assessment and knowledge translation: application to scaling up of training and education for health workers. *Hum Resour Health* 2009; 7: 67.

30. The Cochrane Collaboration. Cochrane Collaboration awarded seat on World Health Assembly. Oxford: The Cochrane Collaboration, 2011. Available at: http://www.cochrane.org/features/cochrane-collaboration-awarded-seat-world-health-assembly.

31. Panisset U. *EVIPNet Evidence-Informed Policy Network for Better Decision Making.* Geneva: World Health Organization, 2009. Available at: http://www.who.int/evidence/en/index.html.

32. Lavis J, Davies H, Oxman A *et al.* Towards systematic reviews that inform healthcare management and policymaking. *J Health Serv Res Policy* 2005; 10 (Suppl 1): 35–48.

33. Waters E, Armstrong R, Swinburn B *et al.* An exploratory cluster randomised controlled trial of knowledge translation strategies to support evidence-informed decision-making in local governments (The KT4LG study). *BMC Public Health* 2011; 11: 34.

34. The Cochrane Collaboration. *Cochrane Summaries*. Oxford: The Cochrane Collaboration, 2012. Available at: http://summaries.cochrane.org/.

35. Canadian Task Force on Preventive Health Care. *Breast Cancer Screening: Patient Algorithm*. Ottawa: Canadian Task Force on Preventive Health Care, 2011. Available at: http://www.canadiantaskforce.ca/docs/Patient_Algorithm_ENG.pdf.

36. Health on the Net Foundation. *Looking for Reliable Health Information?* Chene-Bourg, Switzerland: Health on the Net Foundation, 2011. Available at: http://www.hon.ch/HONcode/Patients/visitor_safeUse2.html.

37. Nutbeam D, Harris E. *Theory in a nutshell: A practical guide to health promotion theories*, 2nd edn. Sydney, Australia: McGraw Hill, 2004.

38. Mavriplis C, Thériault G. The periodic health examination: a comparison of United States and Canadian recommendations (French). *Can Fam Physician* 2006; 52: 58–63.

39. Finkel M. *Understanding the Mammography Controversy: Science, Politics and Breast Cancer Screening*. Westport, CT: Praeger Publishers, 2005.

40. Olsen O, Gøtzsche P. Screening for breast cancer with mammography. *Cochrane Database Syst Rev* 2001;(4):CD001877.

41. Bock K, Borisch B, Cawson J et al. Effect of population-based screening on breast cancer mortality. *Lancet* 2011; 378(9805): 1775–6.

42. Gøtzsche P, Nielsen M. Screening for breast cancer with mammography. *Cochrane Database Syst Rev* 2011;(1):CD001877.

43. Gotzsche P, Hartling O, Nielsen M, Broderson J, Jorgensen K. Breast screening: the facts – or maybe not. *BMJ* 2009; 338: b86. Available at: http://www.bmj.com/content/338/bmj.b86?view=long&pmid=19174442.

44. US Preventive Services Task Force (USPSTF). *Screening for Breast Cancer (2002)*. Rockville, MD: Agency for Healthcare Research and Quality, 2002. Available at: http://www.uspreventiveservicestaskforce.org/uspstf/uspsbrca2002.htm.

45. Moss S, Cuckle H, Evans A *et al.*; Trial Management Group. Effect of mammographic screening from age 40 years on breast cancer mortality at 10 years' follow-up: a randomised controlled trial. *Lancet* 2006; 368: 2053–60.

46. US Preventive Services Task Force (USPSTF). *Screening for Breast Cancer*. Rockville, MD: Agency for Healthcare Research and Quality, 2009. Available at: http://www.uspreventiveservicestaskforce.org/uspstf/uspsbrca.htm.

47. AGREE Collaboration. Development and validation of an international appraisal instrument for assessing the quality of clinical practice guidelines: the AGREE project. *Qual Saf Health Care* 2003; 12: 18–23.

48. Johansson M, Stattin P. Guidelines are too important to be left to clinical experts. *CMAJ* 2012; 184: 159–60.

49. Tong E, Glantz S. Tobacco industry efforts undermining evidence linking secondhand smoke with cardiovascular disease. *Circulation* 2007; 116(16): 1845–54.

50. Barnes D, Bero L. Industry-funded research and conflict of interest: an analysis of research sponsored by the tobacco industry through the Center for Indoor Air Research. *J Health Polit Policy Law* 1996; 21 (3): 515–42.

51. Chapman S, Shatenstein S. The ethics of the cash register: taking tobacco research dollars. *Tob Control* 2001; 10(1): 1–2.

52. Tong E, England L, Glantz S. Changing conclusions on secondhand smoke in a sudden infant death syndrome review funded by the tobacco industry. *Pediatrics* 2005; 115(3): e356–66.

53. Lexchin J. Those who have the gold make the evidence: how the pharmaceutical industry biases the outcomes of clinical trials of medications. *Sci Eng Ethics* 2012; 18(2): 247–61.

54. Muggli M, Forster J, Hurt R, Repace J. The smoke you don't see: uncovering tobacco industry scientific strategies aimed against environmental tobacco smoke policies. *Am J Public Health* 2001; 91(9): 1419–23.

55. Schafer A. Biomedical conflicts of interest: a defence of the sequestration thesis—learning from the cases of Nancy Olivieri and David Healy. *J Med Ethics* 2004; 30(1): 8–24.

56. Lewis S, Baird P, Evans R *et al.* Dancing with the porcupine: rules for governing the university-industry relationship. *CMAJ* 2001; 165(6): 783–5.

57. Genome Canada. Harper Government Invests in Personalized Medicine [press release]. Ottawa: Genome Canada, 2012. Available at: http://www.genomecanada.ca/en/about/news.aspx?i=409.

58. Wade N. A Decade Later, Genetic Map Yields Few New Cures. *The New York Times* June 12, 2010. Available at: http://www.nytimes.com/2010/06/13/health/research/13genome.html.

59. Kazan-Allen L. The asbestos war. *Int J Occup Environ Health* 2003; 9(3): 173–93.

60. Shochat B. Health Canada's Asbestos Advice Rejected by Government. *CBC News,* June 13, 2011. Available at: http://www.cbc.ca/news/canada/story/2011/06/13/asbestos-health-canada.html.

61. Attaran A, Boyd D, Stanbrook M. Asbestos mortality: a Canadian export. *CMAJ* 2008; 179(9): 871–4.

62. Fatal Deception: Is the Federal Government Relying on Junk Science to Justify Its Support for Re-Opening Asbestos Mines in Quebec? *CBC News* February 2, 2012. Available at: http://www.cbc.ca/video/#/Shows/The_National/Health/1274854987/ID=2192550070.

63. Versailles G. Asbestos use at Montreal's new hospital [letter to the editor]. *The Gazette* January 3, 2012. Available at: http://www.montrealgazette.com/business/Asbestos+Montreal+hospital/5941259/story.html.

64. Saganash R. Harper Must Put Lives before Politics on Asbestos: NDP [press release]. *Romeo Saganash MP Blog* June 14, 2011. Available at: http://romeosaganash.ndp.ca/post/harper-must-put-lives-before-politics-on-asbestos-ndp.

65. Schmidt S, De Souza M. Feds Admitted Dangers of Asbestos While Fighting 'Hazardous' Label: Documents. *PostMedia News* June 25, 2012. Available at: http://www2.canada.com/topics/news/story.html?id=6838117.

66. Van Lerberghe W, Evans T, Rasanathan K *et al.* World Health Report 2008 - Primary Health Care: Now More than Ever. Geneva: World Health Organization, 2008.

67. O'Hagan H. Medical Tourists Opting for Sea, Sand, Sun and Surgery. *The National* February 18, 2012. Available at: http://www.thenational.ae/lifestyle/travel/medical-tourists-opting-for-sea-sand-sun-and-surgery.

68. James C, Peabody J, Solon O, Quimbo S, Hanson K. An unhealthy public-private tension: pharmacy ownership, prescribing, and spending in the Philippines. *Health Affairs* 2009; 28: 1022–33.

69. Cromwell J, Mitchell J. Physician-induced demand for surgery. *J Health Econ* 1986; 5: 293–313.

70. Bennett S, Dakpallah G, Garner P, *et al.* Carrot and stick: state mechanisms to influence private provider behaviour. *Health Policy Plan* 1994; 9: 1–13.

71. The World Bank. *Health Policy Toolkit.* Washington DC: The World Bank, 2012. Available at: https://www.wbginvestmentclimate.org/toolkits/public-policy-toolkit/.

72. Hozumi D, Frost L, Suraratdecha C *et al. The Role of the Private Sector in Health: A Landscape Analysis of Global Players' Attitudes toward the Private Sector in Health Systems and Policy Levers That Influence These Attitudes.* NY: The Rockefeller Foundation, 2008. Available at: http://www.resultsfordevelopment.org/sites/resultsfordevelopment.org/files/resources/A%20Landscape%20Analysis%20of%20Global%20Attitudes%20toward%20the%20Private%20Sector.pdf.

73. Whitehead M, Dahlgren G, Evans T. Equity and health sector reforms: can low-income countries escape the medical poverty trap? *Lancet* 2001; 358(9284): 833–6.

74. Tipping G. *The Social Impact of User Fees For Health Care on Poor Households: Commissioned Report to the Ministry of Health.* Hanoi, Vietnam: Health Policy Unit, Ministry of Health, 2000.

75. Stuckler D, King L, McKee M. Mass privatisation and the post-communist mortality crisis: a cross-national analysis. *Lancet* 2009; 373(9661): 399–407.

76. United Nations Research Institute for Social Development (UNRISD). *Visible hands – Taking Responsibility for Social Development.* Geneva: UNRISD, 2000.

Chapter 6

Making evidence-informed decisions

Making evidence-informed decisions with the aim of improving health can be facilitated by using a systematic approach. While there is no single way of summarising or ordering the various elements that should be involved in making such decisions, the algorithm shown in Fig. 6.1 lays out many of the key issues that should be considered. Indeed many different types of evidence and value judgements are needed during the decision-making process to answer a wide range of questions, including: (1) What is the priority health problem? (2) What causes this health problem? (3) What are the different strategies or interventions that can be used to address this health problem? (4) Which of these options as compared to the *status quo* has an added benefit that outweighs the harms? (5) Which options would be acceptable to the individuals or populations involved? (6) What are the costs and opportunity costs? (7) Would these options be feasible in this specific context? (8) What are the ethical, legal and social implications of choosing one option over another? (9) What do different stakeholders stand to gain or lose from each option? And (10) Taking into account the multiple perspectives and considerations involved, which option is most likely to improve health while minimising harms? The remainder of this chapter will go through each of the steps in the algorithm in greater detail.

(1) Define the priority health problem

Whether seeking to improve the health of individuals, populations or our global society, there are generally multiple health problems that could be addressed. Often many of these health problems are inter-related and intertwined. Yet, it is nonetheless helpful to try and identify the priority health problem (or problems) that, if improved, will have the greatest impact on health overall.

For instance, a person may suffer from high blood pressure, anxiety problems and a recent cancer diagnosis. While not downplaying the severity of the other problems, if the issue of cancer is not addressed, then the patient's very survival is threatened. As well, addressing the issue of cancer could also improve the anxiety and high blood pressure. However, if the patient's anxiety problems are so debilitating that the person is paralysed with fear, unable to take any action or even leave the house, then perhaps the anxiety problems would be the priority. Alternatively, if the blood pressure today is 200/100, then this may be the most urgent issue to deal with to prevent stroke and even death. Thus, determining which is the priority health problem often depends on several factors including the severity of the problem, the imminent risk of harm, the potential to intervene and the patient's preferences and expectations.

At a population level, identifying the priority health problems often involves a two-step process as described in Chapter 4. First, an "objective" needs assessment is used to measure

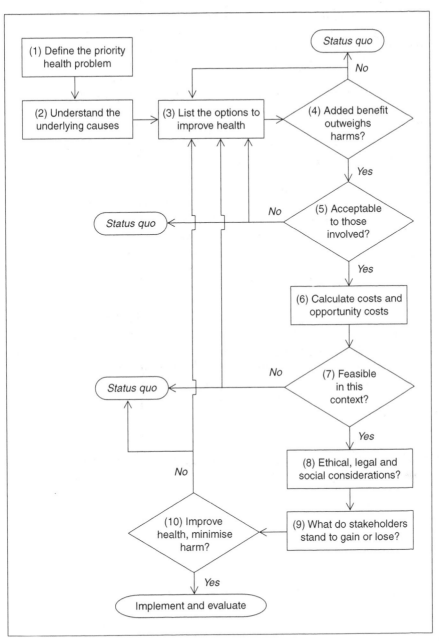

Figure 6.1 Algorithm for making evidence-informed decisions to improve health.

the most common and severe health problems within the population. Next a "subjective" needs assessment is used to elicit the values and preferences of the population.[1] For example, an objective needs assessment based on surveillance data of deaths, disease prevalence, health care utilisation and so forth may determine that the majority of the population suffers from mental health problems, injuries and chronic diseases such as diabetes and heart disease. However, according to the subjective needs assessment, the community may consider the most important priority to be building a school and ensuring that there are excellent teachers who help young people to succeed, thus preventing high rates of substance abuse, violence and suicides among youth. Indeed, mental health problems, injuries and chronic diseases are to a great extent just symptoms of larger underlying social issues such as lack of education, unemployment and low income. Unless these issues are addressed (i.e. the determinants of health), little progress will be made in preventing the other health problems from occurring. Therefore, the combined approach (subjective/objective) helps to determine what are the key issues to focus on for improving health by integrating available data with the perspectives of the community.

At the global level, common approaches for identifying health priorities include the top 10 causes of mortality and the global burden of disease (GBD) list. While not terribly nuanced, the top 10 causes of mortality provide a basic overview of why people are dying. In many countries around the world, the state of health statistics is so limited that even this most basic information is not routinely available. Yet, in spite of these methodological challenges, it is estimated that over half of all deaths around the world can be explained by 10 major causes (Table 6.1).[4] This certainly helps to focus one's attention on which priority problems should be tackled. Notably, heart disease and stroke are in top place. However, the "top 10" includes all deaths at any age. As we all know, everyone will die of something at some point in their lives. In wealthy countries where infectious diseases have declined greatly over the last century and people generally live into their 70s and 80s (also known as the epidemiological transition),[2] about one-third of people die of heart disease, one-third of cancer and one-third due to other causes.[3] Thus, it is not surprising that heart disease, stroke and cancer are high on the list, and the number of deaths continues to rise as an

Table 6.1 Leading causes of death worldwide.

Health problem	Number of deaths (million)	Percentage of overall deaths (%)
1. Heart disease	7.2	12.2
2. Stroke	5.7	9.7
3. Lung infections	4.2	7.1
4. Chronic lung disease	3.0	5.1
5. Diarrhoeal diseases	2.2	3.7
6. HIV / AIDS	2.0	3.5
7. Tuberculosis	1.5	2.5
8. Lung cancer	1.3	2.3
9. Road traffic injuries	1.3	2.2
10. Prematurity	1.2	2.0
TOTAL	**29.6**	**50.3**

Adapted from: World Health Organization. *The Global Burden of Disease: 2004 Update.* Geneva: World Health Organization, 2008.

Table 6.2 Leading causes of burden of disease (DALYs) worldwide.

Health problem	DALYs (million)	Percentage of overall DALYs (%)
1. Lung infections	94.5	6.2
2. Diarrhoeal diseases	72.8	4.8
3. Depression	65.5	4.3
4. Heart disease	62.6	4.1
5. HIV / AIDS	58.5	3.8
6. Stroke	46.6	3.1
7. Prematurity	44.3	2.9
8. Birth asphyxia / trauma	41.7	2.7
9. Road traffic injuries	41.2	2.7
10. Neonatal infections	40.4	2.7
TOTAL	**568.1**	**37.3**

Adapted from: World Health Organization. *The Global Burden of Disease: 2004 Update*. Geneva: World Health Organization, 2008.

ever-increasing number of low- and middle-income countries develop and go through the epidemiological transition. That being said, since infectious diseases are still important causes of death in many countries, most notably in Africa, Latin America and Southeast Asia, diseases such as HIV/AIDS, tuberculosis and malaria are also highly ranked. However, these crude mortality measures do not take into account premature deaths or level of health across the lifespan.

Thus, more nuanced measures were developed to assess the global burden of disease. The disability-adjusted life year (DALY) is a composite measure that combines the years of life lost due to premature death (YLL) and the years lost due to disability (YLD).[4] Unlike mortality statistics which simply measure the number of people who die from a given health-related condition, DALYs factor in the age at death, and also allow for the inclusion of chronic conditions such as mental health problems or hearing loss, which can greatly impact the quality of life even if they do not significantly shorten the length of years lived (Table 6.2).[4] Indeed, by using DALYs to determine the top 10 health problems, depression jumps up to the number three position, accounting for almost 5% of the global burden of disease. Conditions that occur at birth or during childhood are also given more weight. Thus lung infections, diarrhoeal diseases, prematurity, birth asphyxia/trauma and neonatal infections all move up the scale and explain why maternal–child health has received so much attention in recent years, including from the recent G8 summit in Muskoka.[5]

Priority setting is therefore a very important first step. All too often, a great new drug or intervention is discovered and people lobby for its implementation and scale up, when the need for this intervention has not even been demonstrated and it is unclear that it will truly have a widespread impact on the health of the entire population. Therefore it is important in the first instance that we understand what the true health needs are, to be able to then address them in an evidence-informed way.

(2) Understand the underlying causes

As demonstrated by the research cycle described in Chapter 4, it is difficult to tackle a health problem unless there is an understanding of what causes the problem and where it would be possible to intervene to mitigate the problem or ideally to prevent the problem from occurring in the first place. For a long time, we have been mostly focusing on the proximal causes of the problem commonly known as the "risk factors". More recently, Sir Michael Marmot coined the phrase "the causes of the causes" to show how the distribution of risk factors in a population can be influenced by other upstream factors known as the "social determinants of health".[6] Going even further upstream, Jeff Reading, formerly Director of the Institute of Aboriginal People's Health at the Canadian Institutes of Health Research, described the "causes of the causes of the causes" to show how the Aboriginal determinants of health underlie the social determinants, which underlie the distribution of risk factors, leading to the notion that there can be proximal, intermediate and distal causes of poor health.[7]

Causes

When examining why people die or are in poor health, a relatively small number of risk factors explain a large proportion of mortality and morbidity worldwide. Considering that heart disease, stroke and lung disease are the top killers (Table 6.1), it is not surprising that the leading risk factors accounting for these deaths include high blood pressure, tobacco use, high blood sugar, physical inactivity, overweight and obesity, and high cholesterol (Table 6.3).[8] Basically it all boils down to poor diet, lack of exercise and smoking.

If one instead uses the Global Burden of Disease list (Table 6.2), which also includes diarrhoeal diseases, neonatal infections, HIV/AIDS, depression and road traffic injuries, then

Table 6.3 Leading risk-factor causes of death worldwide.

Risk factor	Number of deaths (million)	Percentage of overall deaths (%)
1. High blood pressure	7.5	12.8
2. Tobacco use	5.1	8.7
3. High blood glucose	3.4	5.8
4. Physical inactivity	3.2	5.5
5. Overweight and obesity	2.8	4.8
6. High cholesterol	2.6	4.5
7. Unsafe sex	2.4	4.0
8. Alcohol use	2.3	3.8
9. Childhood underweight	2.2	3.8
10. Indoor smoke from solid fuels	2.0	3.3
TOTAL	**33.5**	**37.0**

Adapted from: World Health Organization. *Global Health Risks: Mortality and Burden of Disease Attributable to Selected Major Risks*. Geneva: World Health Organization, 2009.

Table 6.4 Leading risk-factor causes of burden of disease (DALYs) worldwide.

Risk factor	Number of DALYs (million)	Percentage of overall DALYs (%)
1. Childhood underweight	91	5.9
2. Unsafe sex	70	4.6
3. Alcohol use	69	4.5
4. Unsafe water, poor sanitation	64	4.2
5. High blood pressure	57	3.7
6. Tobacco use	57	3.7
7. Suboptimal breastfeeding	44	2.9
8. High blood glucose	41	2.7
9. Indoor smoke from solid fuels	41	2.7
10. Overweight and obesity	36	2.3
TOTAL	**570**	**37.2**

Adapted from: World Health Organization. *Global Health Risks: Mortality and Burden of Disease Attributable to Selected Major Risks*. Geneva: World Health Organization, 2009.

the risk factors reflect this (Table 6.4).[8] Food insecurity in childhood, suboptimal breastfeeding, unsafe water and poor sanitation are major risk factors for diarrhoeal diseases and neonatal infections, unsafe sex is a major risk factor for HIV/AIDS, and alcohol use is a major risk factor for road traffic injuries and a comorbidity of depression.

Thus it is not uncommon to see people trying to improve health by using a risk-factor approach. By reducing the prevalence of risk factors, it should follow that one can thereby reduce mortality and burden of disease. While it is certainly important to understand the underlying risk factors and protective factors and how they relate and interact, there is an uneven distribution of these factors in the population, and, therefore, it is important to recognise the other upstream causes at play.

Causes of the causes

As described previously in this book, the social determinants of health include factors such as education, employment, family income, housing and social support that influence the health status of populations and can help to explain why some people are healthy and others are not (Fig. 6.2).[9,10]

For instance, people with higher levels of education have more job security, higher incomes, better access to healthy social and physical environments, and a greater sense of control over their life circumstances.[11] In contrast, lack of education and the resulting job insecurity can increase the risk of physical and mental ailments such as cardiovascular disease, anxiety, depression and suicide.[12] It is also linked to an increase in alcohol and tobacco abuse, poor nutrition and physical inactivity. In many cases, people who are suffering from poverty and social exclusion do not even have their most basic physiological needs fulfilled (Fig. 6.3).[13]

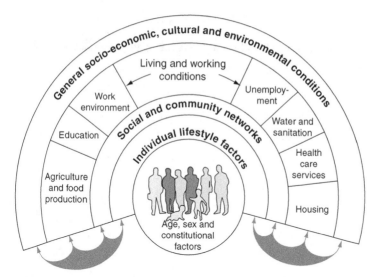

Figure 6.2 The social determinants of health.
Reproduced with permission from Dahlgren G, Whitehead M. *Policies and Strategies to Promote Social Equity in Health*. Stockholm: Institute for Futures Studies, 1991.

These determinants can therefore in part explain why there continues to be a health gap between the rich and the poor. For instance, there is a great deal that has been written about the impact of socio-economic status (SES, i.e. income, education level and social status) on cardiovascular disease risk factors such as smoking, obesity and high blood pressure. Indeed, even in low-income countries, there is evidence that poor people (i.e. low SES) smoke more, are more overweight and have higher blood pressure[14] – all of which increases their risk of dying prematurely from heart disease – as compared to rich people (i.e. high SES). Indeed, Sir Michael Marmot and the Commission on Social Determinants of Health have shown that this SES gradient exists across contexts worldwide. The bottom line is "the lower the socio-economic position, the worse the health".[15]

Thus, we could take a risk-factor approach and attempt to reduce blood pressure, increase physical activity and so forth, or, we could take a social-determinants approach and attempt to tackle the underlying social injustice – namely the unequal distribution of power, income and wealth which determines the disparity in daily living conditions between the rich and the poor, and hence the disparity in health outcomes. However, if we consider, for example, Aboriginal populations in Canada, then adjusting for differences in income, education, housing and so forth does not account for the entire health gap. Indeed, there are other factors at play even further upstream.

Causes of the causes of the causes

In a keynote address at the International Union for Health Promotion and Education (IUHPE) World Conference in 2007, Jeff Reading asked:

> What's the cause of diabetes? Many would say diet and exercise. The cause of that is poverty and lack of choice regarding diet and exercise. And the cause of that is colonization and lack of economic opportunity.[16]

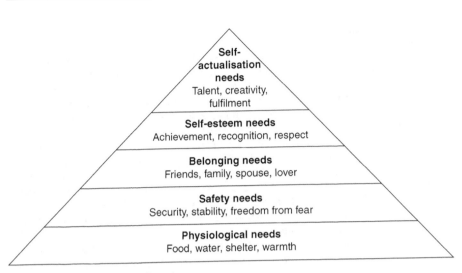

Figure 6.3 Maslow's hierarchy of needs.
Adapted from Maslow A. *Motivation and Personality*, 3rd edn. New York: Addison-Wesley, 1987.

Thus these distal determinants of health – also referred to in this context as Aboriginal determinants of health – help to explain the residual health differences between Aboriginal people and non-Aboriginal people even after adjusting for the common social determinants such as education, employment, income and so forth. I think the notion of the "causes of the causes of the causes" is illustrated best by the story of an Aboriginal elder who explained how the successive waves of historical trauma continue to influence the health and wellbeing of his people (Box 6.1).

Indeed, the residential school system is commonly cited as an important Aboriginal determinant of health:

> Children were forbidden to speak their own languages, and most were emotionally, physically, and sexually abused. This left a legacy of lost language and traditions, destroyed self-esteem, and unestablished parenting skills. As adults, many turned to alcohol and drugs to relieve the mental pain, resulting in fragmented communities and multigenerational trauma. The last residential school closed in 1996, and only in the summer of 2008 did the Canadian government finally offer an apology.[17]

Colonisation, marginalisation and assimilation are therefore important factors that need to be taken into consideration to improve Aboriginal health and reduce health inequities:

> The poor health of Aboriginal peoples has to be seen in connection with the general marginalization that Indigenous peoples suffer from economically and politically ... Critical factors that broadly impact the reduced health status of Aboriginal peoples in Canada include poverty, violence, poor housing and deficient physical environments ... Research has shown that at least three quarters of Aboriginal women have been victims of family violence, and they are three times more likely than non-Aboriginal women to die as a result of that violence ... Access to, and quality of, medical care services is not the main driver of people's health. The concept of social determinants is directed to the factors which help people stay healthy, rather than the services that help people when they are ill.[18]

While increasing access to and quality of clinical services is clearly important, it cannot be the only approach to improving health. Rather, a broad range of strategies is needed, including

Box 6.1 Causes of the causes of the causes

I heard this story told by an Elder when I was at a recent scientific conference on Aboriginal health. The Elder had been invited to perform the ceremonial opening of the meeting. However, unlike many other meetings that I have attended where the Elder concludes the opening and the meeting that follows is then dominated by mostly non-Aboriginal people, in this meeting, the Elder was an active participant in the discussion. He stood up and told the audience about his experiences as a youth on reserve in Canada. How there were no jobs for Aboriginal youth in those days, and how his peers had no hope and no future to look forward to. He explained how his determination led him to find work in the USA, but that he first needed permission to leave the reserve, which was a struggle, but he prevailed. It was only by having this work experience that he was later able to find work back in Canada. His peers who had no such work experience could not find work – it was a "catch 22" for them. For many years he worked in the prison system, helping the young people who had a tendency to gravitate there. Regardless of what offence was committed, it was always the same story. The young Aboriginal men and women found themselves in prison on account of the painful legacy of intergenerational trauma. Even if they were too young to have gone to a residential school, their parents or grandparents had been taken from their families to attend these schools, and the abuse did not stop with the older generations. It is like a "domino effect", the Elder explained, toppling over the generations that follow as well. How different things are today as compared to how things were when he was a boy and the people still lived on the land. Back then, he recalled, the children were the inner circle of the community, nurtured by the mothers, who themselves were supported by the grandmothers, and the outer circle consisted of the men – the protectors and providers. Everyone in the community had an important role to play and everyone was valued. Things are no longer the same now.

engaging community leaders and other key stakeholders to create healthier physical and social environments, as well as incorporating culturally adapted and contextualised solutions to local health problems:

> Unravelling the mysteries of diabetes and why it is so prevalent among Aboriginal people in Canada and around the world requires a renewed exploration of indigenous "ways of knowing," with the integration of innovative ideas derived from ancient traditional practices of Aboriginal healers with the modern scientific methods of inquiry practised by a new generation of researchers ... Diabetes is a complicated disease that is nested in the experience of rapid social and cultural change; thus, its prevention and control may need new ideas that go beyond an individual approach in a clinic or hospital ward. Long-term change will probably require broader community-level action and collaboration between researchers, policy-makers, Aboriginal community organizations, governments, volunteer agencies and health care professionals. In addition, the broader population health determinants need to be addressed and social repercussions of the disease better understood.[19]

Going beyond actions within individual communities, there also needs to be advocacy for improving the relationship between Aboriginal peoples and the Crown – a relationship which has long been fraught with tensions. Even if we have come a long way since the days of Duncan Campbell Scott, Deputy Superintendent of Indian Affairs from 1913 to 1932, who said "I want to get rid of the Indian problem ... Our objective is to continue until there is not a single Indian in Canada that has not been absorbed into the body politic and there is no Indian Question and no Indian Department",[20] there is still a long way to go in improving relations between the government and Aboriginal peoples. Sadly, young Aboriginal people today face the same tough choices as young Aboriginal people over 50 years ago because the same restrictive laws and policies still apply. Either they stay on reserve where there are few jobs and generally inadequate living conditions to preserve what is left of their identity, or else they lose all right to their status by moving away from the reserve to find a job, educate their children and give their family a real chance for the future. Choosing between your job and your identity is not a choice people should have to make. However, changing these distal determinants will require strong advocacy for larger social change and legal reforms, which will only occur if there is buy-in and support from the highest political levels.

(3) List the options to improve health

Once we have defined the health priorities and have understood the underlying causes of these problems at various levels, the next question to ask is "What can we do about it?" There is always more than one option available, but how to choose? The first step is simply identifying what the options are before attempting to weigh the pros and cons of each.

At the individual level, patients are often presented with a series of options but may find it difficult to choose without additional information. Do they truly understand the options that have been presented? Are there other options that were not included in the list but should be added? What about the option to "do nothing?" Isn't that also a possibility? Therefore, it is important to be clear on what the options are and also to have some basis for comparison – i.e. the status quo – to be able to judge later whether there is an added benefit from choosing one or another of these options.

At a population level, there are again many options in terms of what can be done to improve health and reduce health inequities. Generally speaking, as described in Chapter 2, this requires a continuum of strategies (ranging from treatment and rehabilitation to disease prevention, health promotion and action on the social determinants of health), not just one single strategy. All too often, when considering which strategies to choose, people stay within their comfort zone, screening for risk factors and counselling to promote behaviour change. Whether it is the prevention of obesity and heart disease or promoting smoking cessation, there is the notion that people should be making healthy choices, and if they get sick then they are to blame. Yet, these strategies that focus on the more proximal causes fail to adequately address the intermediate and distal causes of poor health, and can even inadvertently increase health inequities. Vineis and Elliott consider that being a "prisoner to the proximate" is "a serious mistake".[21] Mackenbach agrees that we should not be blaming the individual since "human health and disease are the embodiment of the successes and failures of society as a whole".[22] Moreover, there is a growing arsenal of strategies (such as intersectoral action, health in all policies and so forth) that focus on addressing the upstream determinants and changing the environment to make the healthy choices the easy choices. However, if these strategies are not included on the "list of options" they will never be chosen.

For example, rather than simply blaming youth for skipping school and telling them to use condoms to prevent sexually transmitted infections (STIs), the way forward should include a range of strategies that focus more on addressing the upstream determinants of health to get at the root of the problem. Indeed, the young people of today are the parents of tomorrow (maybe quite literally tomorrow). So if a teenage girl is the victim of violence and as a result is abusing alcohol, then as soon as that teenage girl becomes pregnant (perhaps even as a result of violence), it then becomes an issue of alcohol in pregnancy and prevention of fetal alcohol spectrum disorder (FASD). But really it is the same person, a person dealing with multiple problems simultaneously, and it would be important to address these issues before they land on the doorstep of the health system. For instance, if high-school dropout rates are extremely elevated due to a lack of training and retention of qualified teachers, and therefore schools are not able to fulfil their primary mandate of helping students to obtain their high-school leaving certificate, then intersectoral action by partnering with the education sector would be important. Perhaps schools would benefit from improving teacher training programmes and retention packages. This could increase the number of teachers who can act as positive role models and advocates for students, so that they continue their studies to obtain professional or vocational training after high school, which will increase their chances of finding meaningful employment. If overcrowded housing makes it difficult for youth to focus on their studies or if young people must quit school early to support their families, then further intersectoral action is required to partner with government and with employers to address these issues. If youth do not have a safe haven to go to where they can talk about their problems and socialise in a safe environment, then more outreach is needed, whether at sports events or through movie nights, to reach out to young people and help them to navigate through harsh realities that are very often not of their own making and give them the strength to realise their dreams for the future.

Thus the options on the list can address the proximal risk factors (i.e. condom use), or they can address the causes of the causes (i.e. inadequate school system, poverty, poor-quality housing, violence, etc.), and even the causes of the causes of the causes (i.e. colonisation, power differentials, etc.). Tackling these upstream causes will require different ways of working and taking the focus off the health system, but the next question in the algorithm is to determine which option has the greatest added benefits that outweigh the potential harms. Indeed, working "upstream" may actually bring even greater health improvements across a large number of areas by acting on the shared causes of poor health.

(4) Do the added benefits outweigh the harms?

While there are value judgements being made all along – whether to prioritise one health problem over another, whether to focus on the proximal risk factors or more distal determinants of health, whether to list strategies for action that are centred on the health sector or that demand greater intersectoral action – here we come to an important decision node: do the added benefits of a given option or intervention outweigh the harms?

Indeed, this can be further broken down into a few questions. What is the option being considered and what is it being compared to (i.e. to the current gold standard or, if there is no gold standard, to the status quo)? Is there an added benefit at all? And, if so, what are the added benefits? Are there any harms? And, if so, what are the harms? Finally, do these added benefits outweigh the harms? If yes, we can continue on with our algorithm, but, if not, then it is back to the drawing board to look at another option from the list. If we have exhausted all possible options and there are none that have an added benefit that outweighs the harms, then the only logical action would be to stay with the status quo while working on developing better options for the future.

Taking a clinical example, in recent decades, we have seen an onslaught of "me too" drugs which are essentially minor variations on an existing medication that allow the developer to apply for a new patent and continue to sell that product at a high price.[23] Indeed, Goozner and others argue that the true innovation and medical breakthroughs occur mostly through publicly funded research (i.e. paid for by taxpayers), whereas the pharmaceutical and biotech companies then step in and reap the profits.[24] Before patents expire, they "tweak" the medication just enough to put out a "new and improved" patentable version to ensure that their increased revenues continue. Yet, there is no onus to show that this medication is improved at all. So long as it is sufficiently different from what already exists and it works, it can be approved. Before we even begin to look at the issue of cost, what's the point of doing so if there is no added benefit? Whether it is a pill, a policy or a programme, there needs to be some added benefit to justify choosing this option over the current gold standard or status quo. Yet, even if there is an added benefit, that is only the beginning of the process of reflection.

All too often, there is a lack of data on the potential harms. People want to show that something works, but they often overlook the fact that any option has a balance of benefits and harms, and therefore one must also measure the harms to be able to determine whether the balance is favourable or not. In the case of breast cancer screening, the literature on mortality benefit came first. As time went on and national breast screening programmes were being implemented, only then did a new literature start to emerge on the potential harms of screening, ranging from psychological impacts and cancer worries[25] to the effects of radiation related to mammography itself.[26] As a result, this new evidence provided an opportunity for rethinking the balance of benefits and harms.[27]

So, presuming that, out of the initial list of options, there are a few options that have added benefits that appear to outweigh the harms, do we forge ahead and implement these? Not just yet, as there are still many other issues to be considered.

(5) Are the options acceptable to those involved?

Before implementing any treatment, programme or policy, it is important to think about those who will be "on the receiving end". Since we cannot know people's preferences, opinions or concerns unless we ask, it is therefore important that they be involved. Some options will be more or less acceptable depending on what they entail, and this will differ from person to person and from context to context. Understanding individual and population preferences, as well as the local context of implementation, is critical to choosing the best option for that specific person or population at a given place and time. No point thinking about costs if the option is not acceptable in the first place.

For instance, take rectal suppositories. Even though there may be a range of benefits associated with using suppositories,[28] some people prefer not to use rectal suppositories when other routes of medication administration are available, such as taking medicine by mouth or by intravenous injection.[29] Similarly, colon cancer screening programmes that rely upon mailing-in stool samples on a small paper card to test for occult blood have also generally had fairly low acceptability, and therefore low participation rates.[30] Alternative methods such as using a faecal swab that does not involve smearing the sample onto a paper card may prove to be more acceptable.[31] Therefore it is important to take into consideration people's preferences. Otherwise there will be low uptake rates and low impact, money will be wasted and there could even be unintended harms.

For example, some genetic screening programmes entail providing information to be able to make more informed reproductive choices, and, during pregnancy, that could involve the delicate issue of abortion. In some communities, due to religious beliefs or cultural values, having a screening programme which includes the possibility of aborting an unborn child would be quite unacceptable, even if certain individuals within that community may want to have that avenue open to them if it turns out that their child is affected. If the society at large is pro-choice, is it fair to deny couples in this specific community that choice? While a person who is against abortion can decline participation in the screening programme, what if another person chooses to be tested and wants to have an abortion but there are no local health professionals willing to carry out such procedures, on account of their own beliefs or simply out of concern for the uproar that it may cause? Thus the issue of acceptability can become quite tricky, especially when it involves balancing the preferences of individuals with those of the target population and society overall.

Another example of where issues of acceptability are particularly sensitive is when the intervention is delivered to the entire population and there is no real possibility to "opt out". For instance, fluoridation of water is widely recognised as a powerful means of reducing dental caries and improving oral health. Indeed, in the USA, a Centers for Disease Control and Prevention (CDC) working group considered the evidence regarding a range of interventions in terms of their effectiveness in improving oral health, their associated risks of fluorosis, and their cost-effectiveness. Based on this analysis, the working group made a "Grade A" recommendation (i.e. the highest level of recommendation) in support of community water fluoridation across the country.[32] Moreover, as compared to changing personal behaviour (e.g. through taking fluoride supplements), such population-based interventions promote greater equity since everyone receives the intervention equally, regardless of socio-economic status or access to care.[33] Yet, there are those who are vocal opponents to water fluoridation programmes due to concerns about the relatively rare possibility of developing fluorosis or other health problems, as well as issues with respect to freedom of choice.[34] Indeed, one anti-fluoride group has created a list of 50 reasons to oppose community water fluoridation – many of them health related.[35] However, according to Health Canada:

> The weight of evidence from all currently available studies does not support a link between exposure to fluoride in drinking water at 1.5 mg/L and any adverse health effects, including those related to cancer, immunotoxicity, reproductive/developmental toxicity, genotoxicity and/or neurotoxicity. It also does not support a link between fluoride exposure and intelligence quotient deficit, as there are significant concerns regarding the available studies, including quality, credibility, and methodological weaknesses.[36]

Nonetheless, lack of widespread acceptability and outcries from vocal opponents have resulted in millions of people not being protected against dental decay, and even the halting of certain community-based water fluoridation programmes, in spite of evidence of effectiveness in improving oral health.[37]

Therefore, ideally, to proceed to the next step in the algorithm, the options under consideration should be acceptable to all those involved, including the individual, the health workers, the community and society at large. If none of the options are acceptable, then either further information can be provided which may succeed in changing attitudes and generating support for these options, or else it may be a sign to go back to the drawing board and try to think up more options.

(6) Calculate costs and opportunity costs

Presuming that there are a few options which have added benefits that outweigh the harms and where the options are acceptable, can we go ahead? In an ideal world, with infinite resources, one might simply proceed, but we generally find ourselves in a situation where there are limited resources – not enough money to cover the costs, not enough people to do the work, not enough time available to do everything. So, how do we determine which option to choose?

At this stage, people are often quick to point fingers at the government, complaining about the rationing of health services. However, these are the kinds of choices that we make every day. For instance, there are only 24 hours in a day, so what do we choose to do with our time? Will we sacrifice a couple hours of sleep to be able to stay up late and spend more time going out with our friends, or will we arrange to leave work earlier to spend more time with the kids after school, or carve out protected time to spend with one's spouse, or even just for oneself? There are always opportunity costs involved. Doing one thing generally means that you cannot be doing another thing at the exact same time. The fallacy is the belief that more is always better or that the better options are necessarily the more expensive options.

For instance, the focus on the risk-factor approach means that there is a lot of enthusiasm over screening programmes that identify those at high risk in order to focus prevention efforts on this subset of the population. However, screening programmes are often highly costly endeavours, and they do not contribute to improving the health of those at moderate or lower risk.[38] In contrast, population-wide interventions such as building healthy public policies or creating supportive environments for health can have a much greater impact even if there is a smaller effect for each individual because so many more people are implicated. For instance, what is the cost of a policy to ban smoking? There may be some cost to ensuring that the policy is being implemented and fining those who do not adhere to the policy. Even if we also consider the upstream costs of reorienting tobacco growers and manufacturers towards other forms of work, surely this would still be cheaper than simply treating people with lung cancer or even introducing a large-scale lung cancer screening programme (which in any case would not get this far down the algorithm since it has not been shown that screening for lung cancer actually provides any added mortality benefit).

The Disease Control Priorities Project attempts to use cost-effectiveness calculations to determine which interventions to scale up to improve global health and which interventions to scale back (Fig. 6.4).[39] The cost-effectiveness ratios (CERs) are generally much lower for preventive interventions as opposed to curative interventions. For instance, childhood immunisation, insecticide-treated bed nets for malaria prevention and road traffic safety interventions such as speeding laws and speed bumps at busy intersections cost only a few dollars per DALY averted, whereas treating a stroke or heart attack with expensive "clot-busting" medications can cost thousands of dollars per DALY averted. Even action on the social determinants of health to prevent problems at the source (i.e. by improving housing, education, job quality and so forth) are unlikely to be more expensive than treating people once they are ill, with all the health care costs, missed work and suffering that this entails.

Indeed, there is a whole field of health economics that looks at issues of cost and cost-effectiveness to make recommendations on how to get the best value in terms of health returns for your dollar. Yet, there are a great deal of assumptions underlying these calculations that need to be taken into consideration,[40] and often it is difficult to make these calculations for interventions that address the social determinants of health as these tend to involve more complex "clusters" of interventions with less clarity in terms of the specific costs and outcomes.[41] For instance, a recent systematic review of interventions to improve housing conditions found that there was an added benefit for health, with little evidence of harms, but what about the costs?[42] According to the UK's National Institute for Health and Clinical Excellence (NICE), "there is an urgent need for primary research to be undertaken to

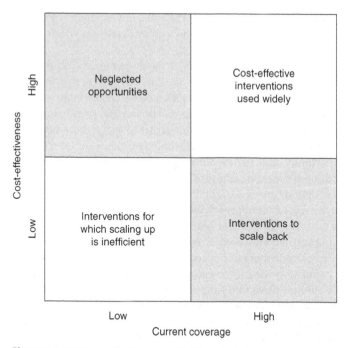

Figure 6.4 Using cost-effectiveness to identify neglected opportunities.
Reproduced with permission from Jamison D, Breman J, Measham A *et al. Disease Control Priorities in Developing Countries,* 2nd edn. Washington DC and Oxford: The World Bank and Oxford University Press, 2006.

examine the cost effectiveness of housing-related interventions to improve health outcomes in both the general population and disadvantaged and vulnerable groups".[43] Thus the evidence base regarding the costs of working more upstream are often lacking, even if evidence of effectiveness is growing. That does not mean that we should not be working more upstream, simply that it is not always so clear what are the costs involved. Moreover, when engaging in intersectoral action and whole-of-government approaches, it also remains to be determined which budgetary envelope these costs will be withdrawn from (i.e. the health budget or the education budget, the national budget or the local budget, and so forth). In any case, while cost issues are clearly important, they are not the only factor in determining the feasibility of one option over another.

(7) Which options are feasible in this context?

If an option is not affordable, it is generally not feasible. Yet, in some countries it may be considered affordable to spend $40,000 per life year saved on dialysis or when using an orphan medication to treat a rare disease, whereas in other countries the health system cannot afford to spend even $10 to save a woman's life in childbirth. Thus what is considered affordable greatly depends upon the context and circumstances. However, even if something is affordable, this does not necessarily mean that it is feasible, since there may be many different kinds of logistical issues involved.

For instance, across many parts of Africa and Southeast Asia, while it may be possible to afford the cost of vaccines against childhood diseases – especially as much of the cost is subsidised by the GAVI alliance through the Expanded Programme on Immunization (EPI) – there are nonetheless various logistical challenges that may remain. Vaccination attempts may be thwarted by social or political unrest, by difficult access to remote areas, and by lapses in the cold chain (i.e. some vaccines become ineffective if they are not continually refrigerated from their site of manufacture to the moment they are delivered to the patient).[44] Alternatively, there may be a great web-based application for improving clinical consultations, but if the local health workers do not have reliable internet access or the required bandwidth to rapidly download the information, then it really is a non-starter.

Thus, beyond issues of acceptability and cost, there are many different kinds of barriers to implementation which result in certain options being less likely to be successful in creating health improvements in specific contexts. Even if in theory it is a great idea, and in a research setting there is proven efficacy in improving health, if it will not work for one reason or another in this particular context, then it is a waste of resources to try – unless, of course, the intervention can be adapted to work in this context. This is always a possibility to consider, but piloting would be needed, sometimes also termed a "feasibility study", to first provide evidence of local effectiveness.

(8) Ethical, legal and social considerations

Presuming there are a couple of options left where the added benefit outweighs the harms, which are acceptable to those involved, as well as cost-effective and feasible in the local context, why can't we simply move ahead already? Well, more often than not, there are ethical, legal and social implications and it is best to consider these from the very outset rather than troubleshooting problems later on once options have been hastily implemented without giving sufficient forethought to potential pitfalls that may lie ahead.

For instance, taking a clinical example, for those who are proponents of euthanasia or physician-assisted suicide, it is a way of dying with dignity, yet, in most parts of the world, it is also illegal. While by definition euthanasia shortens the length of life, it is meant to provide people with terminal illness a reprieve from suffering states that are considered "worse than death". Indeed, while not exactly the same as euthanasia, even the liberal use of narcotic pain medication to the point where this palliative therapy could shorten life if such doses are required to relieve suffering is a fairly new idea. Professor Ron Melzack, also known as the "King of Pain", is a psychology professor who proposed the gate control theory of pain and developed the McGill Pain Questionnaire to rate pain intensity in a more systematic way. In 1990, he wrote an article in *Scientific American* called "The tragedy of needless pain", where he argues that:

> Morphine is the safest, most effective analgesic (painkiller) known for constant, severe pain, but it is also addictive for some people. Consequently, it is typically metered out sparingly, if it is given at all. Indeed, concern over addiction has led many nations in Europe and elsewhere to outlaw virtually any uses of morphine and related substances, including their medical applications. Even where morphine is a legal medical therapy, as it is in Great Britain and the U.S., many care givers, afraid of turning patients into addicts, deliver amounts that are too small or spaced too widely to control pain. Yet the fact is that when patients take morphine to combat pain, it is rare to see addiction ... I do not suggest that morphine be prescribed indiscriminately. I do urge lawmakers, law-enforcement agencies and health-care workers to distinguish between the addict who craves morphine for its mood-altering properties and the psychologically healthy patient who takes the drug only to relieve pain. Particularly when a patient has a terminal Illness, the issue of addiction is

meaningless, and delaying relief is cruel. There is another, more humane way to treat pain, one that is slowly gaining acceptance. In this approach doses are given regularly, according to a schedule that has been actually tailored to prevent recurrence of the individual's pain. Thus, pain is controlled continuously; a patient does not wait for discomfort to return before receiving the next dose.[45]

Yet, even though the notion of adequate pain control is gaining in acceptance, some people nonetheless continue to suffer during the final stages of their illness, in spite of access to these medications. Thus, the ongoing debate over euthanasia continues in many parts of the world. Recently, a well-respected general practitioner and researcher in the UK became an activist for euthanasia when she herself was diagnosed with pancreatic cancer. She founded Healthcare Professionals for Assisted Dying (HPAD) with the mission that "terminally ill, mentally competent adults should have the choice of an assisted death, subject to legal safeguards".[46] After a four-year battle with cancer, which could not be shortened due to existing local laws, her husband writes:

> In her final days, far from seeing the dignity in dying she wanted so desperately for herself and others, I watched my wife of 43 years suffering as she was forced to live in unbearable discomfort. It was Ann's experience of caring for terminally-ill patients that convinced her that the law should be changed, with appropriate safeguards, to allow doctors to end the lives of terminally ill people at a time of their choosing. She had to stand by as her patients were forced to endure a slow, uncomfortable death – and saw the pain such suffering caused their families. She became a vocal campaigner to end 'the cruelty', as she put it, imposed by those who resist the call for new legislation, thereby allowing the dying to suffer so horribly. Yet she found herself fighting a medical establishment that continues to insist that good palliative care and effective pain relief are all that is needed for a good death.[47]

Of course controversial issues such as euthanasia have long been heated topics of debate. Clearly, if something is illegal, that would pose an important barrier to choosing that option – as was the case here. However, when something is illegal, it is because the people who influence and create these laws deem it to be unacceptable. This therefore brings us back to the question of acceptability from a few steps back in the algorithm – demonstrating how decision-making is generally non-linear and often requires an iterative process, going "back and forth" between the various steps, to be able to adequately consider the wide range of issues at stake. It is obvious that euthanasia is a touchy subject, and many members of the medical profession and beyond are more comfortable with palliation as their preferred option, afraid of potential abuses that could occur if euthanasia were legalised, as well as the possible breakdown of trust between patients and their healers. Thus, in situations like these, we are often at an impasse, unable to choose certain options, or else, making these choices and then suffering the consequences, like Dr. Kevorkian, who was sentenced to 10–25 years in prison for his belief that people should be allowed to choose "quality of life, as opposed to maintaining existence".[48] Yet even in this highly controversial area, there is gaining momentum for providing terminally ill patients with more control over the manner and timing of their death, while at the same time ensuring that physicians need not contravene the Hippocratic Oath by using "a system that would remove the physician from direct involvement in the [dying] process".[49]

Euthanasia is certainly a dramatic example, but there are many other areas of medicine and public health that are also fraught with ethical, legal and social (ELSI) issues. Indeed, the acronym "ELSI" is very commonly used by researchers working in the area of new genetic technologies and personalised medicine to describe a range of problems, from concerns about confidentiality and stigmatisation to issues of psychological harm and safeguarding against eugenics.[50] However, it is perhaps even more important to proceed with caution in situations where the ethical, legal and social issues are less obvious and could potentially be overlooked. How about if instead we take a different scenario: improving the health and well-being of an impoverished remote community. The proposed option under consideration is an economic development project to create more jobs in a rural area, thus increasing income and employment among the local population and thereby improving health outcomes. Who could possibly find harm in that? Isn't this exactly the kind of action we should be encouraging to address the social determinants of health? Yes, but things are rarely so simple, particularly when it comes to population-level interventions.

Nancy Kass, who developed an ethics framework for public health, emphasised the importance of ensuring that interventions are fairly implemented and take into consideration the distribution of the benefits and harms.[51] Otherwise, we could find ourselves in a situation where only a small minority reap any benefit, and, even worse, where those who benefit least are burdened with most of the harms. A good example to illustrate this is the *Plan Nord* project currently being launched in Quebec, Canada. This initiative of the provincial government is being touted as:

> One of the biggest economic, social and environmental projects in our time. The *Plan Nord* will be carried out over a period of 25 years. It will lead to over $80 billion in investments during that time and create or consolidate, on average, 20,000 jobs per year.[52]

Whether it will be a success, or not, very much depends on how it will be implemented. There is tremendous potential for improving the health of remote Northern communities, but also great risk of further harming already marginalised and socially disadvantaged groups. Certainly, there will be those with "dollar signs in their eyes" excited about profiting from the gold, diamonds and uranium hidden underground. However, what about the people living in these areas – Aboriginal and non-Aboriginal. Will they see any benefits? Will they be harmed? Will all the profits make a few rich and powerful people even more rich and powerful through backroom deals that further widen existing inequities while others in the population continue to suffer from food insecurity and poor-quality housing? Indeed, one gold mine alone contains over a trillion dollars worth of gold and is expected to make profits of almost a billion dollars each year.[53] That is enough money to solve some major world hunger problems and even contribute to tackling the Millennium Development Goals (MDGs), let alone improve the health status of the relatively small population (about 120,000 people) living in Northern Quebec. But it is not at all clear whether any of that money will be used to improve local health and social services, or find its way into the pockets of local people in need. Thus, while extracting natural resources can make some people wealthier, it also risks negatively impacting local populations. If our main concern is whether or not economic development projects such as this will improve the health of the population and reduce inequities, it is rather doubtful as it currently stands unless this is made an explicit goal that is written into the plan and the budget.

The economic theory of the "trickle down" effect (i.e. if the rich get richer eventually the poor will also see some benefit from a strengthened economy) was debunked by the World Health Organization (WHO) Commission on Macroeconomics and Health in the early 2000s,[54] and was officially "pronounced dead" by the Organisation for Economic Co-operation and Development (OECD) in their recent report *Divided We Stand: Why*

Inequality Keeps Rising.[55] Indeed, it is now common knowledge that the gaps between rich and poor are increasing. But, according to the OECD, this is not inevitable. They recommend the reform of tax laws and benefits to do a better job of redistributing wealth, as well as ensuring that more people are able to secure well-paid stable employment.[56]

Thus, when you scratch beneath the surface, no option is entirely free from ethical, legal and social issues. Depending on the circumstances, these issues can place important limits on the decisions that are made. While there may be high-quality evidence of efficacy and low cost, this in itself is not sufficient to move ahead with one option over another. It is important to consider carefully the ethical, legal and social issues and to systematically examine who is affected and in what way, to ensure that everyone is able to share in the benefits while especially protecting those who are most vulnerable from the harms. This brings us to our penultimate step on understanding what the various stakeholders stand to gain or lose.

(9) What do stakeholders stand to gain or lose?

When considering the potential impacts of any given option, it is important to look at the different groups who could be affected – including various lobby groups, target populations, innocent bystanders and the decision-makers themselves – to better appreciate what each group would gain or lose from implementing this option. Returning to the previous example of an economic development project, it is important to understand the policy-making process which will vary from jurisdiction to jurisdiction. Nonetheless, due to strong activism in the area of the environment and sustainable development since the publication of Rachel Carson's influential book *Silent Spring* in the 1960s,[57] in a large number of jurisdictions around the world, economic development projects must now first be approved by the Ministry of the Environment before being allowed to proceed. The proponent of the project therefore makes a request to the Ministry of the Environment, and the Ministry of the Environment responds by requesting that an environmental impact assessment (EIA) be carried out, which is usually contracted out by the proponent to a team of consultants. The EIA is then submitted to the Ministry of the Environment and, based on a careful examination and further consultations, a decision is made of whether or not to allow the project to proceed and, if so, what modifications to the development plan are required. But what about health in all this? It is true that EIAs systematically examine the potential impact of the project on the environment, but to a much lesser extent, the degree to which there will be human exposures and health effects, not to mention the social impacts on health. Generally some of these concerns will be raised during the consultations and hearings which are part of the process of developing and assessing an EIA. As well, the Ministry of Health may be consulted by the Ministry of the Environment in making their decision, but, ultimately, it is the Ministry of the Environment that decides whether or not the project can proceed.

At this point, some of you might ask, "This is a book about evidence for health, why are we talking about economic development projects and EIAs?" The reason is that projects such as these and any number of other policies outside the health sector (i.e. tax laws, maternity leave policies, etc.) have tremendous potential to greatly benefit and/or harm the health of various groups in society. This is the impetus behind the "Health in All Policies" approach championed by Ilona Kickbush and others (Table 6.5),[58] and also explains the growing interest in conducting health impact assessments (HIAs) to help create more evidence-informed policy,[59] or at the very least adding more on health impacts into EIAs.[60]

Table 6.5 Core principles for "Health in All Policies".

A Health in All Policies approach reflects health as a shared goal of all of government. In particular it:

(1) Recognises the value of health for the well-being of all citizens and for the overall social and economic development. Health is a human right, a vital resource for everyday life and a key factor of sustainability.

(2) Recognises that health is an outcome of a wide range of factors – such as changes to the natural and built environments and to social and work environments – many of which lie outside the activities of the health sector and require a shared responsibility and an integrated and sustained policy response across government.

(3) Acknowledges that all government policies can have positive or negative impacts on the determinants of health and such impacts are reflected both in the health status of the population today and in the health prospects of future generations.

(4) Recognises that the impacts of health determinants are not equally distributed among population groups and aims at closing the health gap, in particular for the Aboriginal peoples [and other marginalised groups].

(5) Recognises that health is central to achieving [the development objectives of a society] – it requires both the identification of potential health impacts and the recognition that good health can contribute to achieving targets.

(6) Acknowledges that efforts to improve the health of all [citizens] will require sustainable mechanisms that support government agencies to work collaboratively to develop integrated solutions to current and future policy challenges.

(7) Acknowledges that many of the most pressing health problems of population health require long-term policy and budgetary commitment as well as innovative budgetary approaches.

(8) Recognises that indicators of success will be equally long term and that regular monitoring and intermediate measures of progress will need to be established and reported back to citizens.

(9) Recognises the need to regularly consult with citizens to link policy changes with wider social and cultural changes around health and well-being.

(10) Recognises the potential of partnerships for policy implementation between government at all levels, science and academia, business, professional organisations and non-governmental organisations to bring about sustained change.

Adapted from Kickbush I, McCann W, Sherbon T. Adelaide revisited: from healthy public policy to Health in All Policies. *Health Promot Int* 2008; 23(1): 1–4.

Returning once again to the example of a mining project being developed in a remote Northern region, who would be the various stakeholders involved? For starters, there is the proponent (i.e. the company) proposing the project and the decision-makers at the Ministry of the Environment. As well, there are the potential workers on the project (e.g. the miners) and their families. There are also workers who will be employed by spin-off businesses (i.e. in transportation, food supply, etc.) and their families. There are the communities (Aboriginal and non-Aboriginal) living in the vicinity of the project and the people who own land near the project site, as well as those who own land near any new infrastructure to support the project (i.e. roads, air strips, etc.). There are also local service providers such as health care workers and youth protection. All of these different groups could be affected in different ways by the project.

Next, once the stakeholders have been identified, what does each group stand to gain or lose from the project? For the proponent (i.e. the company), it is quite clear. They stand to make a lot of money for themselves and for their shareholders, otherwise they wouldn't be investing in this. For the local community leaders and people with property on or near the site of the mine, they are looking to be compensated for the environmental degradation and any inconvenience associated with the project. Depending on the sum of that compensation, they too could make a lot of money. People who own or work for spin-off businesses that depend on the project would also be able to get a (better quality) job and increase their standard of living. The government, as mentioned previously in this book, has a dual mandate to protect the public good, but also to keep the economy running, and therefore they cannot refuse every single project, and particularly not those that could be highly profitable for the government through corporate taxes which could lower the budget deficit, and similarly for projects with a large potential for local job creation which could increase the government's popularity and the likelihood that politicians would be re-elected in future. The mineworkers would benefit from stable employment and increased income for many years while the mine is in operation. This would benefit themselves and their families by increasing their socio-economic status and presumably also their health outcomes. However, under-ground mining is a dangerous job, so workers would also be exposed to a number of occupational hazards including noise pollution, poor air quality, physical strain, minor injuries, and the more unlikely yet more dangerous possibility of serious injury or death in the event of a flood or collapse of the mine, or a large scale spill or leakage of toxic substances used in the mining process (i.e. the extraction of gold involves using hundreds of gallons of cyanide each year in addition to a large number of other chemicals). As well, there are also potential social harms, especially for fly-in mines far from the community requiring long periods of separation and fragmentation of families. Lack of experience in managing a large increase in income could also lead to the possibility of misuse of funds to engage in harmful behaviours involving alcohol, drugs or gambling, as well as difficulties adjusting and finding new employment at the end of the development project. Members of communities living downstream from the mine may also be subject to health risks since certain contaminants can travel far distances by air to be deposited into the water and soil, and other contaminants released directly or indirectly into the water may travel through underground reservoirs to the drinking water of these communities. Thus health and social services workers, often already overburdened and understaffed in these remote areas, may find that they have an increased workload as a result of the potentially far-reaching impacts of the mine.

In terms of the distribution of the benefits and harms, it would certainly be unfair if the proponent retained the bulk of the profits while the workers are paid low wages despite the great potential for physical and social harm. Or even worse, if local people were unqualified to even get a job working for the mining company and all of the jobs went to people from down South. As well, if local community members found that their water supply was contaminated due to the project, that would also be highly unfair since they are not compensated at all, especially if community leaders do not redistribute the wealth from deals signed with the proponent or at the very least use these funds to benefit the local population in some way. Indeed, lack of transparency and coordination with regard to profit-sharing resulting in profits going to a small number of individuals or groups, lack of equal opportunities for employment in the project or lack of access in starting spin-off businesses, as well as failure to reinvest profits into health and social services and tackling the upstream determinants of health (i.e. through improving education, access to child care, building social cohesion, etc.) could all lead to worsening health inequities – in spite of the large influx of money to the region.

Knowing all this, prior to the last step in the algorithm there is an opportunity for refining or even redesigning the proposed option such that the benefits are maximised, the harms are minimised, and the distribution of benefits and harms is fair. For instance, making transparent and respecting agreements for profit-sharing, and providing training and equal opportunities for employment and spin-off economic opportunities, would be one way of maximising benefits. As well, ensuring the highest standards in preventing contamination due to toxic substances and conducting ongoing monitoring at the project site and within communities to detect any breaches early and to provide immediate remediation, even if this entails greater costs and reduced profits for the proponent, would be one way of minimising harms. Thus, once these additional safeguards and adjustments are incorporated, in the spirit of the precautionary principle which aims to prevent harm even in the face of uncertainty,[61] only then is it possible to determine which options have the greatest potential for improving health and reducing inequities.

(10) Which options improve health most and minimise harm?

At the end of the day, a decision must be made that integrates all of the evidence from the various steps in the algorithm and makes a final judgement regarding whether or not to proceed. Surveillance data, cross-sectional surveys and qualitative research may be used to identify the most common and serious health problems. Delphi techniques and other related consensus-building approaches may be used in prioritisation of these health problems. Evidence from various types of research ranging from basic science and epidemiological research to qualitative studies and policy research can help to map out the various causes of the health problem. Evidence of the benefits and harms of an intervention based on RCT data, quasi-experimental studies or natural experiments can help to determine whether there is an added benefit that outweighs the harms. Assessing acceptability can be carried out through the use of surveys (e.g. consumer polls) or qualitative research (e.g. focus groups). Evidence of cost-effectiveness is determined through economic evaluations, and an understanding of feasibility and the ethical, legal and social considerations can be further elucidated based on prior experiences or through consultations with stakeholders and experts. And so forth. Thus, many different types of evidence and expertise are called upon to make an overall decision about which option(s) to choose and how to best proceed. Clearly there will be differences in how one goes about this, depending on whether these are clinical decisions, population-level decisions or global policy decisions. Nonetheless, the ultimate question is "Which options maximise potential health and social benefits, minimise potential harms, and ensure that the distribution of benefits and harms within and between populations is fair?"

While no decision is ever free from value judgements, using a systematic approach at the very least ensures that the final decision is grounded in the best available evidence, in all its facets. As well, by identifying and making explicit the various trade-offs and opportunity costs, and by providing reasons for choosing one way rather than another, there will be the possibility of understanding why certain value judgements were made, as well as being able to challenge the final decision if the underlying reasons are not well founded.

Integration of evidence, values and contextual considerations

Integrating and balancing all of the complex considerations and making a final decision is indeed the most challenging part of the algorithm. In the health field, there can be life or death decisions at stake. The choices that we make really matter. Patients can feel paralysed with fear about taking the wrong turn. Politicians may have visions of their political careers going up in smoke. There is a tendency to try to defer this often-overwhelming responsibility to others: "What would you do, doctor, if you were in my shoes?" But no one else can truly know another person's values or preferences. With all the information at hand, how to take the plunge and transform all of these different considerations into a binary choice – will I choose this option or that option?

To take a clinical example, a pregnant woman has had a previous caesarean section due to prolonged labour with her first delivery. She would have the option of either having a planned repeat caesarean section (i.e. a surgery to deliver the baby by cutting open the uterus) or to have a trial of labour and attempt a vaginal delivery the second time around (also known as a VBAC – vaginal birth after caesarean). Of course, some women would not be eligible for a trial of labour for various reasons that would make this option too risky (i.e. women who have already had two prior caesarean sections, women with a horizontal uterine scar as opposed to a lower transverse scar, lack of facilities for fetal monitoring during delivery, etc.).[62] In these situations, there is no choice. The only safe option is a planned repeat caesarean section. In other settings, for instance in a low-income country if an operating-room generator stopped working or the only surgeon in the area who is qualified to do the procedure has been recruited to work in a high-income country (i.e. a product of the "brain drain" in the global battle for human resources for health), there is also no choice. However, imagine that this woman is eligible for a trial of labour and that the facilities exist to either have a repeat caesarean section or attempt a trial of labour. What should she choose?

Imagine that the woman is making this decision without knowing anything about the growing body of evidence on this topic. Indeed, in practice, women are often not provided with substantive information on the health risks and benefits of the various options.[63] Yet, the woman might nonetheless have many different considerations that could influence her choice. Having gone through the recovery process from a previous caesarean section with her first child, she may prefer a vaginal delivery which has a much shorter and less difficult recovery. Alternatively, she may want to have greater control over her birthing experience, thus opting to "go natural" and avoid a second caesarean section. There may even be financial constraints, and the woman may opt for the vaginal delivery because she cannot afford a second surgery and is still in debt from the first surgery. In contrast, a different woman may not share any of these concerns or constraints but, instead, she may have another important event in her life around the time when the baby is due – such as the marriage of a sibling or an important work-related function. She may therefore prefer having a fixed date set for the delivery by caesarean section to ensure that she would be able to attend this special event rather than leaving it to chance. In some countries, there is even a social norm that surgery is better, and so those who can afford it would prefer a caesarean section in any case, as they are "too posh to push". Thus, even without looking at the evidence, people may have many different reasons for choosing one way or another. All things being equal, these may be relevant reasons for choosing whether to undergo a repeat caesarean section or to have a trial of labour. However, what about the chances of having good health outcomes – for the baby and for the mother? Wouldn't this be an even more important consideration? To better understand these chances, we need to look at the evidence, or else we are deciding "in the dark", so to speak.

Indeed, with 1.5 million women undergoing caesarean deliveries each year, there have been literally thousands of research articles written on the subject of repeat caesarean section versus trial of labour after a previous caesarean section. According to one systematic review, trial of labour significantly increases the rates of uterine rupture as compared to repeat caesarean section (4.7 per 1,000 versus 0.3 per 1,000).[64] While uterine rupture is associated with serious morbidity and even mortality (i.e. the mother and/or the baby could die as a result), poor outcomes are generally very rare overall in both the trial of labour and the planned repeat caesarean section groups, with the risk of maternal mortality from repeat caesarean section being nonetheless somewhat higher at 13.4 deaths per 100,000 as compared to 3.8 deaths per 100,000 for a trial of labour. However, it is important to note that the risk of uterine rupture increases with the number of previous caesarean deliveries (e.g. more than two), with a shorter interval since the last caesarean section (e.g. less than 12 months), and with the use of oxytocin for labour induction or augmentation.[65] In a recent prospective study that followed outcomes over time, out of 7,429 women who delivered a child after a single caesarean section,[66] one-quarter had an elective repeat caesarean section. The remaining three-quarters opted for a trial of labour. However, of these, only two-thirds had a successful VBAC, and one-third nonetheless had to undergo an emergency caesarean section. A successful VBAC is associated with a somewhat lower rate of complications during delivery. Yet patients who have a failed VBAC need an emergency caesarean section and this is associated with "higher risks of uterine disruption and infectious morbidity compared with patients who have successful vaginal birth after caesarean or elective repeat caesarean delivery".[67] Thus, a VBAC has the best chances of a positive health outcome if all goes well, although one cannot entirely predict in advance whether it will succeed or not.

The evidence is therefore helpful in informing the decision even if the decision is being made under uncertainty with regard to whether things will go well or go badly. For those who want to use decision theory to help in making the choice,[68] it is clear that a trial of labour could have the best outcome if the VBAC is successful and the worst outcome if an emergency caesarean section is required, whereas the planned caesarean section would have the second-best outcome if it goes well and, even if it goes poorly, it would have the third-best outcome, but not as bad as the worst outcome with an emergency caesarean section (Table 6.6).[68] Therefore, according to decision theorists, if one is using the "maximin rule", one would want to maximise the worst possible outcome and therefore choose the planned caesarean section. In contrast, with the "maximax rule", one would want to maximise the best possible outcome and therefore choose the trial of labour. So it depends to some extent on whether you are an optimist or a pessimist.

Therefore, even with the evidence and the application of decision rules (if you choose to use these), the various personal values, preferences and contextual considerations must still be integrated into the decision. As well, each individual has their own personal circumstances and prior health record which can also influence the decision. For instance, a woman with a

Table 6.6 Applying decision theory based on the evidence.

	Goes well	Goes badly
Trial of labour	Best outcome	Worst outcome
Planned caesarean section	Second-best outcome	Third-best outcome

Adapted from Table 3.6 in Peterson M. *An Introduction to Decision Theory.* Cambridge: Cambridge University Press, 2009.

pre-existing health condition that is not an outright contraindication to a VBAC may nonetheless be better off opting for an elective repeat caesarean section in a controlled setting if her physician thinks that she would be less able to tolerate a failed VBAC and the ensuing emergency caesarean section. In contrast, if that woman has always dreamed of having a very large family with many children, in spite of the increased risk associated with a failed VBAC, she may nonetheless want a trial of labour and take the chance of being able to have a successful VBAC. Her reasoning would be that having a second caesarean section means that all future deliveries would need to be done in the same way, and her risks of having a poor outcome would therefore greatly increase with each subsequent caesarean section. And then, there are the contextual factors that can also come into play. If there is no availability for a planned caesarean section (i.e. people who have an absolute contraindication to a trial of labour have already taken up all the spots, the local hospital is undergoing construction and the only other hospital is a three-hour drive away, etc.), this can also have an influence. The challenge is therefore integrating the evidence, values and contextual factors to come to a final decision. Indeed, while decision aids have been created to assist women in making such decisions, and while these tools increase women's knowledge and decrease their decisional conflict,[69] quite often women feel that the information is not sufficiently tailored to their individual clinical circumstances and needs.[70] Nonetheless, decision aids with explicit "values-clarification" exercises can lead to more informed choices as well as having a positive effect on patient–practitioner communication.[71] Thus, it is not about labelling a decision as being "right" or "wrong". Rather, the emphasis should be on supporting this particular person (or population) in making the best possible decision under the current circumstances.

Moving beyond checklists to more nuanced decision-making

Now that we have arrived at the end of the algorithm, I am sorry to disappoint those of you who were hoping for a "quick and dirty" checklist to make decisions, or those who believe that the information can simply be plugged into a formula or equation to come up with the best answer. Indeed, following the algorithm outlined in this chapter probably raises even more questions than it answers, but that is the whole point. The idea is to make reflected judgements about improving health and reducing inequities based on the best available evidence and taking into account a multitude of complex considerations. Yet, it is important to strike a balance between making decisions that are not at all thought through versus overthinking every step. The systematic approach can therefore be helpful to avoid becoming too bogged-down in the details to see the big picture, or, even worse, being paralysed by indecision when faced with a large number of perspectives and trade-offs. In the end, decisions must be made, since failing to choose is simply choosing the status quo.

The goal is therefore to foster a dialogue among stakeholders that will promote decisions that are more nuanced, more transparent and ultimately more likely to have an impact on improving health. Nonetheless, decision-making remains an inherently iterative and often somewhat disorganised process, especially as we move towards population-based and global-level decisions. According to one policy analyst:

> I describe public policy making . . . as being a ping pong player in a very large box with many other ping pong players, both public and private. Every once in a while I get to hit the ping pong ball, placing my spin on the public policy ping pong ball topic at hand. Sometimes it is the first imprint, sometimes it is the final spin, but usually the policy goes on to change either through public and industry review or political back lash before or after the next

election. Public policy is messy. If you hold on too tightly to your policy formulation you will wither in this environment. Policy is rarely final and usually changes with every new administration.[72]

Indeed, because decision-making is messy and decisions have a tendency to be revisited over time, there is all the more reason to ensure that decisions are informed by evidence and that the key stakeholders are involved in a meaningful way. The next chapter therefore concludes this book with a discussion of ensuring a fair and participative process in decision-making and a call to action for improving health.

References

1. Green L, Kreuter M. *Health Program Planning: An Educational and Ecological Approach*, 4th edn. New York: McGraw-Hill, 2005.

2. Omran A. The epidemiologic transition: a theory of the epidemiology of population change. *Milbank Q* 2005; 83(4): 731–57. Reprinted from *Milbank* Mem Fund Q 1971; 49(4): 509–38.

3. Organisation for Economic Co-operation and Development. *Health at a Glance 2011*: OECD Indicators. Paris: OECD publishing, 2011. Available at: http://www.oecd.org/dataoecd/6/28/49105858.pdf.

4. World Health Organization. *The Global Burden of Disease: 2004 update*. Geneva: World Health Organization, 2008. Available at: http://www.who.int/healthinfo/global_burden_disease/GBD_report_2004update_full.pdf.

5. *G8 Muskoka Declaration: Recovery and New Beginnings*. Ottawa: Government of Canada, 2012. Available at: http://canadainternational.gc.ca/g8/assets/pdfs/2010-declaration_eng.pdf.

6. Marmot M on behalf of the Commission on Social Determinants of Health. Achieving health equity: from root causes to fair outcomes. *The Lancet* 2007; 370(9593): 1153–63.

7. Reading C, Wien F. *Health Inequalities and Social Determinants of Aboriginal People's Health*. Prince George, BC: National Collaborating Centre for Aboriginal Health, 2009. Available at:http://www.nccah-ccnsa.ca/docs/social%20determinates/NCCAH-Loppie-Wien_Report.pdf.

8. World Health Organization. *Global Health Risks: Mortality and Burden of Disease Attributable to Selected Major Risks*. Geneva: World Health Organization, 2009.

Available at: http://www.who.int/healthinfo/global_burden_disease/GlobalHealthRisks_report_full.pdf.

9. Evans R, Barer M, Marmor T (eds.). *Why Are Some People Healthy and Others Not? The Determinants of Health of Populations*. New York: Aldine de Gruyter, 1994.

10. Dahlgren G, Whitehead M. *Policies and Strategies to Promote Social Equity in Health*. Stockholm: Institute for Futures Studies, 1991.

11. National Collaborating Centre for Aboriginal Health. *Education as a Social Determinant of First Nations, Inuit and Metis Health*. Prince George, BC: National Collaborating Centre for Aboriginal Health, 2009. Available at: http://www.nccah-ccnsa.ca/docs/fact%20sheets/social%20determinates/NCCAH_fs_education_EN.pdf.

12. National Collaborating Centre for Aboriginal Health. *Employment as a Social Determinant of First Nations, Inuit and Metis Health*. Prince George, BC: National Collaborating Centre for Aboriginal Health, 2009. Available at: http://www.nccah-ccnsa.ca/docs/fact%20sheets/social%20determinates/NCCAH_fs_employment_EN.pdf.

13. Maslow A. *Motivation and Personality*, 3rd edn. New York: Addison-Wesley, 1987.

14. Bovet P, Ross A, Gervasoni J et al. Distribution of blood pressure, body mass index and smoking habits in the urban population of Dar es Salaam, Tanzania, and associations with socioeconomic status. *Int J Epidemiol* 2002; 31(1): 240–7.

15. Commission on Social Determinants of Health (CSDH). *Closing the Gap in a Generation: Health Equity through Action on the Social Determinants of Health. Final Report of the Commission on Social Determinants of Health*. Geneva, World

Health Organization, 2008. Available at: http://whqlibdoc.who.int/publications/2008/9789241563703_eng.pdf.

16. Reading J. Keynote address. International Union for Health Promotion and Education (IUHPE) World Conference, Vancouver, 2007.

17. Macaulay A. Improving aboriginal health: how can health care professionals contribute? *Can Fam Physician* 2009; 55: 334–6. Available at: http://www.cfp.ca/content/55/4/334.

18. Commission on Social Determinants of Health (CSDH). *Social Determinants and Indigenous Health: The International Experience and Its Policy Implications*. Geneva: World Health Organization, 2007. Available at: http://www.who.int/social_determinants/resources/indigenous_health_adelaide_report_07.pdf.

19. Reading J. The quest to improve aboriginal health. *CMAJ* 2006; 174(9):1233. Available at: http://www.cmaj.ca/cgi/reprint/174/9/1233.

20. Royal Commission on Aboriginal Peoples. *Final Report*, Vol. 1. Ottawa: Government of Canada, 1996.

21. Vineis P, Elliott P. Why is epidemiology necessary to policy-making? *J Epidemiol Community Health* 2009; 63(3): 186–7.

22. Mackenbach J. Politics is nothing but medicine at a larger scale: reflections on public health's biggest idea. *J Epidemiol Community Health* 2009; 63 (3): 181–4.

23. Angell M. *The Truth About the Drug Companies: How They Deceive Us and What To Do About It*. New York: Random House, 2004.

24. Goozner M. *The $800 Million Pill: The Truth Behind the cost of New Drugs*. Berkeley: University of California Press, 2004.

25. Lerman C, Trock B, Rimer B *et al.* Psychological side effects of breast cancer screening. *Health Psychol* 1991; 10(4): 259–67.

26. Beemsterboer P, Warmerdam P, Boer R *et al.* Radiation risk of mammography related to benefit in screening programmes: a favourable balance? *J Med Screen* 1998; 5(2):81–7.

27. Roberts M. Breast screening: time for a rethink? *BMJ* 1989; 299: 1153–5.

28. Henry C. The advantages of using suppositories. *Nurs Times* 1999; 95(17): 50–1.

29. Colbert S, O'Hanlon D, McAnena O, Flynn N. The attitudes of patients and health care personnel to rectal drug administration following day case surgery. *Eur J Anaesthesiol* 1998; 15(4): 422–6.

30. von Euler-Chelpin M, Brasso K, Lynge E. Determinants of participation in colorectal cancer screening with faecal occult blood testing. *J Public Health* 2010; 32(3): 395–405.

31. Ellis R, Wilson S, Holder R, McManus R. Different faecal sampling methods alter the acceptability of faecal occult blood testing: a cross sectional community survey. *Eur J Cancer* 2007; 43(9): 1437–44.

32. Fluoride Recommendations Work Group. Recommendations for using fluoride to prevent and control dental caries in the united states. *MMWR* 2001; 50(RR14): 1–42.

33. Slade G, Spencer A, Davies M, Stewart J. Influence of exposure to fluoridated water on socioeconomic inequalities in children's caries experience. *Community Dent Oral Epidemiol* 1996; 24(2): 89–100.

34. Cross D, Carton R. Fluoridation: a violation of medical ethics and human rights. *Int J Occup Environ Health* 2003; 9(1): 24–9.

35. Connett P on behalf of the Flouride Action Network. *50 Reasons to Oppose Flouridation*. Flouride Action Network, 2011. Available at: http://www.fluoridealert.org/50-reasons.htm.

36. Federal-Provincial-Territorial Committee on Drinking Water. *Fluoride in Drinking Water*. Ottawa: Health Canada, 2009. Available at: http://www.hc-sc.gc.ca/ewh-semt/alt_formats/hecs-sesc/pdf/consult/_2009/fluoride-fluorure/consult_fluor_water-eau-eng.pdf.

37. Attwood D, Blinkhorn A. Dental health in schoolchildren 5 years after water fluoridation ceased in south-west Scotland. *Int Dent J* 1991; 41(1): 43–8.

38. Rose G. Sick individuals and sick populations. *Int J Epidemiol* 1985; 14: 32–8.

39. Jamison D, Breman J, Measham A *et al.* *Disease Control Priorities in Developing*

Countries. 2nd edn. Washington DC and Oxford: The World Bank and Oxford University Press, 2006. Available at: http://www.dcp2.org/pubs/DCP.

40. Drummond M, Sculpher M, Torrance G, O'Brien B, Stoddart G. *Methods for the Economic Evaluation of Health Care Programmes.* 3rd edn. Oxford: Oxford University Press, 2005.

41. Petticrew M, Whitehead M, Macintyre S, Graham H, Egan M. Evidence for public health policy on inequalities: 1: the reality according to policymakers. *J Epidemiol Community Health* 2004; 58(10): 811–16.

42. Thomson H, Thomas S, Sellstrom E, Petticrew M. The health impacts of housing improvement: a systematic review of intervention studies from 1887 to 2007. *Am J Public Health* 2009; 99 (Suppl 3): S681–92.

43. Taske N, Taylor L, Mulvihill C *et al. Housing and Public Health: A Review of Reviews of Interventions for Improving Health.* London: National Institute for Health and Clinical Excellence, 2005. Available at: http://www.nice.org.uk/niceMedia/pdf/housing_MAIN%20FINAL.pdf.

44. Schoub B, Cameron N. Problems encountered in the delivery and storage of OPV in an African country. *Dev Biol Stand* 1996; 87: 27–32.

45. Melzack R. The tragedy of needless pain. *Sci Am* 1990; 262(2): 27–33.

46. Warlow C. Ann McPherson: Obituary. *BMJ* 2011; 342: d3424.

47. McPherson K. My Wife Championed the Right to Choose When to Die, the Distress Of Her Final Days Proves Her Case. *The Daily Mail* June 14, 2011. Available at: http://www.dailymail.co.uk/health/article-2003269/Euthanasia-Ann-McPherson-championed-right-choose-die.html#ixzz1nudmB5Kr.

48. Nicol N, Wylie H. *Between the Dying and the Dead. Dr. Jack Kevorkian's Life and the Battle to Legalize Euthanasia.* Madison: University of Wisconsin Press, 2006.

49. Julian J, Prokopetz B, Lehmann L. Redefining physicians' role in assisted dying. *N Engl J Med* 2012; 367: 97–9.

50. Nuffield Council on Bioethics. *Genetic Screening: Ethical Issues.* London: Nuffield Council on Bioethics, 1993. Available at: http://www.nuffieldbioethics.org/sites/default/files/Genetic_screening_report.pdf.

51. Kass N. An ethics framework for public health. *Am J Public Health* 2001; 91(11): 1776–82.

52. Government of Quebec. *Plan Nord: Building Northern Quebec Together.* Quebec: Government of Quebec, 2012. Available at: http://plannord.gouv.qc.ca/english/.

53. Financial Post. Goldcorp Gets Approval for Quebec Mine. *Financial Post* November 14, 2011. Available at: http://business.financialpost.com/2011/11/14/goldcorp-gets-approval-for-quebec-mine/.

54. Commission on Macroeconomics and Health (CMH). *Investing in Health: A Summary of the Findings of the Commission on Macroeconomics and Health.* Geneva: World Health Organization, 2002. Available at: http://www.who.int/macrohealth/infocentre/advocacy/en/investinginhealth02052003.pdf.

55. Timmins N. OECD Calls Time on Trickle Down Theory. *The Globe and Mail* December 5, 2011. Available at: http://www.theglobeandmail.com/report-on-business/economy/economy-lab/oecd-calls-time-on-trickle-down-theory/article2260605/.

56. Organisation for Economic Co-operation and Development. *Divided We Stand: Why Inequality Keeps Rising.* Paris: Organization for Economic Co-operation and Development, 2012. Available at: http://www.oecd.org/dataoecd/40/12/49499779.pdf.

57. Carson R. *Silent Spring: 40th Anniversary Edition.* New York, NY: First Mariner Books, 2002.

58. Kickbush I, McCann W, Sherbon T. Adelaide revisited: from healthy public policy to Health in All Policies. *Health Promot Int* 2008; 23(1): 1–4.

59. World Health Organization. *HIA and policy-making.* Geneva: World Health Organization, 2012. Available at: http://www.who.int/hia/policy/en/.

60. Health Canada. *Canadian Handbook on Health Impact Assessment: The Basics.* Ottawa: Health Canada, 1999. Available at: http://publications.gc.ca/collections/Collection/H46-2-99-235E-1.pdf.

61. Kriebel D, Tickner J. Reenergizing public health through precaution. *Am J Public Health* 2001; 91(9): 1351–5.

62. Society of Obstetricians and Gynaecologists of Canada. SOGC clinical practice guidelines for vaginal birth after previous caesarean birth. Number 155 (Replaces guideline Number 147). *Int J Gynaecol Obstet* 2005; 89(3): 319–31.

63. Emmett C, Shaw A, Montgomery A, Murphy D on behalf of the DiAMOND study group. Women's experience of decision making about mode of delivery after a previous caesarean section: the role of health professionals and information about health risks. *BJOG* 2006; 113(12): 1438–45.

64. Guise J, Eden K, Emeis C *et al.* Vaginal birth after cesarean: new insights. *Evid Rep Technol Assess* 2010; 191: 1–397.

65. Fitzpatrick K, Kurinczuk J, Alfirevic Z *et al.* Uterine rupture by intended mode of delivery in the UK: a national case-control study. *PLoS Med* 2012; 9(3): e1001184.

66. Erez O, Novack L, Kleitman-Meir V *et al.* Remote prognosis after primary cesarean delivery: the association of VBACs and recurrent cesarean deliveries with maternal morbidity. *Int J Womens Health* 2012; 4: 93–107.

67. Hibbard J, Ismail M, Wang Y *et al.* Failed vaginal birth after a cesarean section: how risky is it? *Am J Obstet Gynecol* 2001; 184 (7): 1365–71.

68. Peterson M. *An Introduction to Decision Theory.* Cambridge: Cambridge University Press, 2009.

69. Shorten A, Shorten B, Keogh J, West S, Morris J. Making choices for childbirth: a randomized controlled trial of a decision-aid for informed birth after cesarean. *Birth* 2005; 32(4): 252–61.

70. Moffat M, Bell J, Porter M *et al.* Decision making about mode of delivery among pregnant women who have previously had a caesarean section: a qualitative study. *BJOG* 2007; 114(1): 86–93.

71. Stacey D, Bennett C, Barry M *et al.* Decision aids for people facing health treatment or screening decisions. *Cochrane Database Syst Rev* 2011; (10): CD001431.

72. Anderson J. Sausage and the Art of Public Policy-Making. *The Examiner* November 27, 2010. Available at: http://www.examiner.com/ environmental-policy-in-national/ sausage-and-the-art-of-public-policy-making#ixzz1qcwBaGil.

Conclusion

It is easy enough to propose an algorithm for making evidence-informed decisions to improve health, but the real challenge is putting it into practice. We have already discussed in Chapter 5 the various facilitators and barriers to using evidence in making decisions about health, and Chapter 6 describes the key elements that should be considered as part of the overall decision (i.e. the content), but it is important not to overlook *how* decisions are made and, in particular, *who* is involved (i.e. the process). In many ways, the process itself can be just as important as the content. This concluding chapter will therefore look at how to make evidence-informed decisions work in practice, as well as how to ensure that these decisions have the greatest possible impact on improving health.

Making it work in practice

It may appear self-evident, but decisions do not occur in some other realm and then are handed down to us mere mortals to abide by and follow. Rather, everything that structures our lives has been decided by people, and, if we want, these decisions could be changed to create a healthier and more equitable world. Indeed, the recent Rio +20 United Nations (UN) Conference on Sustainable Development asks: *What is the Future We Want?*[1] Once we define our goals for the future, it is possible to change course and make it a reality. For instance, it was recently announced that "the [Millennium Development Goal (MDG)] drinking water target, which calls for halving the proportion of the population without sustainable access to safe drinking water between 1990 and 2015, was met in 2010, five years ahead of schedule".[2] Only two decades ago, almost one-quarter of the population on this planet did not have access to clean drinking water – one of the most basic necessities for health and daily life. Yet, with a concerted effort on the part of our global society, in 2010 there were only 11% left who still relied on unimproved sources of water – and that number is continually decreasing. That is not to say that no challenges remain. Nonetheless, it is quite remarkable what can change when the decision is made to make it happen. However, influencing decisions and ensuring that they are implemented requires involving a range of key players from the very outset.

Ensuring a fair, transparent and participative process

As discussed in Chapter 3, Norman Daniels, Professor of Ethics and Population Health at Harvard University, emphasises the importance of a fair process in decision-making,[3] especially when making complex decisions that contain inherent value judgements requiring that we make trade-offs between competing ethical principles. In situations such as these, Daniels recommends "a fair, deliberative process that is transparent, encourages relevant stakeholders to deliberate on relevant reasons, provides room for revising decisions, and enforces adherence to the process".[4] Therefore, the process itself can encourage a shared

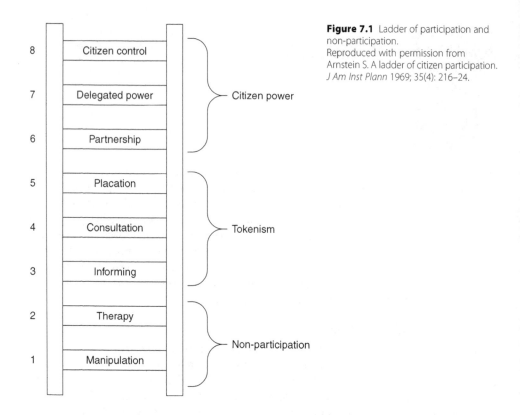

Figure 7.1 Ladder of participation and non-participation.
Reproduced with permission from Arnstein S. A ladder of citizen participation. *J Am Inst Plann* 1969; 35(4): 216–24.

understanding among all stakeholders of: (1) the evidence, (2) the implications, and (3) the intended outcomes. This shared understanding serves to promote informed choices, as well as to reduce decisional conflict and future "undoing" of decisions made.

The idea of participatory decision-making is not new. A great deal has been written on this subject in the area of business and also with respect to local governance and community empowerment.[5] Increasingly, there is a growing interest in participatory decision-making in the health arena as well. Church and colleagues consider that:

> The interest in increased citizen participation reflects an attempt by government to respond to the increasing and widespread view that the major institutions of society are unresponsive and unaccountable to citizens. The effectiveness of traditional mechanisms employed by government to elicit citizen participation in public decision-making are now being increasingly questioned.[6]

Indeed, decision-makers should engage various stakeholders from the outset to provide meaningful input and to take ownership over the decisions that are made – rather than resorting to mere "tokenism". According to Sherry Arnstein, there is a ladder with increasing levels of participation that are possible (Fig. 7.1):[7]

> The bottom rungs of the ladder are (1) Manipulation and (2) Therapy. These two rungs describe levels of "non-participation" that have been contrived by some to substitute for genuine participation. Their real objective is not to enable people to participate in planning or conducting programs, but to enable powerholders to "educate" or "cure" the participants. Rungs 3 and 4 progress to levels of "tokenism" that allow the have-nots to hear and to have a voice: (3) Informing and (4) Consultation. When they are proffered by powerholders as the

total extent of participation, citizens may indeed hear and be heard. But under these conditions they lack the power to insure that their views will be heeded by the powerful. When participation is restricted to these levels, there is no follow-through, no "muscle," hence no assurance of changing the status quo. Rung (5) Placation is simply a higher level tokenism because the ground rules allow have-nots to advise, but retain for the powerholders the continued right to decide. Further up the ladder are levels of citizen power with increasing degrees of decision-making clout. Citizens can enter into a (6) Partnership that enables them to negotiate and engage in trade-offs with traditional power holders. At the topmost rungs, (7) Delegated power and (8) Citizen control, have-not citizens obtain the majority of decision-making seats, or full managerial power. Obviously, the eight-rung ladder is a simplification, but it helps to illustrate the point that so many have missed – that there are significant gradations of citizen participation. Knowing these gradations makes it possible to cut through the hyperbole to understand the increasingly strident demands for participation from the have-nots as well as the gamut of confusing responses from the powerholders.[7]

Therefore, at the very least, there should be a partnership between the various stakeholders and those with decision-making power, to ensure that voices are not only heard, but also acted upon. Making the decision is only the first step. Ensuring that the decision will be widely adopted and implemented requires a great deal of support from various parties involved. Therefore participation can be viewed as both an end in itself (i.e. empowerment and self-determination) as well as a means to an end (i.e. ensuring the widespread adoption and implementation of decisions made). Moreover, using a systematic approach to make these decisions, such as the algorithm described in Chapter 6, allows for greater transparency in terms of the evidence taken into consideration and the reasons why certain choices were made. Thus, as the evidence base or context changes over time, these decisions are more easily revisited to determine whether the reasons previously proposed still apply or whether a different choice may now be warranted.

Indeed, greater participation, transparency and a systematic approach is not only important for population- and global-level decisions, but also for decisions made at the individual or patient level. While paternalism used to be the predominant *modus operandi*, with the physician making most of the decisions on behalf of the patient, those days are now over (although some argue that there is still room for a libertarian paternalist approach when it comes to public health decisions).[8] It is widely recognised that patients have an important role to play in preventing disease, in choosing treatment options for acute care, and in managing chronic health problems. However, ensuring that patients are able to take a more active role in decision-making requires that the necessary conditions are in place to support them in doing so. In a policy brief to promote evidence-informed decision-making by patients, Coulter and colleagues state that:

A number of interventions have been shown to be effective in building health literacy, promoting patient involvement in treatment decisions and educating patients to play an active role in self-management of chronic conditions. These interventions include:

- written information that supplements clinical consultations
- websites and other electronic information sources
- personalised computer-based information and virtual support
- training for health professionals in communication skills
- coaching and question prompts for patients
- decision aids for patients
- self-management education programmes.[9]

Perhaps the most important factor, however, is the attitude and openness of the health care provider. The key players involved in making health-related decisions at the individual level are generally the patient and the health care provider (and sometimes also the patient's family and the extended health care team, depending on the nature and complexity of the problem). Yet, due to the inherent power differential between health care providers and their patients, it is important that the health care provider engages the patient in the decision-making process. Indeed, this is something that needs to be quite explicit in training and evaluating health care workers. For example, to become a family doctor in Canada, among the various require-ments, candidates must pass the Simulated Office Oral (SOO) Examination of the College of Family Physicians of Canada (CFPC). To receive a grade of "superior certificant" (i.e. the highest possible score), the candidate:

> Actively explores the illness experience to arrive at an in-depth understanding of it. This is achieved through the purposeful use of verbal and non-verbal techniques, including both effective questioning and active listening. Actively inquires about the patient's ideas and wishes for management. Purposefully involves the patient in the development of a plan and seeks his or her feedback about it. Encourages the patient's full participation in decision-making.[10]

However, the candidate who "demonstrates only minimal interest in the illness experience and so gains little understanding of it. . . cuts the patient off, [and] does not involve the patient in the development of a plan" fails these sections of the exam (i.e. non-certificant) and, as a result, could fail the entire exam. Therefore it is possible to promote a culture of shared decision-making, and even go so far as to ensure that those who do not make decisions in a participatory and patient-centred way are barred from making any decisions at all.

Overcoming challenges to make it work in practice

Just as there are many barriers to using evidence in practice, as described in Chapter 5, there are also many challenges to using a systematic, evidence-informed approach to decision-making. These include understanding the decision-making process, identifying and involv-ing the key stakeholders and decision-makers from the outset, ensuring that the best available evidence has been reliably collected and synthesised, helping all those involved to better understand probabilistic information through the use of pictures and stories and various other ways of expressing risk rather than only using statistics, avoiding potential bias when framing the information, making trade-offs and opportunity costs explicit and ensuring that the evidence is accessible during the critical window of opportunity so that it can be incorporated into the decision-making process.

However, as we move further upstream to address the social determinants of health, in addition to the many challenges described above, an even greater challenge is getting the issue of health onto the agenda and ensuring that the intersectoral partners who are most able to influence change are at the table. Building healthy public policies and creating supportive environments for health is not an easy process. Improving the health of the population requires taking a fresh look at local issues and problems. Healthy communities need social meeting spaces, places for physical activity, schools that are conducive to learning, local jobs, transportation, adequate housing, good governance, redistribution of power and wealth, and so forth. This may be outside of the comfort zone of health workers who are more familiar with vaccination campaigns and anti-smoking radio announcements, but it will be necessary

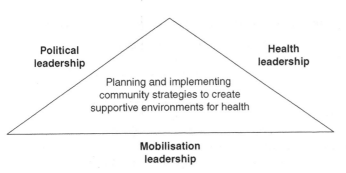

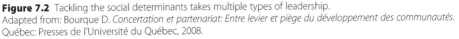

Figure 7.2 Tackling the social determinants takes multiple types of leadership.
Adapted from: Bourque D. *Concertation et partenariat: Entre levier et piège du développement des communautés.*
Québec: Presses de l'Université du Québec, 2008.

to incorporate different ways of working and approaching health issues to make lasting and meaningful improvements to the health of the entire population. Together, all the community partners need to agree upon the collective problems – ranging from health and social issues to environmental sustainability and economic development. Together, all the community partners need to develop a shared vision of the collective solutions and the way forward given the local realities and resources available. This requires strong leadership, not only from health planners and "content experts", but also from elected officials in local and national government as well as community mobilisers who can ensure that the process continues to move forward towards transformative change and does not "run out of steam". According to Bourque, many different types of leadership are therefore required to make these changes happen, including: (1) political leadership, (2) health leadership, and (3) mobilisation leadership (Fig. 7.2).[11]

In terms of political leadership, it is necessary to have buy-in at the highest levels. The politicians and leaders need to be involved as they have the power and authority to make the changes that can influence the health of the population. However, it is also important to have health leadership, which can supply the evidence and recommend which strategies should be implemented to have the greatest impact on improving health. Finally, without mobilisation leadership, these intersectoral processes have a tendency to start off with lots of enthusiasm and quickly fizzle out after a few weeks to months. It will not work if it is not a sustainable process. Of course, in addition to strong leadership and sustainability, another important element is money, and ensuring that the money is being spent in the right places, including in support of intersectoral processes such as these.

Asking the right questions and putting money in the right places

Without dedicated funds for supporting intersectoral action, it is unlikely that much progress will be made. Often it is not an issue of a lack of funds, but more an issue of whether the funds are being spent on strategies that are most likely to improve health. Here is where evidence-informed decision-making is especially critical. In the first instance, it is important to ask ourselves "Are we even asking the right questions, and, if so, are we putting our money in the right places?" There is an old joke about the police officer and the man with the missing keys that illustrates this well (Box 7.1).

Box 7.1 The police officer and the man with the missing keys

A police officer sees a man at night crouched down under a street lamp.

The police officer stops beside him and asks the man "What are you doing?"

The man replies "I am looking for my keys. I dropped them and now I am locked out of my car".

"I can help you look", says the police officer "where did you drop your keys?"

"Over there" says the man, pointing off into the distance.

"So why are you looking for your keys here if you dropped them way over there?" responds the police officer with a puzzled look on his face.

"Because here there is light", says the man. "I wouldn't be able to see anything over there in the dark".

Indeed, it is not possible to improve health by continuing to do what we usually do because it is easy and familiar. Rather, we need to work in new ways so that we can make a meaningful impact on improving health and reducing inequities. For example, to address the growing epidemic of chronic diseases such as obesity, diabetes and heart disease, an Aboriginal community suggests as part of their health plan that they will distribute the Canada Food Guide and then quiz community members on their knowledge of the food guide. As well, they will offer cooking classes on how to prepare healthy meals and give out mugs with the logo "eat healthy – live longer". Finally, they will organise a weight-loss competition which they will advertise on the radio – an Aboriginal version of "the biggest loser" – whoever loses the most weight in 12 weeks wins an all-expenses paid trip for two to the nation's capital. It is not to say that these are bad ideas, but it is not very convincing that these are going to make a real and lasting impact on the health of the population.

We know from Chapters 2 and 3 that individual behaviour change strategies are not very effective. Knowing that something is bad for you (i.e. smoking, fatty foods, etc.) often does very little to stop people from engaging in these unhealthy behaviours. Imagine that "Community A" implements the above strategies targeted towards individual behaviour change. One might expect some increased knowledge about healthy foods. A few motivated people might participate in the cooking classes and the contest. Some people may lose weight in the short term. However, it is extremely unlikely that there will be a population-wide improvement in obesity and diabetes rates in one year or even in five years using these strategies. Why are strategies like this doomed to be ineffective? Suppose you are Daisy, a member of "Community A" who has been obese ever since she was a teenager. Daisy is interested to read about the food guide and she would like to lose weight since many of her relatives already have diabetes and her doctor has warned her several times that she is also at risk. However, when Daisy goes to the grocery store in her remote Northern community there are only shrivelled and rotting fruits and vegetables on sale, and the few that look edible are extremely expensive. At home, Daisy's husband is furious that she spent so much money on the groceries and they get into a big fight in front of the children. As usual, Daisy turns to comfort foods like ice cream and cake to ease her anxiety. The next day, her friends tell her, "Daisy, what are you so unhappy about? 'Big is beautiful.' You don't need to change". Daisy nonetheless wants to win the contest and works hard to lose the weight. While she doesn't win the grand prize, she has lost a few kilograms. However, within the year, with the usual stress of work and family life, she has put back on all the weight and is now even heavier than before. Did Daisy's environment change? No. Did the social norm that "Big is beautiful" change? No. Did health outcomes improve? No. Was the money that went into implementing these strategies well spent? You decide.

So, instead imagine an alternative scenario of how things could be different if we work to change the environment rather than asking people to change their behaviours while their environments are still working against them. There was an elegant study carried out by the US Navy in 1990 which demonstrates this very nicely. Two ships were going out to sea. On "Ship A" the standard navy food was served, but on "Ship B" the chefs were instructed to prepare meals according to specific nutritional guidelines – thus creating a supportive environment for healthy eating. Both ships were out at sea for six months. The sailors on Ship B ate oven-roasted lean meats and baked potatoes in place of fried steaks and mashed potatoes with gravy. Low-fat frozen yogurt and low-fat cookies were offered in place of other higher-fat desserts. Neither ship had any individual counselling or behaviour change interventions. When they returned, the sailors on Ship A gained an average of three kilograms and their waist sizes grew three to five centimetres. Moreover, of those who weighed over 90 kilograms before they left, 74% gained even more weight. However, the sailors on Ship B had lost on average five kilograms and five centimetres from their waist. Of those who weighed over 90 kilograms before they left, 74% actually lost weight – without any special exercise regimen or even changing their eating habits.[12] This is the power of changing the environment.

Therefore, imagine "Community B", where, instead of blaming the victim and putting all the responsibility on the individual, there is an attempt to change the environment and "make the healthy choices the easy choices". Funds are set aside to hire a community mobiliser in Community B, who encourages greater community dialogue and helps to establish an intersectoral action committee to identify shared problems and solutions. The community mobiliser also helps to ensure implementation and follow-up on the recommended solutions. For instance, the community mobiliser meets with local store and restaurant owners encouraging them to provide more healthy options and to stop selling products that are unhealthy (i.e. cigarettes, junk food, etc.). Additional funds are spent to buy a refrigerated truck and to hire two community members previously on income support to run a fresh-food co-op service. Each week they drive to the closest farmer's market (even if it means spending two to three days on the road) to buy a truckload of fruits and vegetables that they distribute at cost to local community households. More funds are then spent building a large greenhouse for a community garden that can operate all year round, as well as a community kitchen, a park, a communal freezer and walking or snowshoeing trails. Another dozen or so community members are hired to operate the garden, to organise activities for children and youth in the park and on the trails, to organise the communal hunting parties which will bring back fresh meat and fish to be stored in the freezer, to run the freezer, to maintain the trails, and to prepare subsidised healthy meals that are distributed throughout the community – addressing both the problem of obesity and chronic disease as well as the concomitant problem of food insecurity (i.e. people not having enough to eat). The new jobs provide a boost to the self-esteem and mental well-being of the community members, and the local government is now considering developing tourism opportunities and the sale of local crafts to bring more external money into the community and to create more local jobs. There has even been talk of establishing a telemarketing centre, which is encouraging students to stay in school, since they would need a high-school diploma to apply to work there. For the first time in a long time, people are hopeful, energised and engaged in their community.

While it is always difficult to divert funds from acute-care health services into prevention (indeed, as mentioned previously, public health receives on average only 3% of the overall health budget), how long will we continue to "put on band-aids" rather than working on the upstream determinants of health and creating supportive environments to prevent health problems from occurring in the first place? This involves mobilising political and social action on the determinants of health, which includes increasing the income of those who are the least well off, improving access to child care services, increasing financing and availability of social housing, strengthening the publicly funded health services system, and so forth.[13] If we want to make a real impact on improving population health, this is the way forward.

From high-quality evidence to best practices and innovative solutions

Perhaps counter intuitively, moving towards greater intersectoral action to address the underlying causes of poor health may actually lead us "into the dark" as in the joke about the police officer and the man with the keys described above. While there is an explosion in the research literature on genetic markers of common diseases, on the efficacy of blood pressure and lipid-lowering drugs, as well as a range of clinical interventions from screening to behaviour change counselling, there is relatively little evidence on larger-scale, population-based interventions for creating supportive environments and health in all policies. That is not to say that there is no evidence. Indeed, the International Union for Health Promotion and Education (IUHPE) produced a compendium of such evidence a decade ago.[14] As well, there are proven community-based interventions included in *The Community Guide*[15] and some of the Cochrane summaries.[16] There is also evidence on strategies for addressing the social causes of poor health compiled by the Commission on Social Determinants of Health,[17] as well as guidance on how to use the evidence provided by SUPPORT tools for evidence-informed policy-making.[18] Yet, there is far less evidence available for making population- and global-level decisions as compared to evidence of what works in clinical settings. As a result, it is not surprising that people are generally focusing on clinical approaches, since that is where the evidence tends to be most developed and robust. However, we are caught in an endless cycle – generating more evidence where we already have strong evidence and neglecting areas where there is little evidence. Nothing will change unless we start to build up the evidence base for a more balanced continuum of approaches that includes the clinic, but also includes outreach work as well as larger community-based strategies and even national and global strategies that support and reinforce local action.

Indeed, according to the Population Health Template Working Tool developed by the Public Health Agency of Canada, the key elements and actions that define a population health approach: (1) focus on the health of populations, (2) address the determinants of health and their interactions, (3) base decisions on evidence, (4) increase upstream investments, (5) apply multiple strategies, (6) collaborate across sectors and levels, (7) employ mechanisms for public involvement, and (8) demonstrate accountability for health outcomes (Fig. 7.3).[19] In particular, this approach emphasises how we cannot only focus on clinic-based strategies – even if that is where we have the highest quality evidence – but rather "population health integrates activities across the wide range of interventions that make up the health continuum: from health care to prevention, protection, health promotion and action on the determinants of health".

Therefore, even when evidence is lacking on which population-based interventions would be most effective, it is nonetheless possible to proceed using best practices and

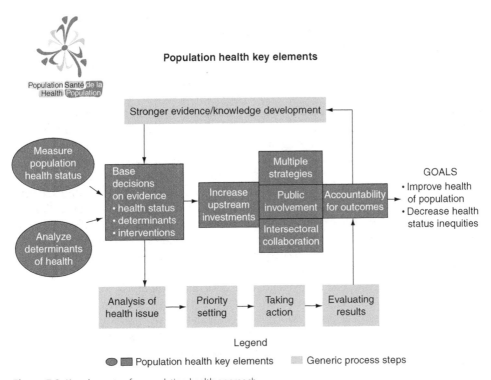

Figure 7.3 Key elements of a population health approach.
Reproduced with permission from: Public Heath Agency of Canada. *The Population Health Template Working Tool.* Ottawa: Public Heath Agency of Canada, 2001.

innovative solutions for improving health. For instance, imagine that, in a given community, all the different partners and stakeholders consider the high rates of family violence to be a major problem. The conviction of the local community members that this should indeed be the main priority was further strengthened when the local health worker presented evidence from the ACE Study demonstrating that childhood experiences of abuse and household dysfunction are associated with increased rates of alcoholism, drug abuse, depression, suicide attempts, sexually transmitted diseases, smoking, obesity and physical inactivity later in life.[20] A link has even been shown with premature death among family members.[21] However, is there anything that can be done to prevent this? Looking to evidence-based resources such as the US Preventive Services Task Force, there is "insufficient evidence to recommend for or against routine screening of parents or guardians for the physical abuse or neglect of children, of women for intimate partner violence, or of older adults or their caregivers for elder abuse".[22] Yet, this is the priority health problem that has been identified, and although there is insufficient evidence at this time to recommend screening, it does not mean that we will simply stop here and avoid addressing the issue altogether. So, we can continue to search for other evidence-based recommendations. For instance, *The Community Guide* also has a section on interventions to address the problem of violence. While there is again "insufficient evidence" for or against most of these interventions, there are nonetheless a few interventions where there is a sufficient evidence base to be able to judge. For example, *The Community Guide* recommends early childhood home visitation programmes to prevent child maltreatment by providing parents with guidance for caring and constructive interaction with their young children, facilitating the development of parental life skills, strengthening social support for parents and linking families with social services.[23] However, imagine that we are interested in a specific sub-population, and that this strategy – though evidence-based – does not resonate with the local culture or setting. In a small Aboriginal community where everyone knows everyone else, and often they are even related to everyone else, a programme whereby a person comes to your home for regular visits during and after your pregnancy to ensure that there is no child maltreatment may not be palatable, both for the person making the visits and the people who are being visited. Thus, implementation of such programmes would require cultural adaptation, or simply rethinking other possible strategies that may work better in the local setting. We could therefore look to the larger body of research literature and attempt to find evidence of interventions specific to this sub-population that have been shown to work. For example, Shea and colleagues conducted a systematic review of interventions and approaches to reduce family violence in Aboriginal communities.[24] However, they found very few studies relating to the Aboriginal context, most of which focused on tertiary prevention rather than primary prevention. As well, the methodological quality of these studies was quite low.

Therefore, in the event that the evidence base does not reveal much, we can also turn to best practices. The Public Health Agency of Canada (PHAC) has assembled a resource called the Canadian Best Practices Portal which "is a compendium of community interventions related to chronic disease prevention and health promotion that have been evaluated, shown to be successful, and have the potential to be adapted and replicated".[25] While not the highest quality evidence, relying on best practices is "the next best thing". For instance, the Portal has a list of programmes and other interventions that have been used to prevent violence in childhood, adulthood and the elderly. While these programmes may or may not be applicable to all contexts, at least one does not have to start from scratch, but can browse existing programmes, consider their strengths and weaknesses, and determine whether to choose one of these to be adapted locally. By further searching the grey literature (i.e. published and unpublished reports that are difficult to find via conventional channels such as peer-reviewed journals or monographs), it is possible to find information more specific to Aboriginal populations. For instance, there are best practices related to running local shelters for victims of family violence.[26] While it is very positive that such shelters exist (a form of tertiary prevention), often these are the only strategies used to address the issue of family violence. In many communities, the social norm is such that family violence is considered to be a "normal" part of daily life.[27] Indeed, Rupert Ross, a Crown Attorney who has worked extensively in Aboriginal communities, describes how family violence has become so pervasive, and explains why we should look to traditional approaches for addressing these issues in a more culturally adapted and holistic way.[28]

The Aboriginal Healing Foundation (AHF) has created a repertory of approaches for dealing with the intergenerational trauma related to residential schools and centuries of colonisation and marginalisation. While the evidence base is limited (i.e. when you search the PubMed database, for instance, you will not find much published on these approaches), in practice there are literally hundreds of interventions that have been implemented to address the issue of family violence and a host of other problems related to the trauma of residential schools, to centuries of colonisation and to the overall breakdown in the social fabric of many communities. The authors of the AHF report categorise these approaches according to three pillars of healing: (1) reclaiming history, (2) cultural interventions, and (3) therapeutic healing.[29] Reclaiming history entails programmes and activities that promote learning about the past as a catalyst for mourning what was lost and being able to put one's personal trauma in a larger social and historical context to avoid self-blame and guilt. Cultural interventions then engage people in a process of recovering and reconnecting with their culture, language, history, spirituality, traditions and ceremonies to reinforce self-esteem and a positive cultural identity. Finally, therapeutic healing encompasses a broad range of traditional, alternative and conventional or Western therapies for recovering from trauma in a way that is holistic and culturally adapted. While very little of this is written up in the research literature, these approaches can nonetheless be very useful for addressing the "causes of the causes of the causes" as described in the previous chapter. However, unless people are made aware of these approaches, it is unlikely they will be widely used to help others.

Notwithstanding the extensive selection of best practices for improving health, nothing stands in the way of also developing new ideas for interventions that may prove to be even more useful in local settings. This is particularly important in a global health context where evidence of intervention effectiveness is often lacking and innovative solutions are urgently needed.[30] Indeed, the Canadian Government has committed $225 million over five years to the Development Innovation Fund administered by Grand Challenges Canada to "support the best minds in the world as they search for breakthroughs in global health and other areas that have the potential to bring about enduring changes in the lives of the millions of people in poor countries".[31]

However, when relying on best practices and innovative solutions, it is particularly important to build up the evidence base by conducting rigorous evaluations on whether and how these interventions had an impact on improving health.[32] The findings of these evaluations should be widely disseminated to decision-makers at all levels so that effective interventions can be adapted and applied to other contexts and settings – rather than the usual scenario where there is a plethora of single-country demonstration projects that never get scaled-up globally.

Evaluating progress in improving health outcomes

The importance of having reliable and comparable data to be able to measure progress in improving the health of individuals and populations cannot be over-emphasised. Indeed, high-quality data is required throughout the decision-making process, starting at the very outset, to be able to determine the priority health needs and to guide the selection of an appropriate combination of strategies that can maximise health improvements. Then, high-quality data is also required after implementing these strategies to be able to determine whether health has improved and how, and to identify new priority areas for the future.

When choosing indicators to measure population health needs and to evaluate progress in improving health and reducing inequities, there is no need to overcomplicate matters. To a great extent, these indicators already exist and are currently being used by various surveillance systems or population-based surveys to collect data. What is therefore important is to use the same indicators, so that it is possible to have comparable data. For instance, if a community wants to know whether there are fewer problems of food insecurity (i.e. lack of access to food) now as compared to five years ago, they could develop their own survey and ask people. Perhaps they will find that 30% of people living in the community experienced food insecurity in 2000 and only 25% in 2010. Is that good? Is that bad? It looks like there has been an improvement, but it is hard to say for sure whether this is good or bad. How can we tell? Well, we need something to compare this to. If instead of doing their own "home grown" survey, the same community joins a national survey that is collecting data on food insecurity across the country (or at least uses the same questions and indicators), then we will have a basis for comparison. If, for example, when answering the very same question, only 20% of the overall population experienced food insecurity in 2000 and 5% in 2010, then we know that the rate of food insecurity is now five times higher in the community as compared to the rest of the country, and that progress in reducing food insecurity has been much slower, resulting in a widening gap (i.e. the rate of food insecurity in the community used to be only 1.5 times higher than the national average in 2000, thus health inequities are getting worse rather than better, even if there have been some improvements in reducing food insecurity). Therefore, to measure the impact of different strategies on improving health, ideally one wants to use existing indicators, which means that it is necessary to know what type of data is already being collected and how to access this data to be able to monitor progress.

For health data to be meaningful and useful very much depends on how the data is collected, analysed and communicated. To assess the health of an individual, one usually relies upon findings from the patient history, the physical examination and any number of clinical tests. However, to assist decision-makers in their role of improving the health of a population, it is common practice to combine many different types of data in creating a "health portrait", which is a snapshot in time of the health of a population. A health portrait generally includes information on:

- demographics (i.e. population size, age distribution, population growth, etc.)
- mortality (i.e. rates and causes of death)
- morbidity (i.e. incidence and prevalence of diseases, rates and causes of hospitalisation)
- health services utilisation (i.e. medical consultations, prescription drug use, etc.)
- risk factors (i.e. smoking, alcohol use, physical inactivity, unhealthy diet, etc.)
- determinants of health (i.e. education, income, employment, etc.).

The health portrait is therefore the primary tool in assessing the "objective" health needs of a population – i.e. how healthy is this population and how does it compare to the rest of the country or to the rest of the world? The health portrait is generally complemented by consultations with the population to determine the "subjective" health needs – i.e. what do local people think are the biggest health problems facing their community? Together, this information is used in setting priorities and in choosing the appropriate combination of interventions to be implemented. On a regular basis (e.g. every 5 or 10 years), another health portrait is then needed to determine how health has improved (or not) over time, and to plan the next round of interventions. For instance, Healthy People is a US initiative that establishes evidence-based national goals and objectives with 10-year targets for improving health. Going back to Healthy People 1990, which was launched in response to the 1979 report entitled *Healthy People: The Surgeon General's Report on Health Promotion and Disease Prevention*,[33] a new set of goals and objectives is released each decade. The most recent iteration is Healthy People 2020, which was launched by the Department of Health and Human Services in December 2010,[34] with each new version building on the successes and shortcomings of the previous attempt to improve health.

When creating health portraits, there are many different types of data from a variety of sources that can be used (Fig. 7.4). However, not all data is reliable and comparable across different groups, which is particularly important when assessing health inequities or health

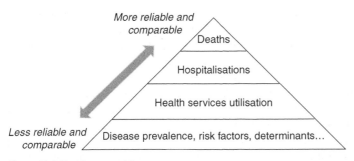

Figure 7.4 The data pyramid.

gaps. At the top of the "data pyramid", we have the most basic and fundamental information about the health of the population: "On average, how many people die each year and what are they dying from?" Countries, such as Canada, the USA and the UK, have long-established vital statistics registries based on death certificates. This mortality data is among the most reliable sources of data which are easily comparable across different groups. In this way, it is possible to determine that, on average, the life expectancy of a given population is higher or lower than the rest of the country. Since the goal is not only to improve health but also to reduce health inequities within and between groups, having comparable data to measure these "gaps" – and to determine whether these gaps are shrinking or growing – is extremely valuable.

Even so, we cannot build a health portrait based on mortality data alone, since it is just the tip of the iceberg. Thankfully, there are far fewer deaths each year as compared to people being hospitalised, for instance. Thus, it is also helpful to look at morbidity data. Once again, many wealthier countries have well-established administrative databases that collect information on hospitalisations using the "discharge summaries" – i.e. the final report filled out at the end of each hospitalisation which records the main reasons why the patient was hospitalised. Therefore, hospitalisation data is another highly reliable source of data which is also easily comparable across different groups.

Going further down the pyramid, we know that not everyone with a disease is necessarily being hospitalised. Especially in this day and age where there is a rise in chronic diseases, many people live for years with a disease and are never hospitalised, but nonetheless have contact with health services. Thus, there are also administrative databases which record the number and reasons for visits to the doctor, or the use of various prescription medications, which can provide us with insights into how many people are suffering from specific diseases or health problems. We can even look at the usage of non-medical services such as the number and reasons for reporting children to youth protection services. All of these different sources of data are helpful in providing a well-rounded portrait of how the population is doing. However, quite often, the further down the pyramid we go, the more difficult it becomes to compare the data across different groups since the data may be collected in different ways. Thus the reliability and comparability is often not as robust as for the mortality and hospitalisation data, which tends to be more standardised.

Indeed, much of the data at the bottom of the pyramid is collected using a variety of surveys or other research designs which may or may not provide reliable and comparable data depending on how these studies are carried out. Among the most reliable and comparable data at this level is from the national census, which is a type of survey that collects information from households across the country on topics such as family income, level of education, housing overcrowding, and so forth. However, many countries around the world do not have a national census and instead rely upon other types of survey methods such as the Demographic and Health Surveys (DHS) funded by the United States Agency for International Development (USAID), which have been used extensively in over 90 low- and middle-income countries since the 1980s.[35] These are nationally representative house- hold surveys that provide data for a wide range of monitoring and impact evaluation indicators in the areas of population, health and nutrition. Nonetheless, there are many other large-scale and small-scale surveys and other types of studies that attempt to capture disease prevalence and exposure to risk factors as well as the interplay of the broader upstream determinants of health – although, once again, reliability and comparability are often an issue. For instance, when attempting to use surveys to assess the prevalence of substance abuse or intimate partner violence (IPV) – including sexual, physical and psycho- logical abuse – it is well known that there are high rates of under-reporting. For instance, a woman may deny that she is a victim of abuse for many reasons. Perhaps she is afraid that the authorities will take away her children. Perhaps she does not trust that the survey is truly confidential. Perhaps she is worried that her husband would find out and hurt her even more. Therefore data from surveys and other sources such as this are certainly better than no data at all, but need to be used and interpreted with caution.

Reliable and comparable health data is therefore essential for being able to measure progress over time. Thus, based on the impact of past decisions, it is important to periodically revisit and revise the decisions that were made (i.e. recalling that, in the health planning cycle in Chapter 2, the next step after "evaluation" is to return to the "needs assessment" and "priority setting", thus beginning the cycle all over again).

Revisiting decisions made

As the saying goes, "If at first you don't succeed, try, try again". While not always possible, in most cases decisions can and should be revisited over time. According to Wharam and Daniels:

> Assessment of new health policies is rarely systematic... Even though the concept of evidence-based decision making is widely accepted in the clinical world, the approach has not fully permeated health policy. Legislation creating policies does not necessarily include "impact assessments," commissioned studies do not use standardized measures, and outcomes examined may be of questionable relevance. Policy change therefore may be based on expert opinion, funding circumstances, or political sentiment rather than evidence of benefits or harm... The lack of systematic and ongoing evaluations of new health policies has led to the discovery of unintended consequences years later... adverse health out- comes also have been documented.[36]

Therefore, it is important not only to evaluate progress in improving health outcomes and reducing health inequities, but also to assess whether there are any unintended consequences or harms arising from the decisions made. If health outcomes are not improving as initially expected, or if there are unintended harms, or if new evidence comes to light, or if the context changes, then these would all be reasons for revising decisions made previously. If a system- atic approach was used, such as the one described in Chapter 6, then it would be quite straightforward to identify which evidence is now changed, which reasons for choosing one option over another have been affected as a result, and what the new decision will be in light of these changes. For instance, one could decide to abandon a policy or programme altogether or simply institute certain modifications and refinements to further maximise the benefits and minimise the harms. Thus decision-making for health is an ongoing, iterative process. Notwithstanding having "missed the boat" in achieving the Declaration of Alma-Ata's target of "Health for All by the year 2000",[37] it nonetheless remains a laudable goal that we should continue to work towards.

A call to action

Three main strategies have been proposed by the World Health Organization (WHO) to make a real impact on improving health and reducing health inequities by influencing the underlying determinants of health: (1) improve the conditions of daily life – the circumstances in which people are born, grow, live, work, and age; (2) tackle the inequitable distribution of power, money, and resources – the structural drivers of those conditions of daily life – globally, nationally, and locally; and (3) measure the problem, evaluate action, expand the knowledge base, develop a workforce that is trained in the social determinants of health, and raise public awareness about the social determinants of health.[38] Thus, addressing the social causes of poor health requires the ability to engage other sectors (education, labour, etc.) in intersectoral action and whole-of-government approaches that extend far beyond the health sector.

Engaging other sectors in addressing the social causes of poor health

History shows how large-scale health improvements are not the result of new technologies but, rather, occur when "the politics of public health could direct collective resources toward the good of the community as a whole".[39] Community mobilisation is therefore a critical step in initiating intersectoral action and making it work.[40] Increasingly it is recognised that the impetus for improving health needs to come from the community, born out of the realities that people face. It is really an issue of problem solving – finding shared solutions to the shared problems that people experience in their day-to-day lives. Community health has been defined as "the collective expression of the health of individuals and groups in a defined community".[41] It is determined by the interaction of multiple factors including personal and family characteristics, social and physical environments, health and social services, cultural and political contexts, and so forth. It may appear self-evident, but planning and implementing interventions to improve the health of the community requires the involvement of the community throughout the process, from conducting an initial health assessment and identifying health needs to measuring the impact of various interventions on health outcomes. When it comes to choosing which interventions to use, one need not always reinvent the wheel. As described previously, even in the absence of evidence-based strategies, there often exists a wide range of potentially useful strategies developed in other contexts and settings that can be adapted and evaluated locally.

Although there are many proponents of community-based approaches such as the Community-Oriented Primary Care (COPC) model, which blends public health and primary care,[42,43] until now, we have generally been focusing too much of our time and effort racing to "put out fires" once health problems appear and people present themselves to the clinic or hospital. Practical solutions are needed that move beyond addressing the symptoms and start acting on the underlying causes in a more evidence-informed and systematic way. Action taken at the local level also needs to be reinforced and supported by complementary actions at the national and global levels to truly promote widespread change. However, despite a rapidly growing literature on intersectoral approaches and health in all policies, this promising field of public health is still very much in its infancy.[44] As Potvin points out:

> Despite the appealing rhetoric of intersectoral action, very few among health promotion professionals and researchers would be able to describe successful initiatives that involve sectors other than education. There would be even fewer people being able to list the conditions of success of such initiatives. The reason for this is quite simple: such projects are not that frequent and only a very small proportion of them have been studied. Although some case reports have been compiled for the WHO Commission on the Social Determinants of Health, there is still a dearth of in-depth analysis of how they come about and the process by which they overcome the formidable obstacles that the normal functioning of public administration represent for intersectoral coordination and intervention.[45]

While action is clearly needed outside of the health sector, it is very unlikely that we will be able to mobilise this action without the concerted efforts of people working on the frontlines within the health sector. They are the ones who witness first-hand how social inequities result in premature death and increased rates of disease. They are the ones who hear the stories of the marginalised and disenfranchised, and, they are the ones who can make these voices heard to engage wider political and social action.

Engaging the health sector in addressing the social causes of poor health

Ironically, while people working within the health sector are the ones most preoccupied with improving health, they often feel disempowered and unable to address the social causes of poor health. It is generally not a subject area that is explicitly being taught to health workers in training, and, once they are working, they are usually very busy and overburdened with the sheer volume of acute care and treatment activities. All this talk of poor housing, poverty, low educational attainment and unemployment can sound very vague and insurmountable to frontline health workers trying to keep up with the demand for health services. Shouldn't someone else be dealing with this?

Yet, frontline health workers are essential to mobilising change. Not only are they well placed to bear witness to the injustice and unfairness in society which leads to poor health and health inequities, but they are also in a strong position to recommend the implementation of a continuum of strategies for improving health (from treatment and rehabilitation to disease prevention, health promotion and addressing the upstream determinants). According to Whitehead and colleagues:

> Any planned response to the gross and pervasive inequities in health must acknowledge right from the start that action involves ethical and political choices – and therefore has to be based on a firm foundation of shared values within a society. Developing value-driven policy action is, however, particularly challenging in the current global context. Economic, social, and health policies have increasingly sacrificed ethical concerns in the race to contain costs and in the pursuit of "efficiency." Therefore, an essential first step is to demonstrate the injustice and unfairness of present economic and social arrangements while making explicit the values on which proposed action is based.[46]

There is certainly a growing body of evidence that justice is good for our health, and that governments such as China, Cuba and Costa Rica, which have systems in place for ensuring social equity, have had greater health gains than countries which focus only on rapid economic growth.[47] As respected members of the community, frontline health workers are able to advocate and encourage political leaders to take action to create larger social change. Even on an individual level, frontline health workers are able to at least ask their patients about the social causes of poor health and document the underlying causes. They can also listen to, respect and care for their patients, particularly those who are the most vulnerable and marginalised. They can even refer patients to social support networks that exist in the community, or help mobilise communities in developing support services to meet the local demand. Addressing the social causes of poor health is therefore integral to practising good medicine and to improving the health of the population.[48]

Even though the majority of the social causes of poor health lie outside the health sector, frontline health workers can nonetheless be powerful change agents in promoting more nuanced and evidence-informed decisions to prevent needless suffering and injustice. Indeed, this should be seen as an important part of their mandate and role. According to Mercer:

> If our goal is to improve health, those within the health sector must move outside class-rooms, laboratories, and hospital walls to embrace a broader approach to health. We cannot be 'neutral'. . . people from many walks of life must be inspired to move out of their 'comfort zones' and step into other worlds, to see the reality of globalization as it affects the lives and health of people today. We need above all to globalize dissent, resistance, and the demand for accountability. We need to envision and project a new reality that will move the globe towards a more just system.[49]

From polarised opinions to nuanced and evidence-informed decisions

This book has attempted to describe the complexity inherent to decision-making and how to make more evidence-informed decisions to improve health. While decision-making rarely follows a purely rational and linear process, evidence nonetheless plays an important role. Stone argues that, when making policy decisions at a population level, one cannot separate reasoned analysis from the political process:

> Political reason is a process of persuasion, it is an enterprise of searching for criteria and justifying choices. . . we may not ever see eye to eye, yet there is a world of difference between a political process in which people honestly try to understand how the world looks from different vantage points, and one in which people claim from the start that their vantage point is the right one.[50]

Thus, in the end, decision-making is really about people. It is no longer considered acceptable to make decisions unless those affected by the decisions made are involved in the decision-making process – whether at the patient level,[51] the population level[52] or the global level.[53] Ensuring that sufficient evidence is generated to support decision-making,[54] and that the evidence is packaged in such a way so as to increase uptake by decision-makers,[55,56] is surely important, but it is not enough. While one might think it obvious that everyone should want to improve health, in reality, this is a highly contentious area fraught with paradoxes. For instance, increased spending on universal health care and education as well as various forms of social protection could entail higher rates of taxation for the rich and powerful. Even if living in a more just and equitable society results in improved quality of life for all members of that society,[57] how many people do you know want to pay more taxes? Indeed, fierce political debates are being waged on a daily basis as to whether governments should do more to help poor and vulnerable groups or whether they should "keep their hands out of our pockets" and infringe as little as possible on individual rights and freedoms – including, some would say, the right to spend your hard-earned money in the way that you want. Therefore, emotions run high and these debates often become very polarised rather than being nuanced and based on evidence.

At a global level, bringing entire countries out of poverty would likely require changing international trade and financial policies. Several years ago, I witnessed a WHO Executive Board meeting where the topic of international trade and health was discussed. According to the report from the Secretariat:

> Four of the multilateral trade agreements of [the World Trade Organization (WTO)] – the leading normative organization on international trade – that may affect public health are of particular importance to WHO's work: the General Agreement on Trade in Services (GATS), and the agreements on Application of Sanitary and Phytosanitary Measures (SPS), on Technical Barriers to Trade (TBT), and on Trade-Related Aspects of Intellectual Property Rights (TRIPS). Significant advances have been made to ensure coherence between trade agreements and health interests. Most notably, the international community's endorsement of the Doha Declaration on the TRIPS Agreement and Public Health in 2001... is a very visible expression of governments' commitment to ensuring that the rules-based trading system is compatible with public health interests... The intersection between the framing of national public-health policies and the need to comply with international trade agreements offers opportunities to find common ground. Policies that minimize possible conflicts between trade and health and maximize mutual benefits will serve both interests. Greater interaction is needed between policy-makers and practitioners in the trade and health sectors in order to improve the coherence of domestic and international policy. In view of current and emerging international trade rules, ministries of health need to become more aware of trade issues under consideration within WTO and other international organizations, and need to help colleagues in the ministries concerned with international trade to understand relevant aspects of public health at both national and international levels.[58]

While this is clearly a very important topic that could have far-reaching implications for global health, the discussion that followed was remarkably short. After a few delegates from low- and middle-income countries expressed their interest on the subject, a delegate from one of the powerful rich countries got up and started to vehemently criticise the Secretariat for even working in this area, complaining that this is not part of WHO's mandate, what business do they have interfering with matters of international trade, and so forth. Then the delegate made a motion to table the discussion, which was quickly seconded by the delegate from another powerful rich country, and the entire group got up to have coffee in the foyer.

To make progress in improving health and reducing health inequities, we need to move away from polarised opinions and power plays towards more balanced and evidence-informed decision-making. It is becoming increasingly clear that the biggest challenge of the twenty-first century will be recognising that we are no longer dealing with individual or population or global decisions, but that all of these decisions are inter-linked. Therefore there needs to be greater solidarity[59] and stronger partnerships,[60] as well as more meaningful involvement of vulnerable and disenfranchised groups.[61] According to Ooms:

> Managing mutual dependence is going to be the biggest challenge of the 21st century, whether it concerns climate change, drug trafficking, tax evasion, money laundering, terrorism, biodiversity, inequitable and environmentally unsustainable economic growth

or health. In each case, the reality that emerges is that no country can address these issues effectively without cooperating with others.[62]

Sen suggests that the way forward involves assuming responsibility and being accountable for the current state of the world, and using this as the starting point for creating change:

> People themselves must have responsibility for the development and change of the world in which they live. . . As competent human beings, we cannot shirk the task of judging how things are and what needs to be done. As reflective creatures, we have the ability to contemplate the lives of others. Our sense of responsibility need not relate only to the afflictions that our own behaviour may have caused (though that can be very important as well), but can also relate more generally to the miseries that we see around us and that lie within our power to help remedy. That responsibility is not, of course, the only consideration that can claim our attention, but to deny the relevance of that general claim would be to miss something central about our social existence. It is not so much a matter of having exact rules about how precisely we ought to behave, as of recognizing the relevance of our shared humanity in making the choices we face.[63]

Indeed, we are now at a particularly critical juncture in our history. With the rapidly ageing population, increasing migration and urbanisation, climate change, and global population growth (projected to reach between 8 and 11 billion by 2050),[64] we need to make important changes to our current course if we want to ensure the future health of our planet. The Club of Rome warns that the very survival of humanity is at stake.[65]

While Maynard Keynes was once quoted as saying "there is nothing a government hates more than to be well-informed, for it makes the process of arriving at decisions much more complicated and difficult",[66] times are now changing. There is a growing recognition that "health is not peripheral to foreign policy and the national interest. . . In many ways, protecting and enhancing the health of its population is one of the most important goals and duties of any state".[67] Yet, improving population health outcomes is more likely to be on the agenda under tax-based health care systems and when centre-left parties are dominant in government.[68] Quite recently, there have been some promising moves in that direction. For instance, after 15 years of house arrest and unrelenting intimidation by the military dictatorship, Aung San Suu Kyi won a landslide victory to become the leader of the opposition in Myanmar (formerly Burma), which is slowly moving towards democratisation even though the parliament is still run by the military-backed ruling party. In this same year, the US President Barack Obama made a surprise visit to Kabul to sign a partnership agreement which marks the beginning of the end of a highly contentious decade-long war in Afghanistan. Still, we cannot afford to continue on the path of unbridled growth and greed, nor on the path of ideological conflicts and holy wars, which are all-too common features in many parts of the world. Politics matter if we are to move in the right direction. In democracies, at least in theory, citizens can choose what direction to move in. Improving health and reducing health inequities will require greater redistribution of wealth, decent work and living conditions for vulnerable groups, empowerment and education of women, universal access to primary health care, the ability to choose from a range of family planning options and freedom from coercion, violence and oppression. This is becoming an urgent matter. These projections regarding the future of our planet, which have been made by highly regarded institutions and think tanks, are not the ravings of doomsday preachers. Nor are these projections centuries away. It is a matter of a few decades.

On the bright side, rapid change is possible. Of the eight million fewer childhood deaths each year as compared to a generation ago, over half of the reduction in mortality has been attributed to the recent increase in educational attainment among women of reproductive age.[69] Thus, while we live in a world of great uncertainty,[70] and while evidence is certainly no panacea,[71] "reliable technical and scientific input is essential to making sound decisions".[72] There is therefore a need for more evidence-informed decision-making at all levels – from local to global.[73] I hope that this book provides some insight on how to go about using the best available evidence in making decisions for health. In this way, when readers enter into the seemingly chaotic realm of decision-making, they will be better equipped to argue in favour of more transparent and informed decisions that promote healthier individuals and more equitable societies.

References

1. Rio +20 Conference on Sustainable Development. *The Future We Want.* New York, NY: United Nations, 2012.

2. World Health Organization, UNICEF. *Progress on Drinking Water and Sanitation: 2012 Update.* Geneva and New York: World Health Organization and UNICEF, 2012. Available at: http://www.who.int/water_sanitation_health/publications/2012/jmp2012.pdf.

3. Daniels N, Sabin J. *Setting Limits Fairly: Can We Learn to Share Medical Resources?* New York: Oxford University Press, 2002.

4. Daniels N. Fair process in patient selection for antiretroviral treatment in WHO's goal of 3 by 5. *Lancet* 2005; 366(9480): 169–71.

5. Kaner S, Lind L. *Facilitator's Guide to Participatory Decision-making.* Gabriola Island, BC: New Society Publishers, 1996.

6. Church J, Saunders D, Wanke M *et al.* Citizen participation in health decision-making: past experience and future prospects. *J Public Health Policy* 2002; 23(1): 12–32.

7. Arnstein S. A ladder of Citizen participation. *J Am Inst Plann* 1969; 35(4): 216–24.

8. Verweij M, Hoven M. Nudges in public health: paternalism is paramount. *Am J Bioeth* 2012; 12(2): 16–17.

9. Coulter A, Parsons S, Askham J. *Where Are the Patients in Decision-Making about Their Own Care?* Geneva: World Health Organization, 2008. Available at: http://www.who.int/management/general/decisionmaking/WhereArePatientsinDecisionMaking.pdf

10. College of Family Physicians of Canada. *Marking Scheme for the SOO Video.* Ottawa: College of Family Physicians of Canada,

2012. Available at: http://www.cfpc.ca/uploadedFiles/Education/Marking%20Scheme.pdf

11. Bourque D. *Concertation et partenariat: Entre levier et piège du développement des communautés.* Québec: Presses de l'Université du Québec, 2008.

12. Dakutis P. Cancer-prevention diet wins praise on navy destroyer. *J Natl Cancer Inst* 1992; 84(5): 297–8. Available at: http://jnci.oxfordjournals.org/content/84/5/297.full.pdf+html.

13. Agence de la santé et des services sociaux de Montréal. *Rapport du Directeur de Santé Publique 2011. Les Inégalités Sociales de Santé à Montréal : Le Chemin Parcouru.* Montréal : Agence de la santé et des services sociaux de Montréal, 2011. Available at: http://publications.santemontreal.qc.ca/uploads/tx_asssmpublications/978-2-89673-115-2.pdf.

14. International Union for Health Promotion and Education. *The Evidence of Health Promotion Effectiveness: Shaping Public Health in a New Europe (Part 1).* Brussels: International Union for Health Promotion and Education, 1999. Available at: http://www.iuhpe.org/uploaded/Publications/Books_Reports/EHP_part1.pdf.

15. Task Force on Community Preventive Services; Zaza S, Briss P, Harris K (ed.). *The Guide to Community Preventive Services: What Works to Promote Health?* Oxford: Oxford University Press, 2005. Available at: http://www.thecommunityguide.org/library/book/index.html.

16. The Cochrane Collaboration. *Cochrane Summaries.* Oxford: The Cochrane Collaboration, 2012. Available at: http://summaries.cochrane.org/

17. Commission on Social Determinants of Health (CSDH). *Closing the Gap in a Generation: Health Equity Through Action on the Social Determinants of Health.* Geneva: World Health Organization, 2008. Available at: http://whqlibdoc.who.int/hq/2008/WHO_IER_CSDH_08.1_eng.pdf.

18. Lavis J, Oxman A, Lewin S, Fretheim A. SUPPORT Tools for evidence-informed health Policymaking (STP). *Health Res Policy Syst* 2009; 7(Suppl 1): I1.

19. Public Heath Agency of Canada. *The Population Health Template Working Tool.* Ottawa: Public Heath Agency of Canada, 2001. Available at: http://www.phac-aspc.gc.ca/ph-sp/pdf/template_tool-eng.pdf.

20. Felitti V, Anda R, Nordenberg D et al. Relationship of childhood abuse and household dysfunction to many of the leading causes of death in adults. The Adverse Childhood Experiences (ACE) Study. *Am J Prev Med* 1998; 14(4): 245–58.

21. Anda R, Dong M, Brown D et al. The relationship of adverse childhood experiences to a history of premature death of family members. *BMC Public Health* 2009; 9: 106.

22. US Preventive Services Task Force. *Screening for Family and Intimate Partner Violence.* Bethesda, MD: US Preventive Services Task Force, 2004. Available at: http://www.uspreventiveservicestaskforce.org/uspstf/uspsfamv.htm.

23. Task Force on Community Preventive Services. Recommendations to reduce violence through early childhood home visitation, therapeutic foster care, and firearms laws. *Am J Prev Med* 2005; 28(2S1): 6–10.

24. Shea B, Nahwegahbow A, Andersson N. Reduction of family violence in aboriginal communities: a systematic review of interventions and approaches. *Pimatisiwin* 2010; 8(2): 35–60.

25. Public Health Agency of Canada. *Canadian Best Practices Portal.* Ottawa: Public Health Agency of Canada, 2012. Available at: http://cbpp-pcpe.phac-aspc.gc.ca/index-eng.html.

26. National Aboriginal Circle Against Family Violence. *Ending Violence in Aboriginal Communities: Best Practices in Aboriginal Shelters and Communities.* Ottawa: National Aboriginal Circle Against Family Violence, 2006. Available at: http://nacafv.ca/report/shelter_practice.pdf.

27. World Health Organization. *Violence Prevention, The Evidence: Changing Cultural and Social Norms Supportive of Violent Behaviour.* Geneva: World Health Organization, 2009. Available at: http://whqlibdoc.who.int/publications/2009/9789241598330_eng.pdf.

28. Ross R. *Returning to the Teachings.* Toronto, ON: Penguin Canada, 1996.

29. Archibald L. *Final Report of the Aboriginal Healing Foundation. Volume III: Promising Healing Practices in Aboriginal Communities.* Ottawa: Aboriginal Healing Foundation, 2006. Available at: http://www.ahf.ca/downloads/final-report-vol-3.pdf.

30. Daar A, Singer P. *The Grandest Challenge: Taking Life Saving Science from Lab to Village.* Toronto: Doubleday Canada, 2011.

31. Grand Challenges Canada. *Who we are.* Toronto: Grand Challenges Canada, 2012. Available at: http://www.grandchallenges.ca/who-we-are/.

32. Oxman A, Bjørndal A, Becerra-Posada F, et al. A framework for mandatory impact evaluation to ensure well informed public policy decisions. *Lancet* 2010; 375(9712): 427–31.

33. Richmond J. *Healthy People: The Surgeon General's Report on Health Promotion and Disease Prevention.* Washington, DC: US Department of Health, Education and Welfare, 1979. Available at: http://profiles.nlm.nih.gov/NN/B/B/G/K/.

34. US Department of Health and Human Services. *History and Development of Healthy People.* Washington, DC: Office of Disease Prevention and Health Promotion, 2011. Available at: http://www.healthypeople.gov/2020/about/history.aspx.

35. Measure DHS. *About DHS.* Calverton, MD: Measure DHS, 2012. Available at: http://www.measuredhs.com/What-We-Do/Survey-Types/DHS.cfm.

36. Wharam J, Daniels N. Toward evidence-based policy making and standardized assessment of health policy reform. *JAMA* 2007; 298(6): 676–9.

37. International Conference on Primary Health Care. *Declaration of Alma-Ata.* Geneva: World Health Organization, 1978.

Available at: http://www.who.int/publications/almaata_declaration_en.pdf.

38. Commission on Social Determinants of Health (CSDH). *Closing the Gap in a Generation: Health Equity through Action on the Social Determinants of Health. Final Report of the Commission on Social Determinants of Health.* Geneva, World Health Organization, 2008. Available at: http://whqlibdoc.who.int/publications/2008/9789241563703_eng.pdf.

39. Szreter S. Economic growth, disruption, deperivation, disease and death: on the importance of the politics of public health for development. *Popul Dev Rev* 1997; 23 (4): 693–728.

40. Minkler M (ed.). *Community Organizing and Community Building for Health*, 2nd edn. New Brunswick, NJ: Rutgers University Press, 2005.

41. Gofin J, Gofin R. *Essentials of Global Community Health*. Sudbury, MA: Jones and Bartlett Learning, 2011.

42. Geiger H. Community-oriented primary care: a path to community development. *Am J Public Health*. 2002; 92: 1713–16.

43. Mullan F, Epstein L. Community-oriented primary care: new relevance in a changing world. *Am J Public Health* 2002; 92(11): 1748–1755.

44. Beaglehole R, Bonita R. Strengthening public health for the new era. In: Beaglehole R, Bonita R (eds.). *Global Public Health: A New Era*, 2nd edn. Oxford: Oxford University Press, 2009, pp. 283–98.

45. Potvin L. Intersectoral action for health: more research is needed! *Int J Public Health* 2012; 57(1): 5–6.

46. Whitehead M, Dahlgren G, Gilson L. Developing the policy response to inequities in Health: a global perspective. In: Evans T, Whitehead M, Diderichsen F, Bhuiya A, Wirth M (eds.). *Challenging Inequities in Health Care: From Ethics to Action*. New York: Oxford University Press, 2001, pp. 308–24.

47. Daniels N, Kennedy B, Kawachi I. Health and inequality, or, why justice is good for our health. In: Anand S, Peter F, Sen A (eds.). *Public Health, Ethics and Equity*. Oxford: Oxford University Press, 2004, pp. 63–92.

48. Andermann A. Addressing the social causes of poor health is integral to practicing good medicine. *CMAJ* 2011; 183(18): 2196.

49. Mercer M. Shall we leave it to the experts? In: *Sickness and Wealth: The Corporate Assault on Global Health*. Fort M, Mercer MA, Gish O (eds.). Cambridge, MA: South End Press, 2004, pp. 167–83.

50. Stone D. *Policy Paradox: The Art of Political Decision Making*. New York, NY: WW Norton & Company, 2002.

51. Coulter A, Collins A. *Making Shared Decision-Making a Reality: No Decision About Me, Without Me*. London: The King's Fund, 2011. Available at: http://www.kingsfund.org.uk/publications/nhs_decisionmaking.html.

52. Moat K, Lavis J. Supporting the Use of Cochrane Reviews in Health Policy and Management Decision-Making: Health Systems Evidence [editorial]. *The Cochrane Library* February 16, 2011. Available at: http://www.thecochranelibrary.com/details/editorial/1018237/Supporting-the-use-of-Cochrane-Reviews-in-health-policy-and-management-decision-.html.

53. Chalkidou K, Levine R, Dillon A. Helping poorer countries make locally informed health decisions. *BMJ* 2010; 341: c3651.

54. Braveman P, Egerter S, Woolf S, Marks J. When do we know enough to recommend action on the social determinants of health? *Am J Prev Med* 2011; 40(1 Suppl 1): S58–66.

55. Rosenbaum S, Glenton C, Wiysonge C, *et al.* Evidence summaries tailored to health policy-makers in low- and middle-income countries. *Bull World Health Organ* 2011; 89(1): 54–61.

56. Directorate-General for Research. *Communicating Research for Evidence-Based Policymaking: A Practical Guide for Researchers in Socio-Economic Sciences and Humanities*. Brussels: European Commission, 2010. Available at: http://ec.europa.eu/research/social-sciences/pdf/guide-communicating-research_en.pdf.

57. Wilkinson R, Pickett K. *The Spirit Level: Why Equality is Better for Everyone*. London: Penguin Books, 2010.

58. WHO Secretariat. *International Trade and Health: Report by the Secretariat* [EB116/4].

Geneva: World Health Organization, 2005. Available at: https://apps.who.int/gb/ebwha/pdf_files/EB116/B116_4-en.pdf.

59. Gostin L, Heywood M, Ooms G, et al. National and global responsibilities for health. *Bull World Health Organ* 2010; 88 (10): 719–719A.

60. Fawcett S, Schultz J, Watson-Thompson J, Fox M, Bremby R. Building multisectoral partnerships for population health and health equity. *Prev Chronic Dis* 2010; 7(6): A118.

61. Department for International Development. *The Politics of Poverty: Elites, Citizens and States*. London: Department for International Development, 2010. Available at: http://www.dfid.gov.uk/Documents/publications1/evaluation/plcy-pltcs-dfid-rsch-synth-ppr.pdf.

62. Ooms G. Managing mutual dependence will be the biggest challenge of the 21st Century. In: Merritt G, House R (eds.); Development Policy Forum. *Creating a Global Health Policy Worthy of the Name*. Brussels: Friends of Europe, 2010, pp. 20–21. Available at: http://www.friendsofeurope.org/Portals/13/Documents/Reports/DPF_Report_Global_Health_11.2010.pdf.

63. Sen A. *Development as Freedom*. New York, NY: Anchor Books, 1999.

64. The Royal Society Science Policy Centre. *People and the Planet*. London: The Royal Society, 2012. Available at: http://royalsociety.org/uploadedFiles/Royal_Society_Content/policy/projects/people-planet/2012-04-25-PeoplePlanet.pdf.

65. Randers J. *2052: A Global Forecast for the Next Forty Years*. White River Junction, VT: Chelsea Green Publishing, 2012. Available at: http://www.clubofrome.org/?p=4211.

66. Hunter D. Evidence-based policy and practice: riding for a fall? *J R Soc Med* 2003; 96: 194–6.

67. Ministers of Foreign Affairs of Brazil, France, Indonesia, Norway, Senegal and Thailand. Why we need a Commission on Global Governance for Health. *Lancet* 2012; 379(9825): 1470–1.

68. Tenbensel T, Eagle S, Ashton T. Comparing health policy agendas across eleven high income countries: islands of difference in a sea of similarity. *Health Policy* 2012; 106(1): 29–36.

69. Gakidou E, Cowling K, Lozano R, Murray C. Increased educational attainment and its effect on child mortality in 175 countries between 1970 and 2009: a systematic analysis. *Lancet* 2010; 376(9745): 959–74.

70. Swanson D, Bhadwal S (eds.). *Creating Adaptive Policies – A Guide for Policy-making in an Uncertain World*. Ottawa: International Development Research Centre, 2009. Available at: http://idl-bnc.idrc.ca/dspace/bitstream/10625/40245/1/128804.pdf.

71. Black N. Evidence based policy: proceed with care. *BMJ* 2001; 323: 275–9.

72. Stern P, Fineberg H (eds.). *Understanding Risk: Informing Decisions in a Democratic Society*. Washington, DC: National Academies Press, 1996.

73. Pang T, Tharyan P. Evaluating the global "Evidence Footprint": how can evidence better serve the needs of global public health? *J Evid Based Med* 2009; 2(1): 44–6.

Index